Praise for <u>Thin for Life</u>

"*Thin for Life* is an excellent book. It makes the difficult journey of lifetime weight control seem possible — and worth taking. Books like this help people like me do their work."

> — Dan Kirschenbaum, Ph.D., Director of the Center for
> Behavioral Medicine & Sport Psychology, Chicago, Illinois,
> Professor, Northwestern University Medical School

"*Thin for Life* combines the rigor of scientific study with the reality of life experiences — a great combination for successful long-term weight control!"

> — Gary D. Foster, Ph.D., Clinical Director, Weight and Eating
> Disorders Program, University of Pennsylvania School
> of Medicine

"There are a number of decent books out there on weight loss (and many more lousy ones), but the thing that makes *Thin for Life* stand out is that you actually want to start eating less as you're going through it. It's that motivating."

> — *Tufts University Health & Nutrition Letter*

"*Thin for Life* has helped thousands of people learn from others' weight-loss experiences. Our clients rate this as the number-one book to help them stay inspired and motivated with their weight management efforts."

> — Jackie Boucher, Registered Dietitian and Certified Diabetes
> Educator, HealthPartners, Minnesota

"I loved the first edition of *Thin for Life* so much that I bought fifty copies and gave them to clients who also loved the book."

> — Marg Alfieri, Registered Dietitian, President,
> Body Balance — Total Nutrition Care, Ontario, Canada

"I recommend *Thin for Life* all the time and have found that for men, it is one of the few resources they will read, and they say it helps motivate them. Most of the commercial programs are directed toward women."
— Lynn Parker Klees, Registered Dietitian and
Certified Diabetes Educator, Pennsylvania

"I recommend your book all the time — it's such a great support to my clients."
— Ann M. Silver, Registered Dietitian and
Certified Diabetes Educator, New York

"*Thin for Life* is one of the most informative, inspirational, interesting and practical diet books that I have seen. I often recommend this book to my patients with weight problems."
— Steven Penkhus, M.D., Minnesota Obstetrician
and Gynecologist

"Now, we have a book that provides the inspiration people need to peacefully maintain their new weight. What a helpful tool for encouraging people to trust that they can lose weight and keep it off!"
— Nancy Clark, Registered Dietitian, Director of Nutrition
Services, Sports Medicine, Brookline, Massachusetts

"By reading about other people with similar weight problems, my clients feel empowered . . . I highly recommend this book for your library."
— Kathy King, Registered Dietitian, in the *Journal of the
American Dietetic Association*

"Your book has had a significantly positive impact on a number of people, including patients of mine who have read it."
— C. Wayne Callaway, M.D., Endocrinologist and
obesity expert, Washington, D.C.

"We like *Thin for Life* because it is not a diet book — instead, it offers a mind-body-spirit approach. Our feedback from patients is, 'This is a great book; it's very practical, and I can relate to it.'"
— Suellyn Crossley, Registered Dietitian, Florida

"Thank you for writing *Thin for Life*. The ideas and insights in your book made the difference. I lost 25 pounds and maintain my goal weight of 105, give or take a pound or two. Even more important is my confidence that I am in charge of my weight — not to mention that my acid reflux condition has disappeared, and my knees have stopped hurting."
— Barbara Keating, Ph.D., Minnesota

"I'm a fan of all three of your weight books. Your books have such a positive impact on so many people."
— Judith Forster-Monson, Minnesota

"I can't even begin to tell you how much your book has helped me. I started at 232 pounds and now weigh 145. I couldn't possibly go back to the weight I used to carry around."
— Helen Bathé, Oklahoma

"Although I had kept off 25 pounds for many years, I still had 40 more to lose and couldn't get the wheels started again until *Thin for Life*. Reading how the masters did it was like talking to each of them face to face. I thought, 'They did it, so can I — and I will.'"
— Mrs. Robert Posner, Arizona

"I had all but given up until I discovered your book. Now I'm encouraged to try again."
— Tonyia J. Tidline, Ohio

Also by Anne M. Fletcher

Eating Thin for Life
Thin for Life Daybook
Sober for Good

Thin for Life

———

10 Keys to Success from People Who Have Lost Weight and Kept It Off

REVISED AND UPDATED

Anne M. Fletcher, M.S., R.D.

Foreword by Jane Brody

Houghton Mifflin Company
Boston   New York
2003

For Steve, Wes, Ty and Julia — my family, who support me

For information about permission to reproduce selections from this book, write
to Permissions, Houghton Mifflin Company, 215 Park Avenue South, New York,
New York 10003. Visit our Web site: www.houghtonmifflinbooks.com.

Library of Congress Cataloging-in-Publication Data
Fletcher, Anne M.
Thin for life : 10 keys to success for people who have lost weight and kept it
off / Anne M. Fletcher ; foreword by Jane Brody. — Rev. & updated ed.
p.   cm.
ISBN 0-618-34055-6
Includes bibliographical references and index.
1. Weight loss — Psychological aspects.   I. Title.
RM222.2.F536   2003
613.2'5 — dc21   2002192154

Printed in the United States of America

Book design by Joyce C. Weston

VB 10 9 8 7 6 5 4 3 2 1

The designations of various organizations, systems, and/or products are claimed by their owners as
trademarks or servicemarks. These include: Ask the Dietitian℠, Cooking Light®, HMR®, Jenny Craig®,
Inc., Lap Band®, Meridia®, Nutricise®, Nutri/System®, Inc., OPTIFAST®, POINTS®, TOPS®, Weight
Watchers® International, Inc., Xenical®

PERMISSIONS: Questionnaire in "Setting a Comfortable Weight Goal" adapted by permission of Kelly
Brownell, Ph.D., from Brownell, K. D., and Wadden, T. A., 1992. Etiology and treatment of obesity:
Understanding a serious, prevalent, and refractory disorder. *Journal of Consulting and Clinical Psychology* 60 (4), page 509. Copyright © The American Psychological Association, Inc. Sections of "Are
You Ready?" adapted from *The Truth About Addiction and Recovery* by Stanton Peele, Ph.D., and
Archie Brodsky with Mary Arnold, pages 203–205. Copyright © 1991 by Stanton Peele and Archie
Brodsky with Mary Arnold. Reprinted by permission of Simon & Schuster, Inc. "Calorie Values for 10
Minutes of Activity" reproduced with permission from *The LEARN® Program for Weight Management — 2000*, by Kelly D. Brownell, Ph.D. Dallas: American Health Publishing Company, page 94. All
rights reserved. For ordering information, call 1-888-LEARN-41 or visit www.TheLifeStyleCompany.
com. "Rosy Red Beet Dip," "Snow Peas and Carrots," and "No-Stir Five-Minute Risotto with
Salmon" adapted from *Quick Harvest: A Vegetarian's Guide to Microwave Cooking* by Pat Baird,
Prentice Hall Press, 1991. Food lists and serving sizes in the Jump-Start Diet are based on the "Exchange Lists for Weight Management." Copyright © 1989 The American Diabetes Association and the
American Dietetic Association.

Acknowledgments

First, I wish to thank the hundreds of people who shared their time, enthusiasm, recipes and, most important, their inspiring stories. My deep appreciation goes also to friends, relatives, weight-loss organizations and professionals who helped recruit the masters.

I am grateful to the weight-control experts who shared their time, opinions and expertise — notably Drs. Kelly Brownell, Susan Ross, Susan Olson, Daniel Kirschenbaum and John Foreyt. Also, Larry Lindner and Gail Zyla, of the *Tufts University Health & Nutrition Letter,* were always available to give feedback and thoughtful advice at various stages of *Thin for Life.* Carla Chesley's recipe-testing skills and willingness to be "on call" were invaluable. I also want to thank Don Mauer for his time and contributions. For help with the revised edition, I am particularly thankful to Drs. Thomas Wadden, Gary Foster, Suzanne Phelan, James Hill, Mary Lou Klem, Robert Jeffery, James Anderson, Susan Bartlett and Richard Atkinson. Tammi Hancock, R.D., owner of Hancock Nutrition Analysis, was most helpful with updating the nutrition information in the book.

For her time and expertise, which she gives way beyond the call of duty, I am indebted to my agent, Chris Tomasino. And for their fine editing and wise ways, I thank my editors, Rux Martin and Lori Galvin-Frost. In addition, I appreciate editor Barry Estabrook's tireless efforts on behalf of *Thin for Life.* Finally, I thank my family members, Steve, Wes, Ty and Julia, for their infinite patience and support for each of my book projects.

Author's Note

As with all diets, weight-loss programs and exercise regimes, you should obtain your physician's permission and seek his or her supervision before and while following the diet, menu plans, recipes and/ or advice in *Thin for Life*. This is particularly important if you have a medical problem, such as diabetes, high blood pressure, heart disease, or an eating disorder. A registered dietitian's counsel is advised as well. If you have psychological distress, such as serious depression or high stress in your life, you should see a licensed mental health professional before following *Thin for Life*'s recommendations.

All masters in *Thin for Life* have given their permission to share information about their weight histories. Some of their names have been changed to protect privacy and anonymity. Sometimes the masters' remarks were edited slightly for clarity.

Contents

Foreword

People who have met me within the last 25 years find it hard to believe that I was once a third bigger than I am now. Like many women in their early 20s, I had become obsessed with weight and quite miserable about the extra pounds that had begun to clutter up my 5-foot frame. So, like millions of others in the same boat, I tried dieting. All kinds of diets. Many commercial programs and gimmicks and a few I made up on my own. And sure, I would lose weight, but then I'd gain it back — and usually some extra pounds to boot — when I got sick and tired of feeling deprived and living on eggs and grapefruit or cottage cheese and carrots or whatever happened to be the popular weight-loss concoction of the day.

Believe me, I tried them all — even the ridiculous drinking man's diet — and all they did was result in an ever-bigger me. As my girth expanded, I got increasingly desperate and tried starving all day and eating only one meal at night. But as soon as I put the first morsel of food in my mouth, I couldn't stop eating. Like the starved person I was, I ate and ate and ate until I would fall asleep, often with unchewed food still in my mouth. And like a starved person, I became increasingly undiscriminating about what I would eat, until I was living on an alternating intake of sweet foods and salty foods, all of questionable nutritional value. I had turned myself into a compulsive eater who knew the locations of every all-night grocery in town.

Then one day I panicked. I was fat. But even more important, I realized, I was probably killing myself with my atrocious eating habits. I vowed to turn over a new leaf. I decided that if I was going to be fat, so be it, but at least I could be healthy and fat.

I gave up diets and gimmicks and cycles of starving and binge-ing, and I started eating: three wholesome meals, with wholesome snacks if I was hungry between meals, and one little "no-no" each day — two cookies, a couple of spoons of ice cream, a thin sliver of cake or pie — something I loved and did not want to miss. No deprivation, no starvation, no bingeing. Only moderation. And I put myself on a regular exercise program. Every day I would do something physically challenging: walking, cycling, skating, swimming, tennis — something that got me breathing hard (I kept thinking about how all that oxygen was restoring my cells to health) and feeling good about my body.

Losing weight wasn't part of this plan, but lose weight I did. Even though I was eating whenever I was hungry and consuming what felt like mountains of food, I lost weight: about 7 pounds the first month and then about 1 or 2 pounds a month thereafter, until my weight stabilized 2 years later at 35 pounds lighter. And there it has stayed, give or take 5 pounds here or there, for a quar-ter-century.

Once I dropped to a normal weight for my size, I had to come to terms with another common obsession: wanting to have a per-fect body. I had to convince myself that I could be the best possi-ble me without wanting to look like a fashion model (and if you could see what fashion models live on, you wouldn't want to look like one either). Of course, I could be thinner. I could stop snack-ing on cereal, bread and pretzels. I could refrain from splurging from time to time on ice cream or frozen yogurt. But in doing so, I could also risk the return of my old fixations on unhealthy foods and of the unwanted pounds that used to drag me down mentally and physically. I long ago decided that being perfect simply wasn't worth it. Besides, as I am writing this, I am in the middle of my 53rd year of life, and I know that people looking at my body find it hard to believe I'm a day over 40. That's largely because daily physical activity has remained an essential ingredient in my pro-gram, for reasons of both health and looks.

I know I would have been a lot happier had this book existed 28 years ago when I was a chunky 24-year-old. In *Thin for Life,* Anne M. Fletcher has produced a weight-control program that can work for anyone and everyone who is really ready to give up on quick gimmicks and false promises about weight loss, anyone who is at least as serious about health as about weight — in other words, anyone with an ounce of good sense. Anne's program is not a prescription, it's an approach that can be molded to individual lifestyles and temperaments. It promises only that you *can* lose weight, not how much you will lose or how fast.

In fact, trying to lose weight fast is probably the single biggest mistake dieters make. Weight that comes off quickly nearly always comes back on even faster. You didn't gain those extra pounds in a fortnight, and you shouldn't be trying to take them off in two weeks, or even necessarily in two months or two years. The idea is to adopt an eating and exercise plan that you can go on and can stay on for the rest of your life, a program that will allow you to lose weight slowly, tone up your body gradually and eventually stabilize at a weight and shape that is right for you.

Thin for Life can lead you down the path of sensible weight control. Anyone faced with a weight problem, and especially anyone who has tried and failed one or more times to lose unwanted pounds and keep them off, should read this book, digest its message and start on a new road to a healthy and practical weight.

— Jane Brody
Personal Health columnist,
New York Times

Introduction

I've long been fond of a cartoon posted on my office wall of a man, his head in the shape of a book, sitting on a physician's examining table. The physician asks him, "So, how long has this book been in your head?" And so it goes with many authors who toy with an idea for years before it comes to fruition. Such was the case with *Thin for Life,* which was germinating in my head for more than 10 years before I wrote it — from the early 1980s, when I counseled overweight patients at a weight-management program in Massachusetts, until the early 1990s, when I sat down to write the first edition of the book. Despite the fact that so many of the people I worked with at the weight program regained their lost pounds, I knew that success stories were out there. Over the years, I have collected more and more facts to support my premise. And for this revised edition of *Thin for Life,* there's even more encouraging news — from both research and success stories. A number of exciting new studies suggest that the odds of being able to lose weight and keep it off are much better than we've been led to believe. I continually meet new people who are maintaining weight loss.

In *Thin for Life,* I set out to prove that people really can lose weight and keep it off. I'd grown weary of conflicting messages we receive — on the one hand, about our society's terrible weight problem (and the constant push for all of us to be slim and fit), on the other, the hopelessness of trying to lose weight and keep it off. I decided it was time to stop hearing about all the horror stories of people who gain weight back and, instead, to start learning about the many individuals who have found success. In a short time, I located 160 masters at weight control — people who had lost at least 20 pounds and kept the weight off for a minimum of 3 years.

Most of them more than met the criteria, and their responses far exceeded my expectations. *Thin for Life* is primarily about the motivational strategies that these people used to take hold of long-standing weight problems and that they continue to use to keep the weight off.

A few years after the first edition of *Thin for Life* was published, I recruited more masters — winding up with a total of 208 people who were included in another book called *Eating Thin for Life: Food Secrets and Recipes from People Who Have Lost Weight and Kept It Off.* Since the results bolster the messages of *Thin for Life,* I have interspersed some of the findings from *Eating Thin for Life* in this revised edition.

What's more, the new *Thin for Life* incorporates exciting recent scientific information that firmly buttresses the book's original findings. *Thin for Life* also includes updated nutrition and diet information, plus more resources for help with weight problems. For instance, there are new sections on high-protein diets, yoga and tai chi, and Internet resources for losing weight.

The *Thin for Life* masters' inspiring stories continue to offer a strong message of encouragement, whether you want to lose just a small amount of weight or a lot. (In my experience, some of those who want to lose 10 or 20 pounds suffer just as much as those who struggle with larger amounts.) The principles of *Thin for Life* will help you get a handle on your weight problem regardless of your size.

Thin for Life is the first book to weave together research-based methods of weight loss and maintenance with tried-and-true practices of masters at weight control. The "10 Keys to Success" encapsulate the critical steps that the masters have taken to become thin for life. *Who better to tell you how to lose weight permanently than the very people who have done it?* Many were eager to tell their stories to help others:

♦ Nancy K., master of 60 pounds: "I am open to sharing my story to help other people lose weight. I was heavy during my high

school and college years. It affected me greatly, and I feel for anyone who is heavy and unhappy about it."

◆ Paul A., master of 51 pounds: "I would be happy to be interviewed by you, as I feel there are plenty of men out there who feel
that weight loss can be achieved by running around the block after a major feast."

◆ Holly L., master of 97 pounds: "I sincerely hope that you can
use my story to encourage other kindred spirits to live a carefree,
healthy lifestyle, away from the burden of being overweight."

It doesn't matter if you've lost weight before and gained it all
back, because most of the masters didn't make it the first, second or even the third time around either. You don't have to starve,
buy fancy foods or potions or stay away from sweets and so-
called "junk" foods. And no, you don't have to turn into a marathon runner! *Thin for Life* demonstrates the sensible, livable approaches the masters take to control their weight.

I've kept in touch with quite a few *Thin for Life* participants
over the years and am pleased with the number who've vol-
unteered that they are still maintaining their weight loss. Ann F.,
for instance, has not only maintained her initial 200-plus-pound
drop from her all-time high of 380 pounds in the early 1980s —
she recently dropped down to 155 pounds. She states, "I have
bought a wonderful new wardrobe — I wanted to get rid of my
A-line dresses and now have more fitted clothes." Dennis H. has
maintained his weight loss of more than 30 pounds for 16 years
and is proud that at the age of 48, he's recently nearly tripled his
monthly running distance. Alyce C., who topped out at more
than 220 pounds three decades ago, still weighs in the 130s.
At the age of 55, she can say, "I am healthier than I think I have
ever been." Then there's Bob W., who lost and has kept off 250
pounds — yes, 250 pounds! — for 30 years. Janice C. is now
mother to a 2-year-old and finds, "I pretty much enjoy eating anything I want. Since getting married, I'm probably up 5 pounds,

but I still weigh 122." Through two pregnancies, 36-year-old Lynda C. has been able to maintain her weight loss of 40 pounds for more than 12 years and still weighs 118. She says of the time when she was heavier, "The other life just isn't an option for me."

The need for an optimistic book about permanent weight loss is more important than ever in today's climate, where "overweight and obesity have reached nationwide epidemic proportions," according to a recent U.S. Surgeon General's report, which adds that, "left unabated, overweight and obesity may soon cause as much preventable disease and death as cigarette smoking." Barely a week passes before yet another report is issued about how overweight and out of shape we are as a society. Indeed, when *Thin for Life* was first published, 1 out of every 4 Americans was considered significantly overweight. Now, it's estimated that 6 out of 10 adults are overweight or obese — in fact, the number of obese people has nearly doubled since the 1980s. Yet *Thin for Life* continues to bridge the gap between these alarming statistics and the need for sensitivity concerning people who are overweight by helping them with nonextreme lifestyle changes, realistic goal-setting and increased self-acceptance — regardless of their current or future weight.

In telling the masters' stories, I am not saying that what any one master does is the "best" way to go about weight control. I'm simply sharing what worked for these people, whose approaches are highly individual. One of the goals of *Thin for Life* is to guide you to find what is right for you.

I am also not saying that anyone *should* lose weight — I'm showing that you *can*. My intent is to prove that the masters do indeed exist and to show you exactly what they have done to win the weight battle.

1

Key to Success #1

Believe That You Can Become Thin for Life

They're out there — the masters at weight control. They're people who have lost a lot of weight and kept it off for a long time. They may be people you've known for years who once had other lives as much heavier people.

Tim H. is one of them. I'd seen him around town — a big guy, but good-looking: muscular-big. I never would have dreamed that 7 years ago, he carried around an extra 40 pounds. Then there's my former neighbor Tami B., a pretty brown-haired slip of a woman who, for 6 years, has kept more than 35 pounds off her tiny 5'1" frame. Doug S. is a master too. Before I met him in person, I often talked to him on the phone when he called to speak with my husband. When I finally came face to face with Doug — the man my husband described as one of the best players in his "A-level" racquetball league — I found it hard to believe that he once weighed more than 300 pounds!

I *knew* the masters were out there; I just didn't know how many of them there really were. In a short period of time, I was able to locate 160 masters at weight control, all of whom have managed to keep off at least 20 pounds for a minimum of 3 years. *The story gets even better:*

1

- The average weight loss for the entire group was 63 pounds.
- 7 out of 10 masters lost 40 pounds or more.
- More than half lost 50 pounds or more.
- 20 people lost 100 pounds or more. Most of them have kept it off for at least 5 years.
- Well over half have maintained at least a 20-pound loss for 5 or more years.
- More than one-third have maintained it for 10-plus years.
- 12 people have maintained it for 20 or more years.

The masters' stories will help you believe in your own power to lose weight and keep it off forever. Permanent weight loss may seem like a long shot, particularly when you hear over and over that 95 percent of all dieters gain back all their weight — and then some. Indeed, as far back as 1958, renowned obesity expert Albert J. Stunkard, M.D., concluded, "Most obese persons will not stay in treatment . . . Of those who stay in treatment most will not lose weight and of those who do lose weight, most will regain it." More recently, the Institute of Medicine summarized the odds of being able to lose weight and keep it off by stating that "those who complete weight-loss programs lose approximately 10 percent of their body weight, only to regain two-thirds of it back within one year and almost all of it back within 5 years."

As the celebrity Roseanne once warned, "Do not even try goin' on no diet because you ain't gonna lose no weight and even if you do, you're gonna gain the whole damn thing back!" How can you hope to have any hope with "failure talk" like this?

You *can* have hope because, as obesity expert Daniel S. Kirschenbaum, Ph.D., puts it, "There are many thousands of people who are success stories." As director of the Center for Behavioral Medicine & Sport Psychology in Chicago and as a professor at Northwestern University Medical School, he has worked with hundreds of them. Dr. Kirschenbaum is one of many experts I interviewed who believes the odds against losing weight and keeping it off are not so grim. I would also argue that, even if it were true that just 5 percent of people are able to keep off lost weight, it's time to start paying more attention to the success stories!

The hundreds of masters I found are living proof that it can be done. Theresa D., who is 5'4" tall and has kept off 28 pounds for 5 years, says, "People need to realize that it isn't impossible to lose weight. I am 100 percent behind your efforts to help people realize that they *can* do it."

In talking with masters again and again, I saw connecting threads in the stories of all people who have lost weight and kept it off. *Thin for Life* weaves together these common themes with the findings of scientific studies on weight maintenance and presents them as Keys to Success. Whether you want to lose 10 pounds or 100 pounds, the Keys — presented in the masters' own stories and words — will enable you to master *your* weight problem.

Support from Thousands

Not long after the first edition of *Thin for Life* was published, when I was contacting the masters for *Eating Thin for Life,* I received an intriguing phone call from two researchers. Dr. Rena Wing, of Brown University, and Dr. James Hill, of the University of Colorado Health Sciences Center, were setting up the National Weight Control Registry, a large, ongoing research study of several thousand people who have maintained weight loss. When I asked him how the study came about, Dr. Hill told me, "One day at lunch, one of us observed that everything we have learned about weight maintenance has come from people who have failed at keeping weight off. We were joking at first, but realized there was something to it. We asked ourselves if there were successes out there."

Drs. Hill and Wing and their colleagues have been involved in the Registry, which is now based at Brown University, since 1994. Those eligible for the Registry have to have lost at least 30 pounds and kept it off for at least 1 year. Most participants were once "considerably overweight," but their success at weight loss and maintenance far exceeds the minimum criteria. Although the numbers keep changing and figures are periodically updated as the Registry expands, the most recently published figures indicate that the average weight loss per person was about 66 pounds. And the average length of time they'd been maintaining at least a 30-pound loss was close to 6 years. (In 2002, the Registry had increased to about 3,500 enrollees.) As you'll see throughout the revised edition of this book, findings of the Registry support much of what the *Thin for Life* masters revealed.

They Break the Rules

As I read letter after letter and talked with person after person, it struck me that many of the masters break many of the "rules" or commonly held notions about weight control and maintenance. What are these notions and how do the masters challenge them?

◆ **Myth #1: If you've been overweight since childhood,
it's next to impossible to lose weight and keep it off.**

About 45 percent of the masters indicated that they'd been heavy since childhood. Close to another quarter of them gained weight as teenagers. Says master Joe M., "I was always extremely overweight as a child and teenager. I do remember weighing at least 300 pounds as a senior in high school." Joe, who is 6'2", now weighs 175 and has for the past 19 years. Likewise, findings from the National Weight Control Registry suggest that 7 out of 10 of its weight maintainers had been overweight as children and teenagers.

◆ **Myth #2: If you've dieted and failed many times before,
there's little hope of ever licking your weight problem.**

Most masters at weight control didn't make it the first time around. On the contrary, nearly 60 percent of them had tried to lose weight at least five times before they were finally successful; close to another 20 percent had dieted three or four times before they finally got it right. This finding is supported by research studies on successful maintainers. For instance, 9 out of 10 maintainers from the National Weight Control Registry reported trying to lose weight previously — in fact, the average lifetime loss of those who tried to lose weight previously was about 270 pounds per person! Alyce C. is a good example of someone who tried nearly everything — from Metrecal to Overeaters Anonymous to diet pills. Finally she came up with her own weight-loss plan, one that was right for her. Since then she's maintained a 90-pound loss for more than 20 years. (She's 5'8" and weighs in the 130s.) (Chapter 3, "Do It Your Way," shows how you can learn from your past attempts and use them to launch yourself to long-term success.)

◆ Myth #3: If you do succeed at losing weight and keeping it off, you'll have to eat like a bird for the rest of your life.

Not so: most masters enjoy food, and the majority eat several meals a day, often with snacks in between. Many told me they really don't deny themselves any foods — including sweets and snack foods. They feel like they eat what they want, but in moderation. In the words of Irene S., who started losing her 77 pounds in 1989, "If I want pie or cake or whatever, I have a controlled amount and that's it!" And the masters certainly don't sound like they're living on carrot and celery sticks — the vast majority told me *they do not feel like they are dieting.* (Chapter 4, "Accept the Food Facts," tells how masters come to grips with a new way of eating and how they learn to control their craving for foods they don't want to give up.)

And contrary to the notion that once-heavy people must suffer to keep their weight down, at least 85 percent of participants in the National Weight Control Registry reported that weight loss led to improvements in their general quality of life, mood, self-confidence, level of energy, physical mobility and health. (Fewer than 2 percent of participants reported a worsening in any of these areas.) Only 1 in 5 people reported thinking about weight more often subsequent to weight loss, and just 14 percent said they think about food more frequently — obviously, a minority. And another study that examined the psychological well-being of Registry members concluded, "There was no evidence that long-term suppression of body weight is associated with psychological distress."

◆ Myth #4: In order to lose weight and keep it off, you have to become an exercise fanatic.

Although most masters at weight control do exercise much more than typical people (North Americans, in general, are quite sedentary), there aren't many who engage in extreme forms. In fact, walking is the most popular form of exercise among the masters. My survey, as well as research studies, suggests that what's most important about exercise is *the consistency with which it's done* — that is, making it a regular part of your life. About 70 percent of the 160 masters told me they exercise three or more times a week. Only about 16 percent of them do so every day. Surprisingly, 15 masters (about 9 percent) said they don't exercise at all. Exercise *is* extremely important for the vast majority of people who want to lose weight and keep it off, but it's encouraging to know that it is possible to be successful if you don't want to or can't exercise. (In Chapter 7, "Move It to Lose It," you'll learn how to customize your own physical activity program, one you can live with for the rest of your life.)

◆ Myth #5: It's really hard to lose weight once you pass the age of 40.

I was surprised at the number of masters who lost their weight when they were older than 40 — there were dozens of them. Holly L., for instance, started to lose her 97 pounds at age 69. And Jean B. started losing her 45 pounds in 1985, when she was 52. At a height of 5'5", she got down to 164, stating that she wanted to lose the weight slowly, so, she says, "I won't wrinkle any faster than I have to — and I'm keeping it off. I'll probably lose another 30 pounds over the next 5 years, but I'll stay healthy so I can be a nice grandma."

◆ Myth #6: You can't lose weight on your own, let alone maintain weight loss.

The masters are quite evenly split between those who lost weight on their own and those who said they found success with formal weight-loss programs and self-help groups. (Again, the Weight Control Registry found the same thing: roughly half lost weight on their own, while the other half had help.) The vast majority of masters maintain their weight loss without the support of a group. Remember, though, that most masters had made many previous attempts at weight loss, often through structured programs. It's likely that the valuable approaches gleaned from these programs contributed to their eventual success. That's how Suzanne T. lost the 70 pounds that she's kept off for 4 years. (She's 5′3″ and weighs 150.) She had been to Weight Watchers in the past, but when she lost weight once and for all, she did it on her own — following the "basic Weight Watchers plan," coupled with exercise. "I did not go to Weight Watchers meetings," she maintains; "I followed their basic ideas." (Chapter 3 tells how you can find a weight-loss approach that's right for you.)

◆ Myth #7: Diets don't work — if you lose weight by going on a diet, you're bound to gain it back.

Diets *do* work for some people. Of the masters who lost weight with a structured program, many followed weight-loss diets. Similarly, the success stories in the National Weight Control Registry commonly shed their excess pounds by dieting. (For more on whether or not you should go on a diet, see Chapter 3.) However, few of the *Thin for Life* masters and the Registry participants reported using extreme weight-loss measures, such as fad diets or eating just 1 or 2 types of foods.

◆ Myth #8: If you hit a plateau while losing weight, there's little hope of moving on.

In fact, a good number of masters lost weight in stages, over a period of years rather than weeks or months. More than a quarter took longer than a year. Some were still losing when I heard from them. Joy B., who became overweight as a child, lost 20 pounds her junior year in high school and kept it off. (Her peak weight was over 150 pounds; she's 5'1".) "Then, after 10 more years of struggling," she admits, "I took off another 10-plus pounds." Joy has held her weight at about 115 for the past 4 years. (See page 85 for the discussion "Give Yourself Time.")

◆ Myth #9: If you start regaining weight, you're bound to gain it all back. You should stay away from the scale.

The most striking finding of my survey is that the vast majority of masters weigh themselves regularly so they can catch themselves when their weight starts creeping up: 98 percent of them keep their weight within a 10-pound range. Most have a specific plan of action if their weight starts to climb. Bonnie R., who's been a weight-control master for 18 years (she's kept 53 pounds off her 5'1" body), maintains her weight within a 1-to-5-pound range. If her weight goes up, she stops snacking, finds healthful substitutes and tries to determine what is causing her to put on the pounds. She says, "I stay conscious of what I gain and never let myself forget my 'being heavy' experience. I refuse to do that to myself again — ever!" My findings about weighing in were again corroborated by those of the Registry: most of their participants weigh themselves at least once a week, and many weigh in daily. (Chapter 5, "Nip It in the Bud," helps you design a plan for stopping small weight gains before they get out of hand.)

◆ **Myth #10: If you don't stay at your original weight goal, then you're a failure.**

Contrary to the notion that you're a failure if you don't stay at your original weight goal, about one-third of the masters in *Thin for Life* have settled for a maintenance weight that is somewhat higher than their original goal. Some have regained a portion of the original weight they lost, but they are still significantly thinner than before. I consider them success stories because they're happier and healthier now than they were at their maximum weights. Lisa B. is a good example. She hit 385, her highest weight ever, in 1985. She dropped all the way down to 140 — quite low for someone who is 5'8" tall. She's regained about 30 pounds, but can now proudly say, "I wanted to get to my lowest low (140 pounds), but it took so much to get to where I am. And I'm truly happy with my appearance. I'm a size 14. I'm thrilled!" (Chapter 2, "Take the Reins," shows how to set your own livable, realistic weight goal and how to accept a less-than-perfect body.)

The list could go on. Masters have overcome other challenges that should put them at odds with becoming thin for life. They've maintained their weight loss through quitting smoking, having babies, losing jobs, dealing with alcohol problems, marital strife and more.

How Did I Know I'd Find the Masters?

My own interest in weight maintenance began almost 20 years ago when I was a clinical nutritionist and assistant director of a sophisticated weight-loss program called the New England Institute of Nutrition and Health. I became discouraged, however, because although we employed what were believed to be state-of-the-art techniques for helping people with weight control, more often than not our patients would regain the pounds they'd worked so hard to lose.

Then I came across a 1982 report by veteran obesity expert Stanley Schachter, Ph.D., of Columbia University, arguing that "obesity's reputation for intractability" is grossly exaggerated. After interviewing 161 individuals, Dr. Schachter found that of the 46 people who had a history of obesity (which he defined rather stringently as being 15 percent or more overweight), 25 were no longer fat. On average, they had lost about 35 pounds and had maintained their losses for 11 years.

Dr. Schachter's findings were soon confirmed by psychologists in the professional journal *Addictive Behaviors*. In just a few months, using advertisements in newspapers and on radio and television in the Phoenix, Arizona, area alone, Robert Colvin, Ph.D., and Susan Olson, Ph.D., tracked down 41 women who had lost and kept off an average of 53 pounds for 6 years. They also located 13 men who had maintained an average 76-pound loss for about the same period of time. (Their findings are summarized in their book, *Keeping It Off*.)

Why the "Failure Talk"?

Why the grim statistics on weight maintenance? I posed this very question to renowned Yale University obesity expert Kelly Brownell, Ph.D., when I first met him in 1984. Dr. Brownell contends that one reason for the depressing statistics is that they are based on the individuals who are likely to be the "hard-core" overweight — people with the most to lose who have failed many times over. Because they've had so much trouble with their weight, they may be drawn to university-based research studies. In contrast, people who are successful — particularly those who lose weight on their own or with commercial weight-loss programs — tend not to wind up in research studies from which the statistics are derived.

I don't mean to suggest that there aren't success stories from research-based weight-loss programs, because there are. And of late, researchers have been able to help people lose more weight over the short term than in the past. However, success at maintaining weight loss has made little progress. One problem with scientific studies is that they usually report averages that may blot out the cases of success. Consider a study by the University of Pennsylvania's Thomas Wadden, Ph.D., and Albert Stunkard, M.D., that compared the long-term effect of three different weight-loss approaches in a group of women and men. Regardless of the type of treatment, at the end of 3 years, most of the people had gained back most of their weight. The authors of the study noted, however, that 6 of the 45 individuals in the study showed "perfect maintenance" of weight loss 3 years after treatment. Typically, though, you don't hear about the success stories — what's reported is the discouraging *average* weight loss of a group like this.

Another problem with drawing broad conclusions from research studies is that the weight-loss methods are selected by experimenters and are similar for every participant in any one segment of a study. More often than not, however, the masters lose weight by coming up with their own personal plans, which vary from person to person.

Actually, there have been far more studies on how to lose weight in the first place than on how and why it's so difficult to maintain weight loss. Hard to believe, when 35 percent of U.S. adults are overweight, and another 26 percent are obese — not to mention the fact that weight problems are estimated to cost more than $100 billion in health-care expenditures and money spent on weight-loss products and services. And although some questions have been raised about just how risky it is to be mildly to moderately obese, several recent government reports have clearly stated that being overweight places you at risk for heart disease, stroke, type 2 diabetes, certain types of cancer, osteoarthritis and breathing problems.

Switching Gears to Find Success

All of this suggested to me that we've been looking for success in the wrong places and going about research in the wrong way. Why not study the people who are the real experts at weight control — those who have succeeded at losing weight and keeping it off? Why not closely examine what the masters do to keep weight off forever? Not only did I find my own group of masters, but I found even more support — from research studies — for my theory that far more people are successful at weight control than we're led to believe:

◆ University of Minnesota researcher Robert W. Jeffery, Ph.D., sent me a study for which he and a colleague located 64 people who had lost an average of 51 pounds and kept them off for an average of 30 months.

◆ In an old file, I came across a mention of an unpublished doctoral dissertation by Susan Ross, Ed.D., R.D., of 23 successful maintainers who had lost at least 20 pounds and kept them off for at least 1 year. Ross discovered that 15 of the people had lost 40 or more pounds and that the same number had maintained that loss for at least 3 years.

◆ A 1992 study on successful dieters, conducted at the University of Iowa College of Medicine, located 82 people who had kept off a significant amount of weight for an average of 4½ years. On average, the men had lost 53 pounds, and the women had lost 60 pounds.

◆ In a nationwide survey of 541 of its leaders, Weight Watchers International found that they had been at or near their goal weights for an average of 6 years. On average, they had lost nearly 50 pounds.

◆ A 1993 *Consumer Reports* survey of some 19,000 readers who had used commercial diet programs revealed that about one-fourth of them kept off more than two-thirds of their weight, on average, 2 years after completing the programs. That's more than 4,700 people.

♦ In 2002, *Consumer Reports* went even further, surveying 32,213 dieters, finding more than 4,000 "superlosers" — people who had lost an average of 37 pounds and kept it off for 5-plus years. (A total of nearly 8,000 people had managed to lose at least 10 percent of their starting weight — an amount considered to have medical benefits — and kept it off for at least a year.)

I'm often asked, "Do we really know how many people in the general population have lost weight and kept it off?" In 1999, University of Pittsburgh Medical Center researcher Maureen McGuire, Ph.D., and her colleagues set out to find the answer by making phone calls to a representative sample of 500 individuals from all across the United States. The findings, reported in the *International Journal of Obesity*, estimate that more than 20 percent of overweight people have achieved successful weight loss maintenance — 4 times the widely reported figure of just 5 percent of dieters who are said to achieve long-term success. On average, the once-overweight people who had lost weight and kept it off had dropped 42 pounds and had been maintaining for 7 years.

Like many of the masters I spoke to, master Ann F. refused to let the "failure talk" get in her way. "Don't pay attention to the odds," she advises. "It's a terrible burden on people to hear that you can't do it — if you think you can't, you won't. You have to ignore people who say you can't do it. I had a terrible weight problem. It wasn't easy; I'm not a superwoman. But I did it." What she did was drop from her all-time high of 380 pounds (she's 5'7") to a weight of about 160, which she has maintained for more than 10 years.

Who Are the Masters?

The masters in *Thin for Life* come from all walks of life. Quite a few are secretaries, teachers and retired people. One is a state senator. They include psychologists, homemakers, lawyers, repairmen, writers, a former showgirl and even a chocolate scientist. How did I find them all? It wasn't hard. Many came my way by word of mouth. In addition, I sent public service announcements to newspapers in many different cities and towns.

Friends and relatives across the country posted flyers about my project in public places like supermarkets and health clubs. Finally, I approached major weight-loss organizations, including Weight Watchers, Health Management Resources (HMR), Nutri/ System, Diet Center, Jenny Craig Weight Loss Centres, Take Off Pounds Sensibly (TOPS) and Overeaters Anonymous (OA) for "success" stories. Wherever I turned, I found masters.

What Exactly Is Maintenance?

For some people, maintenance means sticking to a set number on the scale. For others, it's being able to fit in a particular size of clothing. For the vast majority of masters, however, maintenance means keeping weight within a defined range, most often 1 to 5 pounds.

But maintenance is not just reaching your weight goal. As weight-maintenance expert Michael G. Perri, Ph.D., of the University of Florida, stresses, "Maintenance means much more than *weight* maintenance. It includes the maintenance of other healthy lifestyle behaviors, such as healthy eating patterns, exercise, reducing stress, keeping healthy relationships and more."

I often encountered an all-too-common scenario with my former patients. After weeks or months of dieting, they'd see the scale drop to the number they'd been shooting for. Then, after a few weeks, they would cancel their appointments and tell me that they were fine and "knew what to do." I would call them at several-month intervals to see how they were doing and learn that slowly — but surely — the weight was coming back. Or they wouldn't return my calls, and I'd see them a year later in the supermarket or at a restaurant, just as heavy as before. Why does this happen?

"If you spent six months getting in shape by jogging and lifting weights, how long would you expect the positive effects to last after you'd stopped?" responded Dr. Thomas Wadden, director of the Weight and Eating Disorders Program at the University of Pennsylvania School of Medicine, when I posed the question to him. "Exercise training doesn't last three years later. You have to keep practicing the good habits — or you lose the skills." Master Kerry K. now realizes that. He says that after he lost 100 pounds in 1986 (with the help of Health Management Resources), "I thought I knew it all: exercise, decrease fats, keep food records." But he left the program sooner than was recommended, and over the course of the next 4 years, he gained back half of his weight. "I learned that I didn't learn enough," he says. He went back to HMR and lost weight again, this time staying in the program long enough to learn the critical skills for maintenance. All in all, he's kept 83 pounds off his 5'10" frame for about 5 years.

While you are losing weight, you're in what Dr. Kirschenbaum and his colleagues at Northwestern University Medical School call the "honeymoon stage." You're enthusiastic, optimistic and consistent — a veritable tower of strength. It feels good to take control of a problem, and you delight in seeing the numbers on the scale drop.

But just as in marriage, the honeymoon doesn't last forever. As blues singer B.B. King would say, "The thrill is gone." Often my patients would implore, "If I could just get 'it' back. It was so easy before." This is the frustration stage, a "poor me" frame of mind, when you feel resentful that you have to keep working at it and that you can't go back to your old eating habits. The masters at weight control have accepted this reality and decided it's worth the effort. After maintaining a 32-pound weight loss for 5 years, Liane F. still struggles. She says, "It's the hardest thing I've ever done in my life for myself, but it is also the *very, very* most rewarding thing ever. I love being able to wear so many styles of clothing."

Most masters, however, seem to have moved past the frustration stage into what Dr. Kirschenbaum terms the "tentative acceptance stage." They have a peaceful sense of resolve most of the time: it's not so hard to maintain weight anymore, but there's a tendency to gain some weight in certain situations — say, on vacation, during illness, over the holidays or after an injury that interferes with exercising. As indicated in Chapter 5, however, most masters quickly get a handle on the situation and nip the weight gain in the bud.

Some reach Dr. Kirschenbaum's final stage, "lifestyle change." They are confident they'll never gain the weight back and know what works and what doesn't work for them. Food is less of an emotional issue — they handle life's problems without turning to food, and they even maintain their healthful eating and exercise habits when vacationing. As Kerry K. told me, keeping his weight off does entail a tremendous amount of energy and work. But he insists the effort is minuscule compared with the pain of being at his old, heavy weight of 282.

If You're Fat, It May Not Be Your Fault — But That Doesn't Mean You Can't Do Something About It

What causes people to become fat? According to the U.S. Surgeon General in 2001, "For the vast majority of individuals, overweight and obesity result from excess calorie consumption and/or inadequate physical activity. Unhealthy dietary habits and sedentary behavior together account for approximately 300,000 preventable deaths every year."

On an individual basis, is it true that heavy people "just eat too much" and exercise too little — and, as a remedy, should simply "eat less, and exercise more"? This simplistic view supports the prevailing notion that people become fat from gluttony and lack of willpower; it implies that if you just tried a little harder, it would be so easy to lose weight. This thinking suggests that weight problems are the result of a moral failing — when, in fact, many experts view obesity as a complicated chronic disease. It *is* true that if you're overweight, you're eating more calories than your body needs to maintain a healthy weight. And several studies suggest that obese people tend to underestimate the number of calories they consume by one-third to one-half, as compared with nonobese people who underestimate by about 20 percent. However, research also suggests that many cases of obesity are less the result of an overwhelming lust for food or lack of willpower and more from biological causes.

◆ Why are some people fat, but not others?

The answer, according to a survey of 50 physicians and scientists involved in obesity research, is, in large part, "genetic factors." In other words, the tendency to become overweight is inherited — depending on which studies you consider, weight is determined anywhere from 40 to 70 percent by your genes. How do we know your genetic inheritance plays a powerful role? Isn't it just as likely that you become overweight because you learned bad eating habits or a sedentary way of life from your parents?

One way researchers have attempted to answer this "nature-versus-nurture" question is by studying people who were adopted as infants to see if their adult weights are more similar to weights of their adoptive parents or of their biological parents. Several studies of this sort have revealed that the weights of adoptees are far more similar to those of their biological parents than to those of their adoptive parents.

Another way to determine whether there's an inherited tendency to become overweight is to compare weights of identical twins (who have the same genes) with non-identical twins (who share no more genetic heredity than regular siblings). Again, studies reveal that the genetic influence is powerful: identical twins are much more likely to have similar body weights than are non-identical twins. And several studies indicate that weights of identical twins tend to be the same, whether they are raised apart or together in the same home, again suggesting that weight is determined more by genetic than by environmental factors.

◆ Biological differences appear to determine how efficient your body is at processing calories.

Studies suggest that while one person may need 2,000 calories a day to maintain her weight, another person of the same weight, height, age and activity level may require just 1,600 calories. There is also clear evidence that some people gain more weight than others when they overeat by exactly the same number of calories. As one of my former Cornell professors once said, "Some people seem to have more of an ability to 'waste' calories," while others convert them to body fat. Research also suggests that how physically active you are may be "wired in" to a certain extent, as is the distribution of fat on your body. (Periodically, studies are issued on hormones and other body chemicals that may also explain weight differences, but their practical application remains to be seen.)

It's important to note, however, that for some individuals, overweight may be the result of subtle differences in calorie intake that can really add up. For example, if you were to consume just 30 calories more per day than your body needs to maintain your weight — say, by adding an extra teaspoon of regular mayonnaise, salad dressing or margarine to your food — you'd gain about 30 pounds in 10 years' time. (Conversely, cutting back by small amounts can add up, too.)

Consider a recent study on holiday weight gain reported in the *New England Journal of Medicine,* which revealed that, on average, a group of close to 200 typical Americans gained about a pound between fall and winter. While a far cry from the 5- to 10-pound gain commonly believed to accrue over the holidays, this small gain was not reversed during the spring or summer, as demonstrated by the 165 people who returned for a later weigh-in. Such insidious increments in weight explain why so many adults find their weight climbing as they grow older. But none of these explanations for creeping weight gain seem to explain the degree of overweight in some people.

◆ Could it be that differences in calorie needs are the result of chronic dieting?

Indeed, it is known that dieting can lower your metabolic rate, at least temporarily. (Metabolic rate is the rate at which your body burns calories for energy.) That is, if you cut back on calories, your body protects itself from this state of semi-starvation by slowing down the rate at which it burns food. But after losing weight, is your metabolism slower than it was before simply because your body size is smaller? According to a report published in the *American Journal of Clinical Nutrition* that pooled the results of multiple studies on metabolism after weight loss, average resting metabolism appears to be 3 to 5 percent lower in formerly obese people than in people of the same size who have never been obese. However, a small subset of once-heavy people accounted for the differences, suggesting that most formerly heavy people do not have a slow metabolism. It is not known if the slower metabolism in this subset of once-heavy people was caused by dieting or if it was always there and led to their becoming overweight.

According to a landmark study published in the *New England Journal of Medicine,* some people probably do have a sluggish metabolism before they become heavy. Researchers with the National Institutes of Health kept track of weights and metabolic rates of a group of Pima Indians (a population prone to obesity) over the course of 2 to 4 years and found that people who gained the most weight by the end of the study burned significantly fewer calories at the beginning than did people who gained less or no weight. This study also suggested that slow metabolic rates tend to run in families. However, such metabolic differences account for just a fraction of the variation in weight gain — in other words, the amount that people gain can be only partially explained by differences in metabolism.

In short, weight problems have many different causes, and the extent to which biology versus environment plays a role varies from person to person. Your weight problem is more likely to have a stronger inherited root than an environmental one if (1) you were a child or adolescent when your weight problem began; (2) you have a family history of obesity (e.g., if one parent is obese, it more than doubles the risk that you will be obese as an adult; the risk is higher still if both parents are obese); and/or (3) your weight has bounced up and down a lot — particularly if you were obese, then lost a lot of weight and rapidly regained it. The good news here is that even though a lot of masters had these factors working against them, they were able to lose weight and have kept it off.

Certainly, we cannot blame the recent societal increase in obesity on changes in the genetic composition of Americans — the environment is more the culprit here. In the words of Yale University experts Katherine Battle Horgen, Ph.D., and Kelly Brownell, Ph.D., "Biology permits obesity to occur in individuals, but the environment causes obesity in the culture." Because of feast or famine conditions in prehistoric times, it may be that humans inherited a genetic tendency to store energy in the form of fat — and that some of us have more "thrifty" genes than others. Combine this with the plethora of high-fat, high-calorie foods surrounding us — along with the decline in exercise resulting from labor-saving devices and "seat time" in front of TVs and computers — and you've got a setup for an overweight society.

◆ **So what if you come from a heavy family — and you're a slow burner who doesn't need many calories? Are you doomed to become heavy and doomed to stay that way?**

Not according to Gary D. Foster, Ph.D., clinical director of the Weight and Eating Disorders Program at the University of Pennsylvania School of Medicine. He points out, "Obesity is *not* a trait like eye color, which is determined at the moment of conception and does not change. A *tendency* for obesity is inherited. This tendency needs to have an environment that will nurture its development *before* it becomes a reality . . . Remember, your heredity is not your destiny! Most of the experts agree: providing an environment of low-fat foods and increased physical activity can stifle even the most stubborn genes." Indeed, 46 percent of participants in the National Weight Control Registry reported that one biological parent was overweight, while another 27 percent said that both parents were overweight — so there's hope even if you come from a long line of people with weight problems.

A number of years ago, I had the opportunity to meet with Arlen Price, Ph.D., a geneticist at the University of Pennsylvania. He did some studies on identical twins confirming that if one twin is overweight, it's highly likely that the other will be. He notes, "On balance, genes appear to account for as much as two-thirds of individual differences in obesity in adults," suggesting that the other third is environmental and within an individual's control. As such, he points out that even with identical twins, there can be great variation in the degree of overweight. "One brother might only be 20 percent overweight," Dr. Price states, "while his identical twin is 40 percent overweight." The implication is that, even if you are genetically "programmed" to be overweight, you have control over how overweight you will become or remain, depending on how you eat and how active you are. Such was the case with master Kevin C. Part of what spurred him to do something about his long-standing weight problem was recognizing that he had become 50 pounds heavier than his identical twin brother who had always been the more physically active of the two. (Kevin managed to lose 45 pounds and has kept it off for 7 years.)

The masters at weight control are living proof that weight destiny need not be controlled by your genes or by the fact that you're a "slow burner." Yet the studies on genetic and metabolic causes of overweight provide an understanding of why it's harder for some masters to control their weight than others, and they help to explain why many comfortably settle in at weights higher than their original goals. The studies also provide insight about why so many people lose weight and gain it back. The masters are those who have learned how to "stifle" their genetic legacy.

What Have You Got to Lose?

Losing weight can help you get rid of a lot of health "baggage." In fact, a good number of masters report a health-related reason as the primary motivation for losing weight when they finally did it once and for all. Many of them now report feeling good not only about the way they look but about the way they feel.

You may already know the health benefits of losing weight. One study suggests that for each 10 percent drop in body weight, the incidence of heart disease decreases by 20 percent. Indeed, even modest weight losses can make a difference — just losing 5 to 10 percent of body weight and maintaining it can confer health improvements such as lowering of blood pressure and blood sugar.

A number of the masters also report relief from the emotional pain of being heavy in a society that, rightly or wrongly, reveres thinness. Master Jeffrey B. (he's kept off 55 pounds for 22 years) reports that when you're overweight, "people you don't even know feel free to comment on your size. Friends want to advise you to lose weight 'for your own good.'" He recalls a friend who, when advising him to lose some weight, said, "You'd look better, you'd feel better." Jeffrey asked her where she "got off" talking to him that way if she was his friend. He said to her, "I'll make you a deal — you get a nose job, and I'll lose 50 pounds." After she expressed her indignation, he replied, "Well, you'd look better, you'd feel better."

But not everyone is as forthright as Jeffrey. A report in the *New York Times* described a heavy woman who endured strands of spaghetti being thrown in her face, pig sounds and comments like "wide load." In popular media, heavy people are often the butt of cruel jokes and derogatory depictions. Even physicians appear to discriminate against heavy people, as supported by a recent study in the *International Journal of Obesity*. When 122 doctors were asked to evaluate medical charts of patients who were depicted as average weight, overweight or obese, the heavier the patients were, the more negatively they were perceived by the physicians.

Asked why overweight people are still victims of prejudice in our climate of political correctness, Dr. Susan Olson replied, "People see it as a willpower issue. You can't change the color of your skin, but they think being fat has to do with being lazy and a lack of control."

The "Nondieting" Movement

This discrimination against heavy people — coupled with the information about the inherited aspect of weight problems — has spurred a strong "nondieting" movement. Even some experts argue that continually pressuring overweight individuals to lose weight does more harm than good. The nondieting movement also decries the gain-lose-gain syndrome (also known as yo-yo dieting or "weight cycling") — with some proponents saying that it's harmful to your health and your psyche and may lower metabolic rate, making each new attempt at weight loss more difficult.

Certain aspects of the nondieting movement are laudable, moving people away from unrealistic body images, de-emphasizing the importance of physical appearance, getting them off the dieting merry-go-round, and helping them see that it's possible to be healthy at any size — with lifestyle changes like exercising. (And studies on nondieting approaches do suggest that they favorably affect self-esteem, mood and body image — with little impact on weight.) But the notion that all dieting is bad and causes more problems than it solves appears to be unfounded.

In a thoughtful review of the limited research comparing nondieting with other approaches, Dr. Foster and his colleague, Dr. Brian McGuckin, conclude, "The most significant weakness of nondieting approaches is the lack of scientific support. It is troubling that nondieting books and programs have increased significantly, despite a dearth of studies demonstrating their effectiveness. No approach, no matter how well intentioned or sensible, should be marketed as effective when it has not been adequately studied."

As for the effects of weight cycling, the U.S. government's Weight-control Information Network (WIN) concludes in a recent statement on the subject that most studies show that weight cycling does not affect metabolic rate and therefore should not affect whether or not you'll be able to lose weight next time around. And contrary to what some people think, weight cycling has not been proven to increase the amount of fat tissue in people who lose and regain weight. As for psychological consequences, Dr. Wadden and colleagues concluded in a recent review of studies on the subject that "the literature indicates that neither dieting nor weight cycling has serious adverse effects on the psychosocial functioning or eating habits of the great majority of overweight and obese individuals."

While several studies do not support a once-suspected link between weight cycling and heart disease risk, the jury is still out on whether weight fluctuations are harmful to overall health. However, according to the University of Colorado's Dr. James Hill, who helped write the WIN statement, "People should not use this as an excuse to remain heavy because it's quite clear that being overweight is associated with a host of medical problems." Dr. Hill is one of a number of experts who believe that the probable benefits of weight loss outweigh any conceivable risks of weight cycling for obese people.

In no way do I mean to suggest that yo-yo dieting is a good thing — I can't imagine that it doesn't take a toll on a person's self-esteem. Nor do I feel that anyone should stay on a diet merry-go-round in pursuit of a body weight that can never be or to lose small amounts of weight for cosmetic reasons. The possible negative consequences of yo-yo dieting suggest *not* that you should give up your effort to lose weight, but that *you should take a long, hard look at how serious you are before you make your next attempt at weight loss.* (See "Are You Ready?" on page 53.) Note, too, that while most masters at weight control had been on multiple diets, many now maintain their slimmed-down weights without tremendous difficulty.

The other important message is that *you may need to rethink your weight goal.* You may be better off if you accept a smaller weight loss than your "dream" weight, one that you can comfortably maintain.

Finally, as much as I applaud individuals who free themselves from the notion that self-worth is determined by physical appearance, the sad truth is that most overweight people are not happy being heavy. One study on people who underwent surgery to lose weight reported that nearly all said they'd rather be a normal weight and have a major handicap, such as deafness, severe acne or legal blindness — or even have a leg amputated — than be fat again. All said they'd prefer to be of normal weight than to be an obese multimillionaire.

Master Jeffrey B. shares his feelings about the nondieting movement: "If this were a perfect world, we'd leave fat people alone. But I went through these things. I was the fat man. I think it's impossible to be the happy fat person because of our society. I'd do anything to avoid being fat again."

It's Your Choice

Giving up dieting doesn't have to mean giving up the effort to lose weight. Dr. Susan Olson thinks that people often need permission not to diet. "But," she adds, "the next step is to decide what you *do* want — either love yourself and love your fat or do something about it. It's a choice that you have." And choosing to take control of your weight in a healthful, positive way — as well as developing a more realistic attitude about what you "should" weigh — as the masters have done, can be a freeing experience. It does not mean that you are continuing to be controlled by a world that says everyone should look like a fashion model.

Many of the masters did lose weight with a nondieting approach when they were finally successful. They switched to healthful eating and increased physical activity. Tami B. is a good example of someone who lost weight and keeps it off with a nondieting method. When asked how she finally succeeded, she said, "I had to take control — cleaned up my mac-n-cheese, pizza and ice cream environment. I started eating a balanced diet and exercising." Six years later and 35-plus pounds lighter, she's in control. "I basically eat what I want — I watch the amount and cut back on fat. I eat candy, ice cream and chips on occasion, but it's not on hand at home."

"Learning proper eating habits is not putting someone in a straitjacket," remarks Ronna Kabatznick, Ph.D., a former psychological consultant for Weight Watchers International who has also counseled hundreds of clients concerning weight management. She adds, "Learning how to eat is an empowering thing." (For more on dieting versus the nondieting approach, see Chapter 3.)

It's all a matter of choice. It is possible to become thin for life. But it's up to you to decide if you are happy the way you are or if you want to take the reins and make a change.

If You Think You Can, You Will

If you choose to become thin for life, one of the most important steps is believing in yourself. In her study on successful maintainers (page 12), Dr. Ross saw in many a "newfound belief in themselves as the ultimate authority." They had come to see themselves as people "capable of maintaining a thin body and having no need to return to a heavy one." Master Mindy B., who's lost 84 pounds and kept it off for 7 years, says it well. "Losing weight is hard, but it's always within reach. Take a long look at yourself within and find that inner self-determination. It's there for all of us — use it to your advantage."

You can start to believe in yourself by accepting that your weight condition is not the result of fate: you can control it. Reading about the masters will help you do that. Over and over again, they describe moving from a state of hopelessness to one of self-control and power.

A shining example is Donna C., who says, "When I got to more than 200 pounds, it seemed like so much to lose." But she lost it — 108 pounds to be exact, which she's kept off for 3½ years. Of her final effort, Donna maintains, "This time I felt in control. I knew it was in my hands. It was not an act of fate that I was heavy, not bad luck. I knew it was up to me, within my control. It's exactly the same for keeping the weight off."

Psychologists call this belief in yourself "self-efficacy." It's the sense of how competent you believe yourself to be in any particular situation. You can have a high sense of self-efficacy in some circumstances, but not in others. You may, for instance, have a strong sense of your abilities when it comes to work or being a parent. If you're like many people who struggle with their weight, your belief in your ability to maintain weight loss is likely quite weak. That's because you have little or no experience with weight maintenance.

When I asked the University of Minnesota's Dr. Robert Jeffery,

"Is there any way to increase someone's sense of self-efficacy about weight maintenance?" he replied, "The best way is to show people they can do it." Indeed, Dr. Albert Bandura, the leading authority on self-efficacy, states that one way you can increase self-efficacy is to observe role models — individuals who have struggled to master situations that you fear or see as difficult.

All of these observations firmed my conviction that sharing the experiences of the many masters at weight control could help others who want to be thin for life. I wanted to show how many success stories there are in order to fuel your belief that *"If they can do it, so can I."*

2

Key to Success #2

Take the Reins

How did the masters finally make the choice to do something about their weight? Most of them had tried many times and in many ways before they were finally successful. It struck me that, by virtue of experience, a good number were experts at weight control long before they finally slimmed down. "At least half of the people who want to lose weight could write the whole book on dieting! Knowing never equals doing," maintains Mariah Smith, M.S.W., a weight expert and president of Prescriptions for Health, a company specializing in long-term weight management for individuals and corporate groups.

So, for me, the burning question for each master was, "What was different that last time you lost weight? Why, at this one point in time, were you able to change your life forever?" It soon became clear that, when they decided to take action for that final, successful time, there was one common theme: something happened that spurred them to *take the reins*. They stopped looking to others for all the answers and decided to lose weight for no one other than themselves.

Cindy P.'s Story

"I'm an ex-fatty," Cindy P. wrote me. "I was heavy all my life, from 6 through 21. I got up to 235 pounds and started losing weight when I was 21. Now, I weigh 155, the same weight I've been for over 10 years." (She's 5'8".) The photo she enclosed revealed a stunning, dark-haired woman who looked like she'd never been heavy.

Cindy took the reins — took responsibility for her weight problem — when someone in her life finally accepted her as she was: heavy. Up until that time, she had tried any number of ways to lose weight. But she had been doing it for other people, people who let her know that she wasn't quite worthy as a person because she was fat. She spent most of her early years hearing statements like, "If only you lost weight . . ." However, the more people tried to take control *for* her and nag her about her weight, the less she did about it.

Cindy thinks her weight problem started when she was in kindergarten, living temporarily with an aunt because her parents had gone through a divorce. The aunt had been raised during the Depression and was of the school that "you'd better eat now because you don't know if you'll have it later." Cindy recalls that even at this early age, people would comment, "She's so pretty; it's too bad she's fat."

When Cindy was a teenager, her mother told her, "Men don't like fat girls." So Cindy found another reason to be liked: she developed a great sense of humor. "I was the class clown, and everyone always wanted me to come along. I went to a lot of parties. But I didn't date. I think I developed my sense of humor *because* of my weight. I think it bothered my mother more than me that I wasn't going to proms and out on dates. She had been the cheerleader, the skinny girl, the pretty one that the guys liked."

Cindy wanted to get close to boys, but they often made comments about her weight. "I always had a crush on someone,"

Cindy says, "but as soon as he'd ask, 'How 'bout if you lost some weight?' I'd write him off."

Cindy did try to lose weight many times with over-the-counter diet pills, medically prescribed appetite suppressants and various diets. She thinks that these attempts were for her mother. She always gained the weight back.

Then Cindy went to college and met a guy (on a blind date) who liked her unconditionally — at 235 pounds. For the first time, she was ready to take the reins and lose weight *for herself.* "He never bothered me about my weight. Finally, I had found someone who accepted me *for me.* I didn't need to keep weight on to keep men at a distance anymore." She adds, "I wasn't being bugged. I wasn't doing it for Mom, for Dad, so my brothers wouldn't call me names. I didn't even need a doctor to help me lose weight. I did it because it made me feel good."

Within months, Cindy dropped down to 185 by following the Weight Watchers food plan. (She was too self-conscious about her weight to go to meetings but got the food plan from her mother.) Cindy liked the plan because "it didn't make you starve, and they didn't say you were a bad person if you ate a chocolate chip cookie." Then she hit a plateau. "I got stuck at 185 for 3 or 4 months. I never thought I'd get off that." But she didn't give up.

She realized that to lose more weight, she'd have to begin exercising. So she joined an all-women's health club and started doing aerobics. When her mother asked her, "Aren't you too self-conscious to be wearing a leotard?" her determination was fueled. "That's when I really started becoming my own person." From there, Cindy kept on losing, dropping as low as 140 pounds.

Like many masters, she came up with her own plan for weight control, which is pretty much the same now as when she was losing. (She reads a great deal and has taken courses about food and nutrition.) "I eat a healthy breakfast, snack, lunch, snack, dinner, snack. All very light meals. And I drink a lot of water." She still follows the basic Weight Watchers food plan, which emphasizes fruits, vegetables and grains. She doesn't eat much meat and tries to limit fat to no more than 20 grams a day. She does most of her eating between when she gets up and 1:00 in the afternoon. Typically, she has a salad or something light while her husband eats his supper. When it comes to eating, it's her way, on her terms.

Cindy doesn't have many "shoulds" about food. One morning when I spoke with her, she'd had a tuna sandwich for breakfast. "I suppose some people would say I should have a bowl of cereal or something, but *I* wanted a tuna sandwich." She writes down everything she eats, even if she has a candy bar, but doesn't feel bad about it.

Her exercise consists of working out with aerobic videotapes for 45 minutes three to four times a week. She is also active socially, which she feels is a key to her success. Instead of going out to dinner, she encourages friends to go dancing or horseback riding with her. "I also keep my hands busy with crafts. And I try to avoid sitting in front of the TV because it makes me think of food." When her weight creeps up 5 to 10 pounds, Cindy exercises more, goes back to her original Weight Watchers plan and gives up sweets for a week or so. "It's not easy. Yeah, I'd like to be eating hot fudge sundaes or brownies, but for me the weight is more important."

That doesn't mean Cindy deprives herself of sweets. She's always loved to bake. So about once a week, she whips up a "mound of something," like cookie dough or pralines. But she eats a controlled portion — say, ½ cup of cookie dough, savoring every bite. Then she throws or gives the rest away. Sometimes she'll buy a package of doughnuts, but only eat the centers or the toppings. Again, what's left goes in the trash. She says, "A lot of people can't throw food away. My husband has a hard time with it. So I ask him, 'What am I gonna do: stick it on my hips?'" She listens to her stomach, asking herself, "Do I really want that?" She adds, "I eat until I feel comfortable, not full. I used to stuff myself, but I don't do that anymore. I rarely eat a whole anything." She says to herself, "Okay, now I've had that sensation."

To this day, if someone says to Cindy, "You shouldn't eat that cookie," she wants to eat it all the more. On the other hand, if someone pushes food on her, saying, "You know you want it; go ahead and have some," she can refuse it easily. What's the difference? In the first situation, someone is trying to make the choice for her; Cindy wants to be the one who decides what she can and can't have.

She is the first to admit that the reins get a little slack when she feels someone isn't accepting her as she is. Sometimes, for instance, her husband (not the man she met at college) will comment that she's gained a little weight. Then she'll find herself overeating to spite him, blaming him all the while. "He's not letting me notice my weight and do something about it. I want to be the one to make the decision and do something. If only my husband would just accept me the way I am and think I'm sexy. I want to be liked unconditionally." When he remarked on her weight recently, she caught herself turning to food but gained control by recognizing what was going on. She said to herself, "'Wait a minute. *That's* why I'm eating this instead of taking control. *He* has the problem with my weight.' I see that I'm really hurting myself. I can keep blaming my husband. But I stand back and say, 'I'm the one who's getting hurt.'"

Whatever happened to the guy who enabled Cindy to take the reins by not bothering her about her weight? She says that after she lost the 80 pounds, he "dumped" her because he was not comfortable with other men's attraction to her. Now, she says, "I am happily married and really enjoy being thin."

Look Within

It's striking. It's consistent. The critical starting point for most masters at weight control is *taking the reins*. Like Cindy, they're on top of making the decision to take action, choosing their own way to lose weight and making day-to-day decisions about food. Researchers have found the same phenomenon. For example, Susan Ross, Ph.D., who studied 23 individuals, most of whom had lost at least 40 pounds and kept weight off for a minimum of 3 years, told me, "They seemed to take responsibility from the beginning; they said, 'This is me, this is my problem, and this is how I'm going to do it.'" In addition, "taking responsibility for one's own behavior" was rated as *the* most important skill for losing weight and successfully keeping it off by the 541 Weight Watchers leaders (page 12), who were themselves long-term maintainers.

Psychologists Susan Olson and Robert Colvin (page 10) found, too, that a critical first step for their 54 success stories was taking responsibility. If their people could only make one point, it would be, "You can't hire someone to do it for you," they note in their book, *Keeping It Off.* Dr. Olson told me, "You need to get to where you say, 'No one is going to do it for me; there are no gurus, no magic pills.' Once people are convinced the ball is in their own hands, they can start to do something about their weight."

The masters, like Peppi S., say it best: "I just keep telling myself that no one is going to take care of me except *me.* So I take responsibility for me, which is a far cry from the old days when I would blame everything and everyone for my being overweight." Peppi, who is 5'7", weighed 200 pounds in 1985; she now maintains her weight around 138. She lost her weight with the help of Nutri/System, but realized that, ultimately, weight loss was up to her.

A recent report in the *International Journal of Obesity* on women who belonged to a British weight-loss organization suggests that a person's beliefs about the causes of a weight problem play into his or her ability to take responsibility for it. The study involved 40 obese women who had lost weight and regained it, as well as 44 formerly obese women who had been maintaining weight loss for about 9 years on average. The study also included 58 women whose weight had stabilized at obesity levels. Researchers found that one of the major differences between the maintainers and the other groups was that, when asked what they saw as the causes of obesity, the maintainers were less likely to believe that it is caused by medical factors such as genetics, hormone imbalance or slow metabolism, suggesting that they felt that their weight problem was more within their control than did the others.

In looking within, you have to accept that you may have been dealt a rotten hand of cards when it comes to metabolism or genes. But like the masters, you can overcome what you've been dealt. I recall one of my favorite patients who, before she accepted responsibility for her weight problem, was just about the angriest person I'd ever come across. She literally pounded her fist on my desk and demanded, "Why do I have this problem? It's not fair! Why me?" I responded, "Pat, if I were to tell you that you have a weight problem because your mother stopped breast-feeding you too early — or because your grandmother overfed you as a toddler — where would that get you? How would that help you lose weight? The real question is, *What are you going to do about it?*"

Do It for You

How do you begin to take the reins? Master Lynne C., who has maintained a 77-pound weight loss for 4 years, said it succinctly: "I did it for myself." In other words, start by asking yourself, "Who am I losing weight for?" If the answer isn't, first and foremost, "For me," you may not be ready to lose weight. (See "Are You Ready?" page 53).

Master Jennifer P. describes her old college boyfriend who would tell her she'd be a "10" if only she slimmed down. "I refused to lose weight during the school year, but when I was away from him in the summer, I'd lose and exercise." Eventually, she dropped from 186 to 142, which she's maintained for 7 years. (She's even had two babies in those years.)

Mary Ann K., who's maintained an 84-pound weight loss for 3 years, told me, "Your weight is yours. You have to be responsible for your body. If you are going to lose and keep your weight off, you must be selfish. You do it for you and no one else. I realize I am worth it!"

In the words of Cindy P., if you really want to be thin, "You have to stop listening to your husband and your mother." As a side benefit, you may make your family, colleagues, friends and physician happy. But ultimately, the message from the masters is that *you have to want to lose weight for you.*

Face the Truth

As Dr. Robert Colvin and Dr. Susan Olson stress, before you can take the reins with a weight problem, you first have to *face the truth*. You can't kid yourself about your weight, how you eat or how you look anymore. Master Alisa S. admits she used to rationalize her size by telling herself, "I'm married now, have two kids, am a housewife, and this is all I can expect to be." When she became motivated to lose weight, however, she realized, "It was myself I was unhappy with. I set out to return to the trim, lively person I was." And she did. Alisa has weighed 135 for 7 years, down 66 pounds from her all-time high.

Kathleen H. was forced to face the facts when, at her videotaped 40th birthday party, friends and family goaded her into putting on a T-shirt that said, "This is what 40 looks like." She recalls, "I couldn't stretch it over my (then) 47-inch hips!" As if that weren't bad enough, her children insisted upon watching the tape over and over. "It was different from glancing in a mirror or looking at photos. It was like I really saw myself and how I looked to others. I knew 40 had to look better." Now, at the age of 43, Kathleen weighs 125, very slim for someone who is 5'8" tall.

When you're honest with yourself, Drs. Colvin and Olson believe, you are ready to "own" your weight problem and recognize your responsibility for it. Once the problem belongs to you, you can lose the weight.

The Attitude Shift

In asking each master the question "What was different that last time you lost weight?" I had hoped to discover a miracle — some experience shared by all masters that awakened them to take responsibility. But like others who have studied maintainers, I found that there is not a single answer or experience common to all. I did, however, discover an attitude shift that took place in most masters when they decided to lose weight for the last time. They had undergone a critical change in thinking about themselves and their feelings toward weight control. "It's as if a light bulb goes on, and they do it. Sometimes I think it's like a religious conversion!" notes University of Minnesota researcher Dr. Robert Jeffery, who has studied successful maintainers. In her study, Dr. Susan Ross observed a similar shift: "The attitude was described in different ways but usually reflected a sense of self-responsibility and determination. Most could not describe how they arrived at the decision or what made them shift their attitude, but all were clear as to when it was the right time or decision for them. It seemed that in some way all of them came to realize a 'truth' that had not been in their awareness in that way before."

Jeffrey B. described a striking attitude shift: "I firmly believe that 90 percent of weight loss is mental. When it finally worked, I knew from day one that I was going to lose weight. I had no choice. My eating habits changed naturally, and the weight melted off." He went on to describe a friend who "starved" himself for 2 years but who couldn't seem to lose weight. "I tried to explain to him the almost audible click in the mind when it decides it is time to lose weight. He didn't understand. Then I lost track of him for about 6 months. When I saw him again, he had lost about 80 pounds. The first thing he said to me was, 'Now, I understand.'"

Not every master could articulate the "click" that spurred weight loss, and a number — including Jeffrey B. — were uncertain about why the change took place at that one point in time. But as I went through the answers to the question "What motivated you to do it — once and for all?" I could see that one of five situations had initiated most of their attitude shifts:

◆ **I saw the light** — a single eye-opening experience. For Jim V., it was dramatic. He says he was never too concerned about his weight of 475 pounds — until he almost drowned and couldn't save himself. That near-fatal event started Jim on the course of losing 250 pounds, which he's kept off for 3 years. (Jim is the profiled master in Chapter 7.) For a number of masters, the critical incident involved seeing a photograph or videotape of themselves. For others, turning a certain age triggered the change. Fern C., who has maintained a 28-pound loss (she's 5'2") for 21 years, says she became motivated when "I saw a snapshot of myself and knew that I would be turning 50 on my next birthday."

◆ **I was scared to death** — a worrisome health situation. A number of people expressed general concern about how unhealthy their weight had been. For others, like Kelly D., the situation was far more serious. It took a massive heart attack to get him to lose his 55 pounds nearly 5 years ago. Edith S. became motivated to lose 56 pounds after "a severe angina attack and a serious talk with my cardiologist."

◆ **I couldn't take it anymore** — simply becoming tired of how you look and feel. Bob W., who peaked at 400 pounds in the eighth grade, stated, "I was sick and tired of being sick and tired." He now weighs 150, which he's maintained for 21 years. Says Lou Ann L., "I was tired of being self-destructive and turning my anger inward by eating. I was also tired of being overweight and feeling limited by my weight." That sentiment, 20 years ago, triggered a 43-pound weight loss. Some masters were worn down by their weight-control efforts. Kelly S., who for 6 years has weighed 50 pounds less than her all-time high of 180, responded, "I was tired of having food run my life. I said, 'Enough is enough is enough already.'"

♦ **I liked the new me.** For some masters, the real attitude shift didn't seem to take place until *after* they had lost some weight: they liked what they saw and how they felt, so they kept going. Joseph M., who has kept off 115 pounds for 19 years, states that what motivated him to lose weight once and for all was "seeing results: clothes beginning to loosen, being noticed by females, feeling better physically and mentally." For Cindy P., feeling better about herself began before the weight loss — when a man cared about and accepted her unconditionally, she then gained the confidence to lose weight.

♦ **I wanted to attract the opposite sex.** Not surprisingly, some masters' desire to lose weight was spurred by a wish to find a mate. Eight years ago, Sandy P. was motivated because she wanted to have a boyfriend, like the rest of her friends. "In order to achieve that goal, I had to lose weight." And lose she did — 73 pounds to be exact.

Similarly, the National Weight Control Registry found that the turning points for participants were varied. About a third of them reported either a medical or emotional trigger, with men more commonly reporting medical reasons or that they "just decided to do it" and women more likely to mention emotional reasons for weight loss.

It's More Than a Commitment to Lose Weight

"I looked bad and felt fat."

"The scale kept climbing — it was time, and I had had it."

"My mind was made up."

"*Wait a minute,*" I asked the masters, "*Didn't you want to look better and feel better all those other times you lost weight?*

*And wasn't your mind made up with just as much determination?
Weren't you sick and tired of being heavy before?"* I was *still* left
with that question "Why did you do it — finally?"

When I had the opportunity to speak at length with the masters, as well as interview experts on weight control, I began to realize that much more had taken place in the masters' lives than
just making a commitment to lose weight. Other critical changes
in their lives had taken place — some deliberate, others incidental
— that kept them going after they had made the decision.

Weight-management expert Mariah Smith, M.S.W., says, "It's
not just that something 'clicks.' Several factors take place in the
final attempt to lose weight, and it's different for each person.
But most people who are successful at keeping weight off have
worked at some imperative things that help them live thin in the
world. They may have learned how to solve their problems more
effectively. If they don't exercise because of hecticness at work,
they find a way to do it."

Indeed, the more I talked with the masters and the more I studied other researchers' findings, it became clear that many masters
made *multiple* changes in their lives either before or while they
were losing the weight. Says Dr. Daniel Kirschenbaum, of Chicago's Center for Behavioral Medicine & Sport Psychology, "It
isn't just 'motivation' that last time that makes the difference. For
instance, someone who has worked for years in a candy factory,
where he's exposed to constant temptation, finally changes jobs."
Along the same lines, Dr. Susan Ross found that readiness to lose
weight often relates to changes in life situations, personal matu-
rity or growth, changes in values or some combination of these
changes.

One woman, who had a history of dieting on weekdays then
binge eating all weekend, told me that she literally woke up one
Monday morning and said, "I'm never going on another diet."
That was 12 years ago, and she honored her pledge. Taking her
comment at face value, it would appear that the change in atti-

tude was like some sort of awakening — the "click" that certain people describe. But when she reflected about what else had gone on in her life, she admitted that many aspects of her life had changed so that she was finally ready to give up her compulsive dieting. "Over the course of many years, I learned to like myself better. I had the confidence to change careers and, therefore, became much happier in my work. I also became involved in a supportive rather than a destructive relationship with a man. Part of it, too, was that I had matured and I could accept imperfections about my body; I realized that I was so much more than my weight."

The Keys to Success in subsequent chapters reveal the critical changes made in masters' lives to sustain their weight loss.

Inoculation Concepts

In order to be successful, the masters first had to figure out or accept some things about themselves. Knowing these "inoculation concepts" in the beginning can give you a shot in the arm to take charge of your weight problem *and* can make things easier down the road. (Not all of them will necessarily apply to you.)

◆ **Put yourself first.** You need to get stubborn and develop a kind of selfishness about yourself and your weight. In her book *Alyce's Fat Chance,* master Alyce C. says, "Get ornery. Get stubborn. Figure out what it takes to take care of yourself and *do that*. If you have to carry baked potatoes in your flight bag in order to take the weight off, then *do that*." (She does.) "Stop being concerned about what it looks like." (For more on taking care of your own needs, see Chapter 9, "Get More Out of Life.")

◆ **Get in touch with what your weight is doing for you.** Ask yourself what you're getting out of *not* losing weight. Many people hide behind their weight, allowing it to help them avoid challenges or escape intimacy with the opposite sex. Cindy P. thinks her weight served not only as a statement of anger because boys didn't accept her as she was, but also as a defense to keep them at a distance. "I suppose it had something to do with my parents' divorce. I was afraid of being hurt or left." Being heavy allows some people to put off making decisions or taking action about life. Kelly S. realizes that her weight had something to do with her family's pressure on her to achieve. "It was all assumed. I didn't feel like I had a choice. Food was a coping mechanism to deal with pressure. At some level I must have thought that if I were heavy, maybe people would expect less of me." (You can't always get in touch with what your weight is doing for you. As indicated in Chapter 8, some people need to work with a professional to uncover what their weight really means to them.)

◆ **Prepare for the hardship of being thin.** As Alyce C. puts it, "The world treats you differently at 210, at 185, at 160 and 135." Some of the changes will be positive, others negative — at least initially. People may have different expectations of you, you'll have to deal with buying new kinds and sizes of clothing, and people of the opposite sex may treat you very differently. The praise you get may start to irritate you after a while. You may have trouble accepting yourself as thin. Heavy friends and relatives may resent your success and try to sabotage your efforts. It's important to realize, too, that after you lose weight, you'll still have problems: you'll probably still argue with your husband, have a rebellious teenager to deal with and worry about money. In fact, for some people, certain problems become more acute, particularly if they were hiding behind their weight. Your relationships may change as well. Recall Cindy P., whose boyfriend left her because he couldn't handle other men's interest in her when she slimmed down. Being aware may help you better handle what's ahead. (Subsequent chapters offer guidelines for dealing with these issues.)

◆ **Look forward to what you'll gain.** Masters report more favorable changes in their lives than negative ones. Says Ann F. of her

220-pound weight loss, "It has really changed my life in a positive direction. It is so wonderful to buy clothes in a 'normal' store and not have to deal with all the discrimination, insensitive comments and other humiliations." Donna C. exclaims, "I've enjoyed the compliments (and disbelief) regarding my weight loss and improved appearance. My energy level is better. I'm more active, outgoing and self-assured. I'm attractive to men. And most important, I like myself!" Note, too, that although losing weight will not make your other problems evaporate, you may feel more confident about solving some of them.

• **Accept that it's not easy, it's not always fair.** Losing weight and keeping it off is not a piece of cake — it may be one of the hardest things you ever do. But a number of masters told me that it does get easier with time. As Cindy P. told me, "My weight is something I will have to struggle with all my life. But I've accepted it. It's not 'poor me.' It's just something I have to do. And I care enough about myself to do it. It definitely gets easier with time." (For more on this, see "It Gets Easier with Time" in Chapter 4.) Dr. Kirschenbaum feels that eventually people get to the point where they say, "Yeah, it's unfair that I have this problem, but I'm tired of it." He himself eats only around 1,500 calories a day — not much for a man. "It's not easy," he admits, "but it beats the alternative. There are a lot of things in life that you have to adjust to. It's a choice that you make — instead of fighting it, I accept it."

• **Your motivation for weight control will wax and wane.** Sometimes it's just plain harder than at other times to keep a handle on your weight. It's especially difficult when people stop noticing the "new" you. As Dr. Thomas Wadden, director of the Weight and Eating Disorders Program at the University of Pennsylvania School of Medicine, points out, "*Losing* weight is exciting: your waist gets smaller, and everyone notices. But maintenance is tough because there's no change. And 'no change' is about as exciting as watching paint dry." Although it's important to be prepared for this, note that the masters have not let it get in their way. I was impressed by the enthusiasm and excitement many of them had about their success — long after they'd lost the weight. They seem to develop their own internal incentives, rather than looking to others for praise. One way that Gretchen G. has maintained her 40-pound weight loss for 3 years is, "I try to think thin and visualize myself in a party dress at a social event. I imagine people noticing me and my feeling good about their reactions. This keeps me from binge eating and helps me stay focused on my weight goals." Although Gretchen may seem to be looking to others, she is really engaging in self-praise.

◆ **Give yourself permission to fail.** You *will* make mistakes, and you *will,* from time to time, revert to old habits. But the masters have learned how not to let a "lapse" become a "relapse." (See Chapter 5, "Nip It in the Bud: Break the Relapse Cycle.") They've learned how to pick themselves up after a spill, dust their knees off and start again. As Kevin C., who has lost 45 pounds and kept it off for 7 years, advises, "Learn to forgive yourself. If you mess up, start again tomorrow. You're not going to change overnight." In my experience with counseling overweight people, I found that those who were the most rigid — the ones who never made "mistakes" on their diets — were the most likely to gain the weight back (and gain it rapidly) when they finally did deviate. No one can be a tower of strength all the time.

◆ **Maintenance is not static.** What works at one point in time may not at another. But you'll find new solutions to your problems. Karen S., who's kept 24 pounds off her 5'4" frame for 15 years, says, "I am always trying to improve my eating habits. Some weeks are better than others. Serious overeating is a problem that is always beneath the surface. I must be aware of it in order to prevent it from resurfacing."

◆ **Be persistent.** Although most of the masters had lost and regained weight a number of times before they were finally successful, they didn't give up — they were persistent in their desire to become thin for life. Dorothy C. says, "I feel strongly that many habits leading to overweight can be changed permanently because I achieved drastic changes, but over a long period of time and *gradually*." She lost her 32 pounds over the course of 5 to 6 years and has weighed about 123 for the last 8 years.

How Much Weight Is Too Much Weight?

In the past, overweight people were encouraged to set a goal based on a desirable or ideal weight according to life-insurance company charts. Not only were questions raised about whether these targets were, in fact, ideal from a health standpoint, but they were unrealistically low for many overweight individuals. Now, the gold standard of determining whether you're overweight or obese is a relatively new measure of weight in relation to height, called the "body mass index" (BMI). BMI is determined by taking your weight in pounds, dividing that number by the square of your height in inches, and multiplying that number by 703. The chart on page 46 does the math for you, so you can get an approximate idea of your BMI.

A BMI of 25 to 29.9 puts you in the overweight category, while at a BMI of 30 or above, you're considered obese. When BMI is above 25, your health risks increase compared with someone who has a BMI of less than 25. (The average BMI of American adults is slightly more than 25.)

However, BMI alone is not an indicator of health — in part, because it ignores fitness. One can be physically fit and have a BMI greater than 25. For instance, very muscular people may have a BMI that places them in the overweight category, but this reflects increased body muscle as opposed to fat — and it's excess fat that leads to health problems. On the other hand, going by the BMI may underestimate body fat in elderly people, who tend to lose muscle.

Note, too, that having fat mainly in the abdomen and around

Weight in Pounds

Height	120	130	140	150	160	170	180	190	200	210	220	230	240	250
4'6	29	31	34	36	39	41	43	46	48	51	53	56	58	60
4'8	27	29	31	34	36	38	40	43	45	47	49	52	54	56
4'10	25	27	29	31	34	36	38	40	42	44	46	48	50	52
5'0	23	25	27	29	31	33	35	37	39	41	43	45	47	49
5'2	22	24	26	27	29	31	33	35	37	38	40	42	44	46
5'4	21	22	24	26	28	29	31	33	34	36	38	40	41	43
5'6	19	21	23	24	26	27	29	31	32	34	36	37	39	40
5'8	18	20	21	23	24	26	27	29	30	32	34	35	37	38
5'10	17	19	20	22	23	24	26	27	29	30	32	33	35	36
6'0	16	18	19	20	22	23	24	26	27	28	30	31	33	34
6'2	15	17	18	19	21	22	23	24	26	27	28	30	31	32
6'4	15	16	17	18	20	21	22	23	24	26	27	28	29	30
6'6	14	15	16	17	19	20	21	22	23	24	25	27	28	29
6'8	13	14	15	17	18	19	20	21	22	23	24	25	26	28

Height in Feet and Inches

■ Healthy Weight   ■ Overweight   ■ Obese

Source: *The Surgeon General's Call to Action to Prevent and Decrease Overweight and Obesity 2001,* U.S. Department of Health and Human Services

the waist increases health risks. Men whose waist circumference exceeds 40 inches and women whose waists are over 35 inches are at greater risk of type 2 ("adult") diabetes, high blood pressure and cardiovascular disease than are people with smaller waists. This applies even to people of normal weight who have waists of these measurements. (Measurement should take place around the navel area, after exhaling, and ensuring that the measuring tape is parallel to the floor and snug but doesn't compress the skin.) Both weight loss and exercise can help to reduce abdominal fat. After losing, your waist may still be higher than the cutoff, but University of Pennsylvania weight expert Gary Foster, Ph.D., notes than any improvement is worthwhile.

Thin Is Relative

By using the words "thin for life," I am *not* suggesting that you should pursue the cultural definition of thin or "ideal" body weight. "The prevailing ideal in the United States, particularly for women, is very lean . . . the aesthetic ideal has grown consistently leaner and is now much thinner than the health ideal," Yale University's Dr. Kelly Brownell and the University of Pennsylvania's Dr. Thomas Wadden said in a review article. In other words, American women (and a fair number of men) are obsessed with being *too* thin, thinner than most people — particularly overweight individuals — can ever comfortably be. My definition of "thin" is relative.

In my experience, one of the major reasons many of my former patients regained weight was that they had set their sights on unrealistic goals. Frequently, they would lose about half of their weight, then give up, viewing the cup as half-empty rather than half-full. They couldn't see that even though the charts indicated they should lose 100 pounds, a 50-pound weight loss was a major accomplishment. Many times patients who did meet their goals (based on the charts) would quickly regain because it was too difficult for them to maintain their weight at that level.

As noted earlier, many masters at weight control gained back some weight after they hit their lows. And the National Weight Control Registry study on thousands of weight maintainers has found that most of their success stories are "in the normal to moderately overweight range" after having lost weight. Says *Thin for Life* master Cindy P., "When I weighed 140, I felt like I was in a cage; I had to count everything. I'm definitely not model-thin now, but I figure no matter what you weigh, it could always be another 10 pounds that you want to lose." She has found that not resisting where her body seems to "want" to be is another way of holding the reins — it's easier to control your weight when you're not starving all the time.

Setting a Comfortable Weight Goal

By saying your body "wants" to be at a certain weight, I'm suggesting that I at least partially subscribe to the notion that each person's body has some sort of preset biological weight — one that may or may not fit societal norms — that the body will fight to maintain. If you go much below that weight — for instance, if a 200-pound woman gets down to 135 — your body will fight to be heavier by making you feel constantly hungry and by slowing your metabolism down. Of course, if there is some sort of preset biological weight, it's not necessarily a hard and fast number; there may be a considerable range. And you have control over which end of that range you maintain.

A growing number of experts agree that *any* weight loss is likely to be good for an overweight person. As stated in Chapter 1, research studies suggest that losing just 5 to 10 percent of your body weight (a 10-to 20-pound loss for a 200-pound person) can have beneficial effects on high blood pressure, diabetes and heart-disease risk factors. Sustaining that amount of weight loss for at least a year counts as success from a medical standpoint.

The problem here is that many overweight people don't feel satisfied with such small losses. Indeed, a study headed by the University of Pennsylvania's Dr. Foster, in which nearly 400 obese people were asked to define their "happy weight," "acceptable weight" or "disappointed weight," revealed that, on average, a weight loss of about 16 percent or 42 pounds was considered disappointing, a 64-pound loss was considered acceptable, and a loss of 79 pounds would have made them happy.

So how do you set a comfortable weight goal — one that you're likely to maintain — low enough that you feel successful, but not so low that you feel like you're suffering? Based on guidelines by weight-control experts Drs. Kelly Brownell, Judith Rodin and Thomas Wadden, I put together the following to help you come up with a *comfortable* weight goal, one you can live with:

1. Were/are either your parents or grandparents considerably overweight? If you have a family history of obesity, it may be harder for you to maintain a low weight. Furthermore, if you are very heavy and have been that way for a long time, it makes sense to start with a higher weight goal.
2. As an adult, what is the least you have weighed — and maintained — for at least 1 year? It may be difficult to comfortably maintain a weight any lower than that.
3. What weight would you be if you fit in the largest size clothing that you feel comfortable in? At what point can you say, "I look quite good given where I've been"? (Yes, it might be nice to wear a size 10, but aren't size 14's better than the "plus sizes" you're wearing now?)
4. Think of a few friends or family members of your approximate age and body frame — people who look "normal" to you, not like models. Ask what they weigh.
5. At what weight can you live with the required changes in eating and/or exercise? If you feel constantly hungry at your dream weight and/or you have to exercise more than is realistic, your reasonable weight is higher. You really have to ask yourself whether weighing what a chart says you "should" is worth the price you'd have to pay to stay there.

Consider petite Cathy C., who, at her current weight of 117, has kept off 38 pounds for about 11 years. "Although I'm 5'1", I have a sturdy frame. I wear large-size hats, gloves and shoes. I used to compare my weight with a friend's (she is the same height as I), but found she wears small hats, gloves and tiny shoes. It's hardly a reasonable comparison." Similarly, Chuck F., who's 5'6" and once weighed 205, admits his maintenance weight of 140 to 145 is about 10 pounds more than he originally intended. "I realized that my earlier goal was unrealistically hard to maintain."

In short, a reasonable weight is one that you can maintain without undue suffering, at which you feel quite good about the way you look, and at which you have no serious medical problems caused by weight. Dr. Kelly Brownell suggests that after you've lost the first 10 pounds, you ask yourself if you're willing to continue the food and activity changes you've been making. If so, set your goal at another 10-pound loss, and so on. That's how Ann Q. lost 49 pounds. Starting out at 245, she lost in 10-pound increments. Over the course of several years, she got down to 196.

Accepting a Less-Than-Perfect Body

I have to admit that I've never liked the way I look in a bathing suit. But one summer afternoon, while I was lying on a beach, I took a long, hard look at the bodies around me. Where were all those beautiful women that I see on TV? Instead, I saw one body after another that was far from perfect. My guess is that, at best, 1 in 50 people really look terrific in a bathing suit. Who was I to think that I could — or should — be one of them?

Most people do not have perfect bodies — even after they lose weight. Says dietitian and obesity expert Melanie Polk, M.M.Sc., R.D., "If a person is genetically destined to be shaped like a pear, if she loses weight, she will still be shaped like a pear. She will just be a smaller pear. The same thing is true for a person shaped like an apple."

You can accept your flaws better if you don't focus on your imperfect body parts and instead try to see yourself as a whole. One woman who was obsessed with the "saddle bags" on the outside of her thighs started to see herself differently after her husband told her, "You know, when you walk into a room, people are not staring and thinking, 'Oh my God, look at her thighs.' Instead, they see you as a total person, and the overall impression you give is of a tall, trim woman."

Karen S. told me, "It was important for me to realize that I will never have long, thin legs, nor will I ever look like a fashion model." Karen is one of my dearest friends, and she looks great at 127. (She's kept off 24 pounds for 15 years.) And Linda W., who has been 39 pounds lighter for 6 years, says, "By heritage, I have very heavy calves. For years I tried to diminish their size only to finally find out that all I was doing was building more muscle. I get compliments on my size, so apparently my weight of 126 suits me." (They're both 5′4″ tall.)

Male masters had to learn to accept their shortcomings as well. Ernie L., the profiled master in Chapter 3, maintains, "We have to face up to what we are. No matter how hard I work out, I will never have a body that looks muscular." He adds, "But it's great to have a healthy cardiovascular system."

Once you lose the weight, you do have to be aware of the possibility of what body-image expert Thomas F. Cash, Ph.D., calls "phantom fat." Cindy P. alludes to this when she says, "I don't know if I'll ever look in the mirror and say, 'Gee, I look good.'" According to Dr. Cash, phantom fat occurs when someone who's lost weight has a sense that his or her body is still unacceptable. More often than not, however, masters are able to rejoice in their new bodies. And, like Cindy, even those with phantom fat are much happier with themselves now.

More Than a Weight Goal

Dr. Susan Ross found that many of the successful people in her study lost weight with an attitude of taking one day or one week at a time without an expectation of what the end point would be. Likewise, some masters told me they never set a weight goal. "For me, contentment and normal eating were my goals — not a specific weight," maintains master Claudia B., a philosophy professor who has done research on women's body images. "I'm worried about the amount of attention we give to our bodies. Thus I have *worked* to develop an attitude toward my body that says, 'It's fine just where it wants to be.'" At 5'7½", her body "wants" to be at 135, down 35 pounds for 6½ years.

Some masters had better health and fitness as their goals rather than a set weight. Tom F., profiled in Chapter 8, said, "My motivation was not to lose weight but to become a runner." So at the age of 28 and at a weight of 230 (he's 6' tall), he quit smoking and started running. Within 2 years, he had lost 80 pounds, which was too thin for comfort. He now weighs 185 and has maintained that weight for many years.

A number of experts agree that it's actually better to set health and improved eating habits as your goals rather than a predetermined number on the scale. John Foreyt, Ph.D., coauthor of *Living Without Dieting,* maintains, "The focus should be on healthy lifestyle change. The more you focus on the scale, the worse the outcome." He stresses, "Weight is *part* of one's life; it is *not* one's life." Think, too, about some other benefits of weight loss that are not measured by what the scale says: being able to do more activities with your children or grandchildren, being able to sleep and breathe more easily, or being able to do things you could do before you became heavy — say, playing basketball with your buddies or dancing without getting out of breath.

Indeed, I found that many masters in my survey approached their weight as a symptom of an undesirable lifestyle. Says Irene S., now at a reduced weight of 153 (down from 230), "It's not a matter of dieting. It's a lifetime change. It's a personal change. It's focusing on eating behavior, choices and the rewards of a better quality of life."

Master Becky M. apparently agrees. "When I quit dieting and decided to lead a healthier lifestyle with exercise and good eating, the weight was no longer a struggle. I quit 'living' to eat and hating myself for it." Becky is 5'5" and weighs 120, down 40 pounds from her all-time high. Kelly S. says that what motivated her to lose weight once and for all was the realization that her entire life and self-worth were tied to her weight. "I decided that the weight was not going to be a barrier to feeling good about myself and pursuing my goals." (Be sure to see "You Are Much More Than Your Weight," page 280.)

"You can't just change your lifestyle all at once," points out psychologist Ronna Kabatznick, author of the book *The Zen of Eating*. "That would be like trying to get your Ph.D. in a week. People who are successful meet many small, gradual goals that add up to total lifestyle change." In the following chapters, you'll see the many strategies the masters used to change their lifestyles.

Remember you don't *have* to do anything. You have a choice. It's up to you to decide if you're ready to become thin for life.

Are You Ready?

Are you ready to take the reins, to make the attitude shift? So far, experts have not come up with any reliable tests for readiness to lose weight that will predict the likelihood of success. However, in their book *The Truth About Addiction and Recovery*, psychologist Stanton Peele, Ph.D., and coauthor Archie Brodsky suggest that people trying to overcome weight, alcohol or smoking problems consider the following questions to determine if they're ready to change:

How much do I want to quit the negative behavior — overeating and underexercising?

__ very much   __ a little

__ a good deal   __ not at all

__ somewhat   __ I don't know

Am I ready to change now?

__ ready to change   __ not ready to change

If you are unresolved about these questions, you are not likely to succeed, at least at this point. (Don't give up, though, because the answers can change with time.) Dr. Peele thinks, too, that you can sometimes "light the right kind of fire under yourself" by reflecting on the information you place on the following two lists (sample responses are included):

Reasons for not changing	Reasons for changing
I like to eat.	I'd have more energy.
My husband has never known me thin.	My legs and feet would ache less.
I need food when I'm tense.	I could wear more fashionable clothing.
I hate to exercise.	I'd feel proud of myself.
I'd have to buy all new clothes.	I'd feel less bloated.
	My blood sugar would come down.

The book points out, "It doesn't really matter which list is longer — the one on the right just has to be better." Dr. Peele believes that carefully reflecting on these lists and keeping the positive reasons for change in the forefront of consciousness can motivate some people to change. But if your right-hand list includes few "I's" and "my's" — suggesting you want to lose for others — you probably are not losing the weight for yourself and may not be ready to take the reins.

If you *are* ready, you need to be able to endure some discomfort. Indeed, not every master experienced a mystical attitude shift before losing weight that made the process easy. Some had to really work at changing, and the work was hard. To see if you can handle the discomfort, Dr. Peele suggests asking yourself the following:

If quitting or changing my eating and exercise habits is uncomfortable or painful, how prepared am I to endure this discomfort in order to make the change?

__ very   __ somewhat   __ slightly

You also need to accept the fact that you're in it for the long haul — that this will not be just another couple of weeks of dieting. Can you envision yourself continuing to work on your weight 6 months or a year from now? If the answer is no, now may not be the right time for you to do something about your weight.

Another important consideration in assessing your readiness is looking at your life circumstances. If you have a number of problems right now — or if you've experienced or anticipate any major changes in your life — then it may be better to wait until life is less stressful. The fewer roadblocks in your way, the better, for there is some evidence that if you get off to a good start with weight loss, the more likely you are to be successful over the long haul. Ask yourself the following questions:

- Is my financial situation reasonably stable?
- Is my (or my spouse's) job likely to stay the same for at least the next year?
- Is my workload manageable and will it likely stay that way?
- Am I willing to find time to devote to weight control?
- Are my family members reasonably healthy from a physical standpoint?
- Are my relationships with my spouse, friends and relatives reasonably healthy?
- Can I find a way to become more physically active?
- Are my family members and friends supportive of my desire to lose weight?
- Overall, am I pretty happy right now?
- Am I ready to accept the fact that there is no magic answer — that I have to come up with a plan that works for me in order to lose weight?

In general, the more yeses you have to the questions above, the closer you are to being ready to do something about your weight. Sometimes people do lose weight in the midst of personal crises — it may be one aspect of their lives they feel they can control. And, as Dr. Brownell points out, for some individuals, "life is *always* complicated." Sometimes complications can be the impetus for losing weight, as was the case for several masters who had ended bad relationships and wanted to start "new" lives.

Only you can decide if the time is right.

3

Key to Success #3

Do It Your Way

How did the masters lose their weight? Let me count the ways! The more I looked at their answers to the question "When you were finally successful, how did you do it?" the more I was struck by the diversity of their answers. They lost weight using everything from a macrobiotic diet to a diet high in alcoholic beverages (not recommended!) to a high-fish diet. But it soon became apparent that there was a common theme in how the masters took it off that last time. *Their message — loud and clear — is that if you want to lose weight, you have to find what's best for you. You have to do it your way.*

Ernie L.'s Story

"I am convinced that permanent weight loss is something that each individual must work out for himself," Ernie L. wrote. "For me, it was a combination of exercise, psychological and philosophical enlightenment and healthy diet — low-fat, low-protein, low-alcohol and high-carbohydrate." Ernie came up with this weight-loss plan on his own, but not without years of trial and error. It took him 27 years to find his own way. At a height of 5'11", Ernie weighs 185, down 45 pounds from his all-time high. For the past 12 years or so, his self-styled plan has worked for him.

Until he was 16, Ernie was a skinny kid. That summer, after he started working at a gas station, he explains, "I had money and access to candy and soda machines. I went to drive-ins and loaded up on foods like burgers and shakes. I went from 135 to 180 pounds in one summer."

After high school, he spent 7 years in the Navy, where people always "got on him" because his weight was at the upper limit. (He stayed in the 205 to 215 range; his frame is small, so he can't carry a lot of weight.) "Every diet that came out, I went on. But I'd only lose 4 to 5 pounds." Then, at age 25, Ernie "got very serious" and went on prescription diet pills. "After 6 months on amphetamines, I crashed and ended up in the naval hospital for 2 weeks." He gave up the pills but not the quest to lose weight. Yet he never lost much. In fact, he gained.

After finishing his term in the Navy and completing graduate school, Ernie got a job as a college administrator. With all the sitting around and the two-martini business lunches, his weight soared to 230. Still, Ernie was one of those people who was *always* on a diet. "If anyone asked me, I'd say I'd been on a diet since I was 16 years old." Then, at age 35, Ernie found short-term success by following the Weight Watchers diet and recipes. (He never attended meetings.) He got down to 175 but slowly regained the weight.

The beginnings of what finally did work for Ernie took place about 5 years later. It was his own combination of exercise and a sensible food plan that suited his lifestyle. First, he discovered the value of exercise. He started out with swimming, which did little for his weight but firmed him up. Several years later, he decided to try running. "I hated running, so I started out with one minute a day for the first week. The second week, it was two minutes a day." Within 3 to 4 months, Ernie had worked up to 25 to 30 miles a week. That really slimmed him — all the way down to 175, where he stayed for about 8 years. (Ernie's weight crept up some after he had to give up running because of knee and ankle problems. He now takes a one-hour step aerobics class four times a week as well as doing some long-distance bicycling.)

"When I started running, I became nutritionally aware. I read a lot and discovered that the foods I loved in life might actually be good for me. Over the past 12 years or so, I've structured a diet that works for me. The way I eat now is basically the same way I ate while I was losing weight." When Ernie reflects on his long history of diets, he now sees that they worked for just four or five days. He believes that it was because most of the fad diets at the time were high-protein, low-carbohydrate. "I was raised Italian, on an almost total carbohydrate diet: we had pasta at least two or three times a week, lots of bread, plenty of vegetables, and cereal in the morning. Whenever I went on diets, I went off them because I craved carbohydrates. I realized that the way I ate had to match where I came from culturally.

"So about 10 years ago, when dietitians started talking about increasing carbohydrates, I decided to try it." To this day, Ernie eats lots of pasta and vegetables and views meat more as a condiment or flavoring for foods than as the main part of the meal. He makes an effort to choose chicken or fish, but when he does have meats, they're very lean. He adds, "I had to face up to what I could and couldn't do. I love barbecued spareribs, so I have them once a month. But there are some things I decided to change for the rest of my life — for instance, I gave up butter on bread because it wasn't a big deal to me. I also pretty much gave up beer: I used to drink maybe a six-pack a week. Now, I might have a six-pack in a year."

Ernie also mapped out a daily food plan that works for him. He eats a large, healthful breakfast — say, juice, cereal, banana and 2 percent milk. He finds no need to eat during the day and often works out during his lunch hour. His supper typically is a small portion of broiled meat, chicken or fish, pasta, salad and lots of vegetables. "Then I hit my danger period — from 8 to 10:00 P.M. It's my grazing time. I take care of it with herbal tea or no-sugar European coffees, maybe some cocoa, a piece of fruit or popcorn."

Ernie adds, "This strictly pertains to me. You have to ask yourself *not* 'What diet can I go on?' but 'How can I change my eating habits permanently?' If you live 30 more years, what can you do for the rest of your life?" For Ernie, it's an ongoing process. He says, "My diet gets better and better; it's changing today."

Ernie also believes there's a strong psychological component to losing weight permanently. He says every heavy person needs to start by asking, "Is there any possibility I'm getting a payoff for being fat?" For him, there was a positive component to being overweight. "I wouldn't have to mow my lawn on a hot day because I was afraid of having a heart attack. I couldn't do so many things because of my weight. You have to ask yourself if there's a less neurotic way to get what you want. If you don't want to mow the lawn, you don't have to stay heavy to get out of it. Maybe you could hire a kid to do it."

On a deeper level, Ernie feels that his weight shielded him from competition. "There's a whole physical nature in being masculine, and being heavy meant I didn't have to compete in the same way as if I were not heavy. Then, when I realized I could be physical without being competitive, I saw that there were things other than basketball and football. With running, I could compete with myself."

Over and over, Ernie stressed, "I'm convinced that this is my own thing. Of all the issues, weight control ranks as one of the most complex. Of all the things that need absolute, individual attention, it is weight."

Self-Styled vs. Program People

At times, I was tempted to call this chapter "Get It Off, I Don't Care How." But as I talked with masters like Ernie L., I realized that *how* you lose weight *is* important. It's a matter of finding a healthful plan or program that's right for you, that's safe to follow, that you can tailor to meet your own needs and that prepares you for maintenance. "When it comes to weight-loss success stories, just about any program will work for someone, but no one thing will work for everybody," notes registered dietitian Gail A. Levey.

There were, as always with the masters, common themes. Most of their weight-loss plans fell into one of two categories:

• The *self-styled* masters — people who lost weight on their own. Responses from nearly half the masters indicated they lost their weight as Ernie L. did, by following self-styled schemes, commonly consisting of low-fat, low-calorie food plans and increased exercise. It was a rare self-styled master who lost weight by following any sort of stringent diet. In fact, many used a nondieting approach similar to that which starts on page 128. (Chapter 4, "Accept the Food Facts," offers plenty of ideas for becoming a self-styled master.)

• The *program* people. Nearly half the masters lost weight with the aid of some sort of structured weight-loss program or self-help group, such as Take Off Pounds Sensibly (TOPS), Weight Watchers, Health Management Resources, Nutri/System, Jenny Craig or Diet Center.* (Six people in this category lost weight primarily with the help of a dietitian, behavior-modification class or physician.)

As mentioned in Chapter 1, findings from the National Weight Control Registry are similar: 55 percent of its members used a formal program or professional assistance to lose weight, while the other 45 percent said they had lost on their own. And like the many *Thin for Life* masters who stressed that exercise played a pivotal role in their final weight-loss attempt (see Chapter 7),

---

*Most of these programs are quite different now than they were when the masters lost their weight. For an overview of some popular weight-loss programs, see pages 90–95.

nearly every Registry member reported using a combination of diet plus exercise to both lose weight and maintain weight loss.

When asked how they finally lost weight, *self-styled* masters gave me responses like:

◆ "I threw out the scale and changed my daily activities and attitudes about food."

◆ "No fat, no meat, eating tiny meals and lots of willpower."

◆ "Regular exercise, eating low-fat healthy foods (fruits, vegetables, whole grains) and eating only when hungry."

◆ "Watched diet closely and exercised. No seconds at meals, no bread, no soft drinks and sweets. Plus, I had a friend to do it with me, and we gave each other encouragement."

There were lots of individual techniques that helped masters lose weight. Some mentioned such simple things as eating smaller portions, counting calories and keeping diet diaries. For one person, the key was eating the majority of calories before 5:00 P.M. Another said her secret was not getting upset if she gained a pound. Another drank a lot of the diet beverage Tab. *Very few masters lost weight by following fad diets. None attributed their success to diet pills.*

Of the *program* people, some simply used the programs as a tool for losing weight, but now they maintain on their own. Others continue to attend group meetings faithfully and/or go back to the program when they start to gain weight. (See Chapter 10, "Don't Go It Alone," for more on group support.) Here's what some of the program people had to say:

◆ "I was nearly 40 pounds overweight when I joined Weight Watchers. When my sister-in-law found I had signed up for the program, she said, 'I've never known anyone who was in the Weight Watchers system who didn't gain all the weight back.'

Those were fighting words for me!" (She lost 57 pounds with Weight Watchers and has kept it off for 19 years.)

◆ "For the most part, I have kept my weight either below or around 200 pounds for the past 5 years." (This 6′ man once weighed 382.) "I truly credit my weekly attendance at Health Management Resources maintenance classes."

◆ "I get tremendous support from TOPS — my chapter and state-wide. You talk about what's bothering you. There's a family feeling." This woman lost 62 pounds, which she's kept off for 4 years.

Some program people lost their weight in stages, with a variety of methods:

◆ "10 pounds through Shaklee, 10 through Omnitrition, the other 15 through better eating and exercise." (It took this woman 6½ years to lose 35 pounds, but she did it.)

◆ "I started with Nutri/System, and it was a very good program for me to start with . . . I signed up to lose 30 pounds, and I did [3 years ago]. I joined Diet Center 7 months ago to lose the last 15 pounds."

As much as I'd like to tell you that there is one "right" way to lose weight, the bottom line, when it comes to selecting a plan to get the weight off, is that the process is highly individual.

What Do the Studies Show?

Before discussing how to find a weight-loss plan that's right for you, let's look at some research findings on success stories. Findings from the National Weight Control Registry confirm that successful maintainers use a wide variety of methods to lose weight and to keep it off. Its researchers state, "This great diversity in strategies suggests that individuals may be more likely to lose weight and maintain weight if, rather than attempting to use one standard set of strategies, they selectively choose their means of restricting dietary intake and increasing activity levels."

In this same vein, one of the strongest findings of the large 2002 *Consumer Reports* survey, which identified 4,056 "super-losers" who had lost an average of 37 pounds and kept it off for at least 5 years, was, "When it comes to losing weight, one size definitely does not fit all . . . Diets that work match an individual's personal needs and preferences."

In a fascinating study comparing a group of women who had maintained weight loss with women who had gained back lost weight, researchers at Kaiser Permanente Medical Center offices in Fremont, California, found that the maintainers shed pounds by devising personal "plans to fit their lives." The plans usually included regular exercise and a new eating style that consisted of consuming less fat, less sugar, more fruits and vegetables and much less food than previously. Like Ernie L., with his occasional spareribs, the maintainers did not completely restrict their favorite foods and made efforts to avoid feeling deprived.

In contrast, regainers were far less likely to have exercised to lose weight and were instead more likely to have lost weight by taking appetite suppressants and shots, fasting, going to weight-control groups or to hypnosis or by going on diets described in books or magazines. While dieting, they denied themselves foods they enjoyed, and they felt deprived. Compared with the regainers, the successful women seemed to have more of an ability to "look within" and to depend less on outside help. They also used dietary strategies they could live with permanently.

As Ernie L. puts it, "You have to look at your eating style and see what you crave and, within that style, what will work for you. What are you willing to do?"

How do people personalize commercial weight-loss programs to meet their individual needs? I got some insights from Ed Grattan, M.A., who interviewed each of the 82 weight maintainers in the University of Iowa College of Medicine study (page 12) for

1½ hours. "What was critical was when people took ownership, and a weight-loss program became *their* program," he said. "For instance, even though Mary may have gone to Diet Center, it became her program because she individualized it, making subtle changes in portions or foods." By changing the program, people became responsible for anything that might happen in the future.

Take master Violet Y., who, at the age of 64, went to Weight Watchers. That was 20 years ago, when the food plan was much stricter. "I attended meetings quite regularly and usually lost at least a pound or two. I did not fully comply with Weight Watchers suggestions. Also I am a 'chocoholic,' so every day I ate three chocolate chips!" She lost 57 pounds, which she's kept off to this day. But she did it her way.

Whatever method you choose, you have to find a way to make it your own — so it's your plan and you're in control. Ernie L. believes that one of the reasons he was ready to lose weight once and for all was that he resolved some spiritual issues that led him to take control of his life. After deciding to leave behind his religious ties, he found, "I then became responsible for me. No church or parents were guiding my life."

This was Ernie's way. But it's important to realize that the very act of devising your own weight-loss plan is a way of taking responsibility for your life and your weight problem. It's also a means of increasing your sense of self-efficacy, that sense of how competent and effective you really can be at controlling your weight.

Learn from the Past

Not another diet! When you think about trying to lose weight *again,* you're faced with your past history — that long line of diets and other methods through which you tried unsuccessfully to control your weight. These efforts can serve as cruel reminders of failure. Or, as psychologists Brenda L. Wolfe, Ph.D., and G. Alan Marlatt, Ph.D., propose in *The Weight Control Digest,* you can use your past attempts at weight loss as "a rich library of what worked and what did not." (They note, too, that past weight-loss attempts show your potential for change.) *No matter what you weigh, how many times you've lost and regained weight — you are more knowledgeable now than you were before each weight-loss effort of the past.* Ernie L. says, "You get to be an expert only because you had so many failures."

As Dr. Ronna Kabatznick, author of *The Zen of Eating,* puts it, "When you're learning to ride a bike, it's highly unlikely that you'll do it right the first time. And it's human to fall and scrape your knees. It's the same way with trying to lose weight — you'll have setbacks, but you learn something with each attempt." Look to your past experiences to identify what did and didn't work for you. Says master Sam E., who's lost 35 pounds and kept them off for 10 years, "If you hate fish, don't eat it just to lose weight."

Since you already have a sense of what will and won't work for you, start out by making two lists. Here's a sample:

What worked	What didn't work
occasionally having a treat	strict dieting
having 3 meals a day	skipping lunch
saving up calories for parties	denying myself bread
limiting red meat	eating grapefruit 5 times a day
packing my lunch the night before	

For more help in figuring out what worked and didn't work, ask yourself the following questions while reflecting on your last two or three attempts at weight loss:

◆ Think about the food plan or diet you used — was the calorie level too high or too low? What foods could you have? What foods couldn't you have? Was this just right or too restrictive for you? Was there much food preparation or shopping involved?

What did you do to make the food plan work for you? (For example, did you make a special effort to keep plenty of fruits and vegetables on hand?) Would any of this be right for you now?

◆ How did you feel — both physically and mentally — on past weight-loss plans? Think about what made you feel good and bad.

◆ What sort of exercise plan did you follow? Was it realistic, one you could fit into your current routine? How could you modify it?

◆ What were the most difficult and easiest aspects of this plan?

◆ How did you modify your daily routine? Were there new activities you adopted that were helpful? (For instance, did you stop going grocery shopping right before dinner, when temptation levels are high?)

Call your answers to these questions into play as you finally decide upon a weight-loss program. If, like Ernie L., you love carbohydrates, don't choose a food plan that eliminates them. If you feel you can't lose weight on a plan that allows you to eat sweets, then choose one that temporarily cuts them out. (Remember, though, that most successful maintainers do not deny themselves favorite foods; they eventually learn how to control them.) If you hated swimming the last time you lost weight — it took too much time to drive to the pool — then you might want to consider an at-home exercise program or something you can do outside your front door, like walking. (For more on exercise, see Chapter 7, "Move It to Lose It.")

Consider the possibility of returning to a plan that worked for you in the past. If it helped you before, it may help you again. Moreover, you may find that a weight-loss program you attended in the past is better than before, since good programs change with the times.

In reflecting on her past weight-loss attempts, Donna C. says,

"My problem was that I focused on 'the diet' and what you had to give up. I was either 'going on' or 'going off.' It was feast or famine. I needed the lifestyle-change aspect." And that's how she finally lost her 108 pounds: by attending a several-month class on behavior modification and lifestyle change taught by a registered dietitian.

Ann F. also learned a great deal from her past experiences. (She had plenty to draw from: she estimates that she tried to lose weight 20 to 30 times before she finally lost her 220 pounds.) She had been on many diets that were highly restrictive. She told me, "The more extreme the diet, the more I failed. These diets made me feel physically sick and depressed, probably because I did a lot of them." Ann also learned that "eat-only-one-food, strict-rules diets" set her up for failure. "I wanted whatever I couldn't have. Now I feel there's no such thing as good and bad food." Looking back on her experiences, she found Overeaters Anonymous to be too focused on food and binge eating for her liking. With Weight Watchers, she acknowledges that although she did not lose weight and keep it off with their program, "their reasonable diet may have helped to establish my current habits." Because of her massive weight problem (she once weighed 380), Ann finally had gastric surgery (see page 86). But she still has to do what most of the other masters do to keep the weight off: eat less and engage in more physical activity. Her secret of success is, "I eat what I like, eat moderately and exercise. I try to eat a low-fat, balanced diet."

Think about your past experiences and draw from them as you make the decision about your final weight-loss plan.

Finding the Right Match

The problem with some weight-loss books and regimens is that they try to make you think there is one right way to lose weight. As we've established, however, the approaches used by the masters were highly variable.

I can't even tell you that the experts are always right in their recommendations about what approaches will work for what people. For instance, some experts tend to favor more aggressive approaches, such as medically supervised diets (see page 78) or residential weight-loss programs, for people who have large amounts of weight to lose. Indeed, for someone with more than 100 pounds to take off, it can be far more motivating to follow a plan that allows for more rapid weight loss than one that allows just half-a-pound-a-week weight loss.

Nevertheless, some "big losers" among the masters did just fine on less extreme plans. Bob W. credits his 250-pound loss to Weight Watchers. (He's kept it off for 21 years.) "They taught me what to eat and how to cook low-calorie meals. Through the Weight Watchers program, I received much moral support." Then there's Joseph M., who, 19 years ago, lost 115 pounds by following his own self-styled diet based on Weight Watchers that included lots of fish (twice a day), vegetables and fruit. "I never went to Weight Watchers [although his mother did, and sent him diet information]. I'm not into 'rah, rah' stuff."

It would be ideal to find a way to match people with weight-loss programs personalized *for them,* based on past weight-loss experiences, medical history and other individual differences. In most studies, however, people are randomly assigned to various types of weight-loss treatment groups rather than preassessed and matched to an approach that would fit them, notes Dr. Daniel Kirschenbaum. He also cites evidence that although many people are unlikely to function well in groups, most weight-loss studies offer treatment in group settings.

So how do *you* find the right match? Says Joseph M., "You have to search it out." That is, you have to do some investigation, some research to sort out what you like and don't like about various weight-loss approaches. When Alisa S. was ready to lose weight once and for all, she did her homework by touring her local library diet section. "I found one book that talked about the emotional side of being fat, the purposes of eating and not eating and a diet-for-life plan. That gave me the grounds for a 25-pound loss for the past 7 years."

Diets Can (and Do) Work for Some People

Although a number of masters said that they did best when they threw away all diets, planned diets did work for many masters, either through commercial weight-loss programs or strict medically supervised plans. However, as suggested in Chapter 1, diets — when defined as purposeful and sustained efforts to restrict your calorie intake so you lose weight and/or change your body shape — are spurned by a number of experts and consumer advocacy groups who claim that most people regain the lost weight, that dieting causes more problems than the excess weight itself and that overweight people should give up dieting, then accept themselves as they are. Some also say that dieting leads to emotional problems and eating disorders such as binge eating. Research studies do not support these concerns.

In the first place, according to Gary Foster, Ph.D., clinical director of the Weight and Eating Disorders Program at the University of Pennsylvania School of Medicine, "concerns that dieting is universally harmful are based largely on studies of normal-weight college-age women who have restrictive eating habits." Second, after reviewing studies on the subject, the National Task Force on the Prevention and Treatment of Obesity concluded recently, "Concerns that dieting induces eating disorders or other psychological dysfunction in overweight and obese adults are generally not supported by empirical studies." (These findings do not apply to average-weight people, such as teenage girls who diet to look like models and for whom dieting could be a forerunner to an eating disorder.)

Rena Wing, Ph.D., cofounder of the National Weight Control Registry, told me, "If anything, participants will say that, when they finally lost weight, their diets were stricter than in the past."

In fact, more than 6 out of 10 of the Registry participants essentially said that. Moreover, about 20 percent of the Registry participants used liquid formula as part of their successful weight-loss effort. (At this writing, the Registry researchers are doing an analysis to see how many of these people used liquid formulas as part of medically supervised programs and how many used over-the-counter formulas like SlimFast.) So while many experts are telling people to feel happy losing weight slowly and dropping just 10 percent of their weight — and there definitely are medical benefits from such modest weight loss — it seems that many people who are successful go at it more aggressively.

None of this is to say that crash diets are good for you. (As you'll see later in this chapter, strict diets that lead to loss of more than a pound or two of weight per week require medical supervision.) Nor am I advocating diets for all would-be "masters." Says obesity expert Dr. Susan Olson, "A diet for a short period of time can be a motivation. If it doesn't work, chuck it." Diets do not necessarily set you up for failure — it's how you perceive them and use them. It's important that diets be viewed as tools — not long-term solutions to weight problems. (See Chapter 4, "Food Fact #1: The masters stop seeing the way they eat as dieting.")

If you opt for a formal diet plan — as did a number of the masters — you may want to consider the Jump-Start Diet on page 360. It will allow you to lose weight fairly quickly in the beginning, so that you become motivated to keep losing. But if you decide on the nondieting weight-loss route, then check out the 6-Week Nondieting Weight-Control Plan on page 128. Whatever route you choose, the Weight-control Information Network, which is part of the National Institutes of Health, advises, "If you plan to lose more than 15 to 20 pounds, have any health problems, or take medication on a regular basis, you should be evaluated by your doctor before beginning your weight-loss program."

Doing It <u>Your</u> Way

Following are some questions you can ask yourself to help figure out what's right for you as you investigate various approaches:

◆ **Are you a "program" person or a "self-styler"?** A group person or a loner? Do you find it helpful to be with others who have the same problem or do you prefer to deal with things on your own? If you lean toward groups, does the one you're considering have enough members of each sex to suit you?

◆ **Do you do well on diets or have you had it with dieting?** Decide whether you want to go the dieting route, the nondieting route or something in between.

◆ **If you choose a dieting approach, can you tailor or modify the diet to suit your own needs,** if not in the beginning, later? Does the approach or program discourage this?

◆ **How much freedom of choice do you need?** If you can't bear the thought of liquid meals or prepackaged foods and know you've gone off them quickly in the past, try something different this time. On the other hand, some people prefer a more stringent and structured approach to get them started.

◆ **How much money do you want to spend?** The most expensive programs tend to be residential programs, medically supervised very-low-calorie plans and those that supply you with food. "The good news for dieters is that there is no association between cost and effectiveness," note Tufts University Medical School's Johanna Dwyer, D.Sc., R.D., and Diana Lu, M.S., R.D., in a review of popular diets. When comparing costs, be sure to get a written estimate of the entire program, including up-front and fixed costs, periodic costs, optional costs, the cost of the maintenance program and any refundable costs.

◆ **Does the program or plan in question support your personal weight goal** (see page 48)? If an unrealistically low goal is imposed upon you in any way, it's a tip-off that the approach is less than ideal.

◆ **To what extent is exercise emphasized?** Are the suggestions realistic for your lifestyle? Is medical supervision of exercise encouraged?

◆ **Do you prefer working with professionals,** such as psychologists, dietitians, nurses and physicians? (Don't be afraid to ask for the credentials or weight-management experience of the staff.) Or do you find groups led by laypeople to be more helpful?

◆ **If you're considering a program, how frequent are the sessions?** Is this compatible with your lifestyle?

◆ **What is the maintenance component of the plan?** (Some experts advise you to spend at least one month in a maintenance program for each month that you spend losing weight.) Will you be taught skills for life? Do you go back for group meetings or appointments? Is this included in the original cost?

◆ **Does the plan have the right emphasis on nutrition and food preparation for you?** If you rarely cook for yourself, then a program with a heavy emphasis on food preparation may not be for you.

◆ **If you are an emotional and/or binge eater, does the plan offer a way to help you?** Will the plan enable you to develop more positive thinking and coping skills?

There are no right answers. You have to decide if any one particular approach suits you and your needs. (For overviews of weight-loss programs, consult the list on pages 90–95.)

Be aware that many medical insurance companies do not pay for treatment of weight problems, although they may cover at least part of the program if you have another weight-related health problem, such as high blood pressure. On the good news front, in 2002, the U.S. Internal Revenue Service determined that obesity is a disease and now allows treatment (such as nutrition counseling and obesity surgery) to be tax-deductible as part of medical expenses, whether or not you have a related health problem. However, you must have an official diagnosis of obesity by a physician. Check with an accountant for the details.

Is It Legit?

The following are tip-offs that a weight-loss plan may be less than reputable:

◆ **Suggestions that weight loss will be quick and easy.** For most people, it's not. Unless you're in a medically supervised program, steer clear of programs that promise more than 2 pounds' loss per week after the first week or two.

◆ **Diets that overemphasize one food or food group.** They may be unbalanced, and you won't be likely to stick with them.

◆ **Claims that you can eat all you want and still lose weight.** That's impossible.

◆ **"Guaranteed, forever" results.** There are no guarantees, even with the best of programs.

◆ **Claims that dealing with sensitivities or allergies will "cure" your weight problem.** There is no sound evidence that overweight is caused by sensitivities or allergies.

◆ **Offers of foods or supplements that burn off fat.** There are no known combinations of foods or special supplements that you can take to burn off fat.

◆ **Unscientific remedies, such as body wraps, injections, herbs and cellulite treatments.**

◆ **Promises of secret or breakthrough findings.** If there were a breakthrough, you'd see it on the front page of your local newspaper — and not as an ad.

The Mathematics of Weight Loss

Simplistic as it sounds, if you want to lose weight, you have to eat fewer calories than you burn off each day. You can do it by cutting back on calories or by increasing your activity level so you expend more calories. But the best method is some combination of the two.

Most American women eat about 1,800 calories a day; for men the figure is 2,800 calories. (Men tend to have higher calorie needs because their bodies have a greater percentage of muscle tissue and less fat than those of women; muscle tissue burns more calories than fat.) Assuming that a woman is maintaining her weight on 1,800 calories a day, how much will she lose on a 1,000-calorie-a-day diet? Since she's burning off an extra 800 calories each day — above and beyond the calories she's consuming — her calorie deficit for 1 week would be 7 days x 800 = 5,600 calories. Divide 5,600 by 3,500 (the approximate number of calories in a pound of body fat), and she should lose about 1½ pounds of body fat per week on her 1,000-calorie diet. Of course, weight loss is often greater in the beginning, presumably because of body-water losses. (A major National Institutes of Health report that issued guidelines for managing weight problems recommended that weight loss be achieved by cutting back by 500 to 1,000 calories a day, which theoretically should result in weight loss of a pound or two per week.)

Be aware, however, that weight loss is highly variable from one person to the next — depending on one's overall size, activity level and metabolic rate. Thus, some people on the same diet lose more weight than others do. In one study, published in the *American Journal of Clinical Nutrition,* a group of 108 obese women who were placed on an 800-calorie-a-day diet for 21 days lost anywhere from 2 pounds to 28 pounds. Some women did not lose any weight at all until day 13 of the diet.

Where do the calories you expend each day go? Fully 60 to 70 percent of them are used for your resting metabolic rate (RMR).

RMR is the energy required to run the body at rest — to do the bare minimum: breathe, keep your heart pumping and regulate body temperature. Another 5 to 15 percent of your calories are used to digest and process food that you eat. The remaining component of calorie expenditure — physical activity — is the one over which you have the most influence. Even if you're not physically active, 20 to 30 percent of calories are used on everyday activities.

In Chapter 1, I mentioned that a low metabolic rate may play a role in the development of a weight problem and that this rate can vary greatly among people of similar size. Consider a University of Pennsylvania study in which RMR was measured in a group of overweight women of the same weight, age and height. Individual RMRs for these 5 women were: 1,263, 1,523, 1,778, 1,979 and 2,152 calories per day. "If these 5 women consumed a 1,200-calorie diet for 3 months, their weight losses would be 11, 20, 28, 35 and 40 pounds, respectively," says Dr. Gary Foster, who directed the study.

The differences in RMR explain in large part why some people lose weight so much more easily than others. Just as certain individuals have thick, shiny hair while others have thin, limp locks, some people have slower metabolisms than others. If you're a slow loser, Dr. Kabatznick points out, "You have to learn to see small amounts of weight loss on a steady basis as success — at least you didn't gain." Of course, as mentioned earlier, even if you have a low RMR (which you have little influence over), you still have control over the number of calories you expend in exercise.

We've also talked about how metabolic rate drops with dieting — it's the body's way of adapting to a state of semi-starvation. As an act of self-preservation, the body, in effect, says, "You're not feeding me enough calories, so I'll slow down the rate at which I burn them." RMR also decreases after you lose weight because you weigh less. (It should make sense, for instance, that if you maintained your old 200-pound weight on 2,400 calories a day, you won't be able to eat that much if you want to maintain your weight at 150 pounds.) And unfortunately, RMR drops as most people age, mainly because the body contains proportionately more fat tissue, which is metabolically less active than muscle tissue. A major reason that calorie needs tend to drop in older people is that they are often less physically active. The good news is that exercise may offset at least some of this change.

The Question of Safety

If you choose to follow a formal diet, how can you be certain of its safety — be it a "program" diet or a "self-styled" diet? Let's start with the least aggressive diets, which are the logical starting point for the self-styled dieter and/or for someone who doesn't have a lot of weight to lose, who is relatively new to dieting or who just doesn't opt for a more intensive approach.

Diets providing 1,200 or more daily calories are likely to be nutritionally adequate if they're carefully planned according to the Food Guide Pyramid (see page 129). In general, such diets should provide the following amounts of these nutrients each day:

◆ Protein — about 15 percent of calories, which would mean 45 grams for a 1,200-calorie diet and 56 grams for a 1,500-calorie diet (from lean animal sources, like skinless poultry and fish, and vegetable sources such as legumes [dried beans])

◆ Carbohydrate — at least 100 grams (ideally, 55 percent or more of total calories), predominantly from complex carbohydrate foods (for instance, root vegetables, pasta or rice rather than sweets), whole-grain products, as well as a variety of fruits and vegetables

◆ Water — as a general rule of thumb, 8 eight-ounce cups of liquid (A number of masters told me that drinking lots of water helps them control their weight, although there is no scientific explanation for this.)

◆ Calcium — 1,000 to 1,500 milligrams from foods and/or supplements

◆ Fiber — the "adequate intake" for women is 21 to 25 grams per day; for men, it is 30 to 38 grams.

Moreover, no more than 30 percent of your calories should come from fat. To play it safe, it doesn't hurt to take a multivitamin-mineral supplement when on such a diet. (Note, however, that there is no reason to consume excessive levels of any vitamin or mineral.) Also, many women may need a calcium supplement, and premenopausal women may need extra iron as well — so check with your doctor. (A growing body of studies suggests that, in addition to protecting bones, calcium plays a role in preventing weight gain and may also help with weight loss. However, calcium from pills may not be as effective as calcium from food sources.)

Low-calorie diets — those in the 800-to-1,200-calorie-per-day range — should be undertaken with a physician's approval and ongoing supervision, particularly if you have a lot of weight to lose and/or medical problems. The lower the calorie level, the less likely the diet is to be nutritionally adequate. Multivitamin-mineral supplements are usually recommended, as are iron and calcium supplements for many women. Some commercial weight-loss programs start out with low-calorie diets the first few weeks, then increase calories to 1,200 or more per day.

Very-low-calorie diets (VLCDs), the most aggressive types, proved effective for a number of the masters. Meant for people with BMIs of 30 or more, VLCDs can be particularly helpful when someone needs to lose weight quickly because of urgent health problems. Because they can have serious side effects, *VLCDs should be followed only under careful medical supervision; they are not meant for self-styled dieters.*

VLCDs provide fewer than 800 calories per day, and include relatively large amounts of protein from either animal protein foods or high-protein liquid formulas. Special supplements are needed as well. (VLCDs are a modification of total fasting; protein is added to prevent your body from breaking down its own protein, which can be dangerous. Total fasting is not recommended under any circumstances because of the excessive losses of body protein, water and nutrients.) VLCDs appear to be safe for periods up to 16 weeks when taken with appropriate supplements and used under supervision of experienced medical professionals. (Note that the risk of gallstones increases with any significant weight loss, which is one reason why medical supervision is required on VLCDs.)

Because they require medical oversight, VLCDs are more expensive than less-intensive weight-loss approaches. They should be used as only one part of a comprehensive program that includes behavior modification, cognitive restructuring, exercise, education about nutrition and the transition back to "real foods," and a strong maintenance program. The ideal staff for such a program includes a physician, registered dietitian, psychologist, nurse and exercise physiologist — all specially trained in the treatment of overweight people.

Generally, VLCDs do result in much greater weight losses than low-calorie diets, but there is conflicting information about whether, on average, people on these diets keep off more weight over the long run than do dieters on programs that are somewhat more liberal. Concluding that they do not, a 1998 government report discouraged use of VLCDs. Yet one recent review of 29 studies involving thousands of people compared results from studies involving people on VLCDs with results from studies of people on low-calorie diets and concluded that 5 years after being on the diets, those who had lost weight on the VLCDs tended to have better maintenance of weight loss. Says lead author James Anderson, M.D., a renowned weight and diabetes expert at the University of Kentucky, "There just isn't evidence that slow weight loss results in better maintenance of weight loss."

Nevertheless, acting on the results of several studies suggesting that there is no weight-loss advantage to consuming fewer than 800 calories per day, Dr. Wadden's group at the University of Pennsylvania has stopped using VLCDs in favor of a 900-to-1,000-calorie diet consisting of four liquid meal supplements per day, plus one evening frozen-food entree along with a fruit and vegetable serving. Indeed, some studies suggest that liquid meal replacements and structured meal plans with portion-controlled foods might work better than conventional self-selected diets of the same calorie level for people who have a lot of weight to lose.

Despite the lack of consensus about the one best diet for weight loss, it does appear that we have a much better sense of the ideal diet for weight maintenance: as you'll see in Chapter 4, the diets of most Thin for Life *masters are inconsistent with the popular low-carbohydrate diets so popular today. And fewer than 1 percent of National Weight Control Registry participants said they consumed a low-carbohydrate diet.*

The Skinny on Low-Carb Diets

The most popular diets today advocate cutting way back on carbohydrates that come from simple sugars (in foods like table sugar, syrup, honey, fruits and desserts), as well as starches, which are found in foods like pasta, root vegetables, breads, rice and cereals. Most of these diets also advocate liberal protein consumption. *But in sharp contrast to the low-carb, high-protein fad, almost no masters said they lost weight the low-carb way.*

In the 1980s and 1990s, it was widely believed that as long as you kept your fat intake way down, you could eat unlimited amounts of carbohydrate-rich foods (carbs) and still lose weight. Since this approach failed for many people, it now seems attractive to turn to diets that promise you will lose weight while eating whatever you want of protein-rich foods such as steak and eggs — as long as you strictly limit your carbs.

Mainstream nutrition experts discourage such diets because they are based on faulty assumptions about metabolism, limit foods that supply needed nutrients and endorse levels of protein and fat that might be harmful. Indeed, high-protein diets are often also high in fat and saturated fat, the kind of fat that can lead to cardiovascular disease. In fact, numerous health organizations, including the American Heart Association, steer people away from high-protein diets because of health concerns.

The potential negatives aside, do high-protein, low-carbohydrate diets work for weight control? While there hasn't been much research on the effectiveness of these diets, the truth is that all diets work for some people. You *can* lose body fat on these diets, but that appears to be primarily because you consume fewer calories when following them. People tend to eat between 1,200 and 1,500 calories a day when on a high-protein, low-carb diet, which is low enough for most people to lose weight. (If you give up breads, pasta and sweets as well as many vegetables and fruits, it follows that you will reduce calories, since you can only eat just so much steak, eggs, chicken and cheese.) But are people more likely to lose weight on high-protein plans than on traditional diets?

Several ongoing studies comparing more conventional low-fat, high-carb diets with low-carb, high-protein diets suggest that the high-protein diets might have an edge — at least over the short term. In one of them, respected Danish researcher Dr. Arne Astrup and colleagues conducted a 6-month study in which 65 obese people were allowed to eat freely of either of two fat-reduced diets — one of the diets was high in carbohydrate, the other high in protein. People on the high-protein diets lost more weight — an average of almost 20 pounds versus 11 on the high-carb diet. On average, people on the high-protein diet were eating about 450 fewer calories per day than were the high-carbohydrate eaters. Dr. Astrup suspects that the explanation may lie in the fact that the high-protein meals tend to make people feel full sooner than do high-carb meals. Also, the high-carb eaters were allowed to eat sweets like candy, on which they might have gone overboard. (At the one-year mark, both groups had essentially maintained their weight losses.) It's worth noting, however, that these studies involve only small numbers of people and whether or not they continue to keep the weight off remains to be seen.

Quite a bit of research does suggest that on a calorie-for-calorie basis, if you compare carbohydrate or fat with protein, protein has greater satiating power. (Satiation is the capacity of a food to tell you that you've had enough to eat at a meal and it's time to stop eating.) Dr. Astrup feels that some dieters would do best with a diet that's liberal in *low-fat* high-protein foods, such as lean meats, skinless poultry, fish and low-fat milk products, but also rich in complex carbohydrate foods such as whole-grain breads and cereal as well as vegetables. Indeed, if you do go the more liberal protein route, it's wise to veer away from the high-fat types like regular cheeses, steaks, and fatty processed meats like bacon and salami.

Insulin Resistance

Another premise behind a number of popular low-carb approaches is that a high-carb diet will lead to increased levels of the hormone insulin, which, in turn, is said to lead to weight gain, particularly in "insulin-resistant people." It's true that foods rich in carbohydrates cause the highest spikes in blood-insulin levels because after carbohydrates are eaten and broken down into blood glucose, insulin is needed to transport the glucose out of the bloodstream into the body's cells, where it is used for energy. Those with insulin resistance cannot efficiently dispose of glucose, even though their bodies still make the hormone. As a result, their blood glucose can become elevated, and they may wind up with type 2 diabetes. According to some low-carb-diet proponents, the excess insulin and dietary carbohydrate team up to make you fat. If you restrict carbohydrates, they say, you will lower insulin levels and lose weight.

But according to a review of studies on the effects of sugar, published in 2002 in the *Journal of the American Dietetic Association,* there is no direct link between carbohydrate foods (including sugar) and obesity *or* diabetes, unless excessive consumption of such foods leads to weight gain. In other words, it's *being overweight* that causes insulin resistance to manifest itself and cause problems — not carbohydrates. Nor does scientific evidence substantiate the belief that people with insulin resistance are particularly prone to become obese if they eat a high-carbohydrate diet. Losing weight *in the way that's right for you* is the best way to do away with insulin resistance.

Glycemic Index

Another weight-loss trend that has to do with restricting carbohydrates of certain types is based on "glycemic index," a concept originally designed to help people with diabetes control their blood sugar. Essentially, GI is a way of ranking carbohydrate-containing foods according to how much blood glucose goes up right after you eat them. In general, high-GI foods include sweets and refined starchy foods like cakes, cookies, white rice and white bread. Low-GI foods are generally high in fiber and include certain whole-grain products, as well as many (but not all) fruits and vegetables such as legumes.

Supposedly, foods with lower numbers are best for weight control because — compared with higher-GI foods — they cause less of a peak in both blood sugar and insulin. This, in turn, means that glucose should leave the bloodstream more gradually, which should leave you feeling more satisfied until the next meal.

In contrast, high-GI foods — ones that cause a quick, high elevation of blood sugar — cause a surge in insulin, which then "gobbles up" the blood glucose, causing blood glucose levels to plummet — supposedly leaving you feeling hungrier sooner than you would if you had eaten lower-GI foods. When put to the scientific test, however, some studies have suggested that eating low-GI foods and meals might help with weight loss, while other studies have not. While there is reason to believe that there might be something to GI — not only for weight control but also for controlling diabetes and heart disease — most of the studies have been short-term and do not show whether eating according to GI helps with weight control over time.

A recent issue of the *Tufts University Health & Nutrition Letter* points out that there are a number of practical problems with letting GI guide your food choices. In the first place, many things just don't make sense. For instance, sugar-frosted flakes have a lower GI than fiber-rich bran flakes — and nutritious carrots come out higher still in GI. Whole-wheat bread has about the same GI as white bread, and white potatoes have a higher GI than sweet potatoes. Also, when you combine foods, as in putting butter on a baked potato, the GI of the combined foods is different than that of the food alone.

Some health professionals who feel that GI does influence weight offer guidance that just makes good nutritional sense: eat more whole-grain foods instead of processed versions; eat meals with a variety of foods, including carbohydrate, protein and a little fat; don't eat too many sugary and sweet foods; and eat more fruits, vegetables and legumes.

According to a recent review on popular diets by the North American Association for the Study of Obesity (NAASO), the bottom line when it comes to hunger and satisfaction on diets is this: "There does not seem to be an optimal diet for reducing hunger." The group maintains that whether or not you can stick with a weight-loss plan has more to do with *psychological* issues (such as coping with emotional eating) than the balance of carbohydrates, proteins and fats. It may have to do, too, with individual differences that we don't yet fully understand.

I would not be at all surprised if someday we find out that the ideal diet for weight *loss* is not necessarily the same as the ideal diet for weight *maintenance*. And the "ideal" weight-loss diet for one person may differ from that of another. For some people, that might be a diet that's high in complex carbohydrates, for others it might be a diet more liberal in low-fat protein foods. To help you plan a diet that meets your individual needs and allows you to be healthy while shedding weight, your best bet is to see a registered dietitian and/or physician who specializes in weight management or to go to a program that offers sound dietary approaches.

Give Yourself Time

Whatever means you choose to get the weight off, it's important to be patient. You didn't gain the weight overnight, and you can't expect to lose it overnight (or in a week or a month) either. In fact, the vast majority of masters took 6 or more months to reach their goal weights. Many took 2 or more years.

If you decide you're a program person, the longer you stick with it, the more weight you're likely to lose. A review of 105 studies on behavioral weight-control programs revealed that duration of treatment was the single most important factor positively associated with weight loss. (Often run by local hospitals and university research programs, behavioral programs typically offer weekly sessions of varying duration and are for small groups of participants. Such programs may be led by dietitians, psychologists, nurses, exercise specialists or some combination of those, and they usually include behavior-modification (sometimes called lifestyle modification) techniques (see page 120), positive-thinking strategies (see Chapter 6), and sensible diet and exercise guidelines. After reviewing 13 studies in which behavioral treatment was extended beyond 6 months through the use of weekly or biweekly sessions, weight-maintenance expert Michael G. Perri, Ph.D., and colleague Joyce Corsica, Ph.D., from the University of Florida, Gainesville, concluded that the data "strongly suggest that extended treatment improves maintenance of weight loss . . . that continuing treatment beyond 6 months, through the use of weekly or bi-weekly sessions, improves the maintenance of weight loss." The idea is that a longer program gives you more time to practice the skills necessary for maintenance before you venture out on your own.

Surgery and Drugs

Someone with a body mass index of 40 or above (about 100 pounds overweight for a man, 80 pounds for a woman) who has failed on more conventional weight-loss plans may be a candidate for surgery for weight loss. You could also be a surgery candidate if your BMI is between 35 and 40 and you have obesity-related problems such as type 2 diabetes or heart disease. Two of the masters I interviewed lost weight with surgery. Ann F. once weighed 380 pounds, and Lisa B. was once as heavy as 385. Both have kept off more than 200 pounds. (Note, too, that just a small percentage of National Weight Control Registry members lost weight through surgery.)

Two types of operations have been proven to be effective. "Vertical banded gastroplasty" (VBG) in essence "shrinks" the stomach (with both a band and staples) so you can't eat as much, while the "Roux-en-Y gastric bypass" (RGB) not only creates a smaller stomach, but also creates a "bypass" of part of the small intestine so your body absorbs fewer calories. About 30 percent of people who undergo VBG get down to normal weight, while 80 percent lose at least some weight. The more commonly done RGB operation typically results in more weight loss than VGB — you could expect to lose about two-thirds of your excess weight within 2 years. However, it is important to note that it is possible to regain weight after these operations, so dietary vigilance and exercise are still required to keep the weight off. Although their weight loss resulted primarily from the surgery, both Ann F. and Lisa B. exercise regularly and are careful about what they eat to maintain their new weights.

According to Richard Atkinson, M.D., professor of Medicine and Nutritional Sciences at the University of Wisconsin, Madison, the surgery should be done only by an experienced surgeon who does several such operations per month. You also need to know what kind of follow-up care you'll receive. "If the surgeon tells you, 'I'll do it, then you'll be seen by your local doctor,' that's not good enough." You will need regular follow-up visits with a physician who is knowledgeable about the procedure — be it the surgeon himself or an internist who has a formal collaboration with the surgeon. In fact, if you undergo such surgery, you'll need lifelong medical monitoring. (The main concerns, says Dr. Atkinson, are possible nutrient deficiencies, which can be prevented by taking supplements.) Because success depends on your willingness to change eating habits and to exercise regularly, it is critical that your return visits include education about nutrition, exercise, lifestyle change and behavior modification.

Dr. Atkinson adds that you should talk with people who have had the surgery. "It's a serious step. It should be done only if you can't lose weight any other way or if you have critical medical problems like diabetes or high blood pressure. It's serious surgery, and there are some unpleasant side effects. You'll never be able to eat huge meals again." Surgery for obesity is expensive, too, running as high as $25,000 in 2002. (Medical coverage varies by state and insurance provider.)

In 2001, the U.S. Food and Drug Administration (FDA) approved a new surgical device, called the Lap-Band Adjustable Gastric Banding System, for the treatment of severe obesity. A reversible procedure, it offers some benefits over traditional gastric bypass surgery, but it may not be as effective.

Surgery for weight loss is definitely on the rise — 62,400 such operations were projected by the American Society for Bariatric

Surgery for the year 2002 — up from 23,100 such surgeries estimated to have been done five years earlier. Drs. Thomas Wadden and Suzette Osei note, in the *Handbook of Obesity Treatment,* that surgery for obesity, which was once considered "bordering on the barbaric," is now in their opinion an "underutilized" approach. Indeed, for some people suffering from extreme overweight who have tried everything else and failed, who have serious medical problems caused by their weight, and/or who have lost and regained large amounts of weight, obesity surgery offers hope and may be the treatment of choice.

Like surgery, prescription weight-loss medications are meant for people who are at increased medical risk because of their weight — not for those who want to lose 10 or 20 pounds for cosmetic reasons. These drugs are approved for those whose BMI is 30 or more, as well as for people with a BMI of 27 or above if they have other risk factors, like high blood pressure. And like surgery, these drugs are for individuals who have had little or no success with diet and exercise to control their weight.

As of mid-2002, the only drugs approved by the U.S. Food and Drug Administration for long-term treatment of obesity are sibutramine (Meridia) and orlistat (Xenical), two drugs that were approved for use *after* the masters lost their weight and so were not available to them. Many masters mentioned that they'd tried appetite suppressant drugs in the past, but none said they found long-term success with them. And only about 4 percent of Registry members used medications to help with their final weight-loss effort.

Orlistat works by reducing the body's absorption of dietary fat — by about one-third. Sibutramine, on the other hand, works by increasing the levels of certain brain chemicals that help reduce appetite. Both drugs can have side effects and require medical supervision. If you think you're a candidate for either weight-loss medication, you have to be realistic about what these drugs can do for you. Studies show that, 2 years after beginning these drugs, people can expect to lose as much as 8 to 10 percent of their starting weight (or 4 to 22 pounds), although some lose much more than that. And most of the weight is lost within the first 6 months. (These drugs don't work for everyone — if you don't lose 4 to 5 pounds during the first month of taking them, you should discuss with your physician the possibility of stopping them and considering some other course of action.)

These drugs work by controlling what goes on "inside" the person, while behavior modification helps people control their outside world by learning ways to watch portion size, avoiding high-calorie foods and learning how to manage stress without overeating. So putting the two strategies together — and adding exercise — makes sense. In fact, the major role of medications is that they seem to help you stick with a diet and exercise plan, possibly making your job a bit easier. Even though weight loss tapers off after 4 to 6 months on these drugs, they can help you maintain the weight you've lost. Note, however, that discontinuing medication usually results in gaining back the pounds. (A book that offers a comprehensive weight-loss plan involving Xenical is *The Xenical Advantage* by Dr. John Foreyt, published by Simon & Schuster.)

Both sibutramine and orlistat appear to be generally safe for long-term use, as long as possible side effects are monitored by a physician. However, there is little information on how safe and effective weight-loss medications are when used for many years. (At this writing, the FDA is reassessing the risk-benefit profile for Meridia because of some concerns that a consumer group raised about the drug's safety.) Other prescription drugs are approved for the treatment of obesity, but they are to be used only for a few weeks.

As for weight-loss products claiming that they are "natural" or "herbal," be skeptical — according to the *FDA Consumer* magazine, "This does not necessarily mean they're safe." In fact, a

2002 statement on weight management in the *Journal of the American Dietetic Association* concluded that "over-the-counter and herbal preparations [for weight loss] are currently not recommended." (The FDA is also reviewing the safety and efficacy of ephedra, a chemical compound found in some herbal products promoted for weight loss and currently sold as dietary supplements.)

With the increasingly accepted view that obesity is a disease requiring lifelong vigilance and treatment — and exciting new discoveries about the causes of obesity — it's likely that the future will bring about the approval of additional drugs that will help people win the weight battle. For more information about surgery and medications for obesity, visit the Web site of the Weight-control Information Network at www.gov/health/nutrit/win.htm.

For more information on surgery for obesity (also called bariatric surgery), contact:

American Society for Bariatric Surgery
7328 West University Avenue, Suite F
Gainesville, FL 32607
Phone: 352-331-4900
Web site: www.asbs.org

Some Weight-Loss Programs Used by the Masters

After doing a survey of more than 32,000 dieters in 2002, *Consumer Reports* concluded that you don't need diet programs to lose weight. However, many masters, as well as National Weight Control Registry members, *did* find success with commercial and self-help weight-loss programs. The following list includes some of the more popular programs used by the masters — programs that are worth checking out if you're seeking help for weight loss. Note that programs change from time to time — as such, the descriptions below are of the programs as they exist at this writing. (Nutri/System, for instance, is a different program now than it was when some of the masters found success with it.) Contact each program directly or visit its Web site for details on its dietary approaches, behavioral and exercise components, Internet support programs, maintenance plan, costs and any research studies on its success rates.

(This list is not exhaustive, and exclusion from the list does not signify rejection of a particular program.)

Weight Watchers is the largest commercial weight-loss program, both in the United States and the world. It combines group support with a program consisting of a balanced, low-calorie diet, behavior modification and exercise, at a relatively low cost. The current Weight Watchers eating plan is based on a system in which foods are assigned POINTS, and participants are allotted so many each day to "spend" as they choose. Members who follow the plan as directed should wind up eating between 1,200 and 1,500 calories per day. Costs to join the program vary at different times of the year, but weekly meetings run about $12.00 per session. Weekly meetings are led by company-trained leaders who have successfully been through the program.

Weight Watchers International, Inc.
175 Crossways Park West
Woodbury, NY 11797
Phone: 516-390-1400
Web site: www.WeightWatchers.com

(To locate the nearest meeting, call 800-651-6000 or use the meeting finder at the Web site.)

Jenny Craig offers a one-on-one program in which clients have brief weekly meetings with a company-trained consultant who may or may not have personal or professional experience with weight management. The consultant helps you implement the program menus and educational materials as designed by staff registered dietitians. Menus are low in fat and range from 1,200 to 2,300 calories per day. Clients have the option of choosing from 7 days' worth of Jenny Craig cuisine or a combination of company foods and home-prepared and/or restaurant meals. The 7-day menu option costs between $10 and $12 per day. Jenny Craig's overall program costs, in addition to the foods, vary because the company offers a number of packages of different duration.

Jenny Craig, Inc.
5770 Fleet Street
Carlsbad, CA 92008
Phone: 760-696-4000
Web site: www.jennycraig.com

(To locate the nearest Jenny Craig Centre: call 800-JENNY20 or use the locator at the Web site.)

Nutri/System, Inc. had many franchises when many of the masters lost their weight. In 1999, however, the company reestablished itself as nutrisystem.com, an Internet-based weight-loss company. (The company notes that a small number of franchises still offer the same program and products as nutrisystem.com. But there are also many Nutri/System "distribution centers," which, in addition to the Nutri/System products and program, can offer weight-loss products and services that have nothing to do with and are not endorsed by Nutri/System.) The nutrisystem.com weight-loss program consists of portion-controlled, low-fat meal packages, delivered by ground service to the home, which add up to 1,200 to 1,500 calories per day. In 2002, a week's worth of food (3 meals per day, plus 1 snack) cost $54.95, the only fee for the program. The program includes Internet counseling sessions with a company-trained counselor who may or may not have personal or professional experience with weight loss. For people who don't have access to the Internet, the program is available by telephone.

Nutri/System, Inc.
202 Welsh Road
Horsham, PA 19044
Phone: 800-585-5483
Web site: www. nutrisystem.com

TOPS, or Take Off Pounds Sensibly, is a nonprofit, noncommercial self-help weight-loss support group program with 10,300 chapters worldwide. (More than 8,500 of them are in the United States.) Although TOPS offers a healthy lifestyle guide, the group recommends that participants obtain food and exercise plans from their personal physicians. Aside from a confidential weigh-in at the beginning of each weekly chapter meeting, there is no set program or format for the meetings, which are run by volunteer leaders who are also program members. Headquarters supplies leaders with many different programs, covering a variety of weight-loss issues. Yearly membership in TOPS is $20, and there are also local dues, which vary but typically cost less than $5 per month. A TOPS interactive program was recently introduced on its Web site, which gives members access to professional consultants, including registered dietitians, and allows users to create personalized eating and exercise plans.

TOPS Club, Inc.
4575 S. Fifth Street
Milwaukee, WI 53207
Phone: 800-932-8677
Web site: www.tops.org

OPTIFAST weight management programs are medically supervised and designed for obese people who have health risks because of their weight. The typical OPTIFAST program includes at least 20 weeks of treatment, beginning with 12 weeks of active weight loss during which most clients solely consume OPTIFAST meal replacement formulas in addition to bars and soups. (There are 800-, 950- and 1,200-calorie options. The 1,200-calorie option may include a frozen or self-prepared diet entree.) During the next 6 to 8 weeks, self-prepared meals are gradually introduced, after which patients begin an open-ended maintenance program. Ongoing monitoring by a physician is required during active weight loss and transition to self-prepared meals. Participants are required to attend 60- to 90-minute weekly lifestyle education classes conducted by healthcare professionals of various disciplines including nutrition, lifestyle change and exercise. Costs of the OPTIFAST program vary depending on the calorie level of the diet, health status of the participant and length of treatment. The typical range is between $1,500 and $3,000.

Novartis Nutrition
Box 370
Minneapolis, MN 55440-0370
Phone: 800-662-2540
Web site: www.optifast.com

HMR, or Health Management Resources HMR, or Health Management Resources offers several dieting options, including a physician-directed very-low-calorie diet (500 to 800+ calories) consisting only of HMR weight-loss shakes and entrees, for people who want to lose 30 or more pounds. Another more liberal HMR diet (1,200 to 1,400 calories) that promotes slower weight loss allows fruits and vegetables in addition to the HMR shakes and entrees. In both options, HMR clients meet in weekly group classes led by trained health professionals and receive individualized counseling from a personal weight-loss "coach." HMR is known for its intense maintenance program, which focuses on retraining lifestyle habits, including practicing ways to lower fat and calories, eat more fruits and vegetables and expend calories through physical activity — again, provided through group classes and personal coaching. For people who don't have an HMR program in their area, HMR offers a mail-order catalog of its meal replacements as well as an "at-home" version of its program that provides coaching and group meetings by telephone. Costs of HMR programs vary according to the diet chosen, but typically range from $13 to $20 a week, plus the weekly cost of meal replacements, which runs from $62 to $85. (Price does not include medical supervision.)

Health Management Resources
59 Temple Place, Suite 704
Boston, MA 02111-1346
Phone: 617-357-9876
Web site: www.hmrprogram.com

Books

These books are all written by reputable experts and take the subject of weight control from varying perspectives. Check them out to see if they meet your individual needs. *Note: This is by no means an exhaustive list. There are other legitimate weight-loss books.* (For more recommended books, see page 386.)

The American Dietetic Association Complete Food and Nutrition Guide, 2nd edition by Roberta Larson Duyff. 2002. New York: John Wiley & Sons. (Not a weight-loss book per se, but a good all-around guide to healthy eating.)

The Art & Science of Rational Eating by Albert Ellis, Michael Abrams, and Lidia Dengelegi. 1992. Fort Lee, NJ: Barricade Books.

Dieting for Dummies by Jane Kirby. 1998. Hoboken, NJ: John Wiley & Sons.

Dr. Jo's How to Stay Healthy & Fit on the Road and *Dining Lean: How to Eat Healthy in Your Favorite Restaurants* (2 books) by Joanne V. Lichten. 2001 and 1998, respectively. Houston: Nutrifit Publishing. (1-888-431-5326)

Eating Thin for Life: Food Secrets and Recipes from People Who Have Lost Weight and Kept It Off by Anne M. Fletcher. 1997. Boston: Houghton Mifflin.

Handbook of Obesity Treatment by Thomas A. Wadden and Albert J. Stunkard. 2002. New York: Guilford Press. (Note that this is an advanced guide for professionals.)

The LEARN Program for Weight Management — 2000 by Kelly D. Brownell. 2000. Dallas: American Health Publishing Co. (1-888-LEARN-41)

Living Without Dieting by John P. Foreyt and G. Ken Goodrick. 1994. New York: Warner Books.

Maximize Your Body Potential by Joyce D. Nash. 2003. Palo Alto: Bull Publishing Co.

Mayo Clinic on Healthy Weight by Donald D. Hensrud. 2000. New York: Kensington Publishing Corporation.

The 9 Truths About Weight Loss by Daniel Kirschenbaum. 1999. New York: Henry Holt & Company.

Now That You've Lost It by Joyce D. Nash. 2000. iUniverse.com.

101 Weight Loss Tips for Preventing and Controlling Diabetes by Ann Daly, Linda Delahanty and Judith Wylie-Rosett. 2002. Alexandria, VA: American Diabetes Association.

Thin for Life Daybook by Anne M. Fletcher. 1998. Boston: Houghton Mifflin.

The Truth About Addiction and Recovery by Stanton Peele and Archie Brodsky. 1992. New York: Fireside Books. (Not a weight-loss book, but a good guide to lifestyle change.)

The Weight Maintenance Survival Guide by Kelly D. Brownell and Judith Rodin. 1990. Dallas: American Health Publishing Co.

4

Key to Success #4

Accept the Food Facts: Featuring a 6-Week Nondieting Weight-Control Plan

Most masters peacefully accept their new way of eating: they know they can't eat whatever they want, and they know they can't go back to their old food habits. They have learned how to make low-fat eating enjoyable, and they have accepted certain food facts.

Susan C.'s Story

As I interviewed Susan C., I had a hard time distinguishing the difference between how she ate while she was losing her 100-plus pounds and how she eats now. There are many similarities. When Susan lost weight, she cut way back on meat. She still eats little meat. While losing, she "religiously" ate three regular meals a day. Same behavior now. With every 10-pound drop, Susan would treat herself to a favorite food. Now, at maintenance, she includes plenty of treats. "Yes," she says, "I eat pies, cookies, cakes, drink wine and Scotch — but in moderation." Today, she weighs 132. Fifteen years ago, she carried about 250 pounds on her 5'7" frame.

In retrospect, Susan C. says that her 31-year difficulty with her weight was the result of eating at every time *except* mealtime. "At the age of 9, I was given a cookbook and told to cook for the family when my mother went to work. I could never understand why I had a weight problem because I never ate much at the table. But as I cooked, I would eat. As I cleaned up, I would eat some more. If I made cookies, half of the dough would be gone before it hit the sheets. But I never ate the cookies."

Susan also attributes her former weight problem to her Scandinavian and Portuguese food heritage. "Meat was usually eaten three times a day. It was meat, potatoes and gravy." That tradition, along with her penchant for picking as she cooked, landed Susan in size-18 dresses by the time she was a freshman in high school. "Can you imagine being 16 and wearing a size 44-D bra?" she asked.

From her earliest memories, Susan was heavy. "I have a picture of me as a baby from when I won a contest. I was the happiest, most chubby baby." She recalls many hardships as a child. "My brothers and sisters were slender, and I could never eat the foods they did because I was too fat. I always had to bring my lunch to school because I couldn't eat what the other kids did. My mother would pick me up after school, and I'd go home and eat cottage cheese." Children called her names, and she wore "sack" dresses. "Once my mother made me a crinoline dress, but I looked like a flying hippopotamus in it."

By the time she was in college, Susan weighed 250 pounds. She met a man who wasn't concerned about her weight and married him in her sophomore year. "I would diet, and it never worked out. But it didn't bother him." Like most masters, Susan tried to shed pounds many times and in many ways before she found success. "I tried all the current fad diets available at the time: egg diets, grapefruit diets, eat-everything diets, liquid diets, cottage-cheese diets and so on." But she never lost more than 5 pounds with any of these schemes.

"I was thoroughly convinced that I'd be fat for the rest of my life. I was sure it was the result of an outside problem — my metabolism, my thyroid, a medical problem that would never be resolved. I believe I know all of the excuses for being heavy and most of the avoidance methods for facing the truth."

What finally turned the tide for Susan? She says, "There didn't seem to be any one particular thing or event. I really believe that psychologically I was ready. Something finally clicked in my head." (There's that "click" again.) Her weight loss began when she happened to drop several pounds right before she and her husband moved from Oregon to Southern California, where Susan had access to a swimming pool. She started to swim, which she loves, and noticed some more weight coming off. A spiral began. "I found that it was really possible to lose weight, and I decided to keep up the momentum through exercise and a change in my eating habits."

Exercise was critical to Susan's weight-loss efforts. "I bought a 10-speed bicycle and rode it for 10 miles early every morning. Then I'd swim 50 laps a day — rain or shine — and I did floor exercises two to three times a day." She kept all that up for about a year, the length of time it took to lose most of the weight. What about now? Susan says, "I exercise, but not fanatically." Actually, Susan is one of a minority of masters who has no formal exercise program. But she makes an effort to be physically active: "I walk a little more, climb more stairs, stretch a little more, and sometimes I do floor exercises. In the winter, I shovel snow a lot and wash my car. I try not to sit around. In the summer, I get up early and do work in the garden and yard. I'm conscious of not sitting on my rear end all day."

How did she eat when she was losing weight? Much the way she does now. "I stopped eating a lot of meat and concentrated on vegetables, fruits, fish, chicken and cottage cheese. I never would have dreamed that cutting out meat would make a difference. I also love dairy products: cream, cheese and butter. But gradually, I cut back and learned I could live with less. I also ate at very specific times, three meals a day. My husband would take me for a pizza or ice cream soda once a month. I eagerly anticipated that treat. After a while, I no longer needed that incentive, and as my eating habits changed, so did my longing for certain foods.

"This worked for me but may not for someone else. You have to ask yourself what will suit your lifestyle. Then keeping the weight off will come easier." Susan found that strict diets of the past, "where I ate half a cup of cottage cheese, half a grapefruit, 3 ounces of meat and half a cup of beans, and having to be the only one eating like that made me feel like I was punished. You don't need to be regimented — just have some discipline and stop cheating on yourself."

In general, Susan has cut down on fats and tries to stay away from fried foods of any sort. She eats mostly vegetables, grains and some cheese, like part-skim mozzarella or farmer cheese. She eats meat only about once a week. Breakfast typically consists of cereal, fruit and bread. Lunch might be cottage cheese and fruit, a salad and fresh vegetables. Dinner is usually whatever she cooks for her husband — Italian, Indian, Thai — but Susan doesn't eat as much as he does. She also finds drinking water to be helpful in controlling her weight: she consumes 8 to 10 glasses a day.

Susan's childhood penchant for cooking is still with her. She makes her own bread, cakes, cookies, jams and jellies, pasta and sauces. "My husband is Italian, so we eat a lot of pasta — but not with cream. I might make homemade sausage, but I'll just eat a few pieces. If we have Parmesan cheese, which is full of calories, it's not in the recipe, just sprinkled on top." Lately, Susan has been enjoying Indian cookery. "It calls for quite a bit of oil, so I let the finished dish sit and remove the fat from the top." But Susan loves chicken skin, so she broils the chicken and allows herself the skin. And she eats real butter, but only in small amounts.

As she cooks, Susan has learned not to taste any more than is essential to the success of a recipe in an effort to overcome her old habit of eating a whole meal before she ever got to the table. "When I'm clearing the table, if I feel tempted to eat something left behind, I dump it in the garbage disposal quickly."

I was surprised at the number of tempting foods Susan is able to keep around. "At the moment, there's a jar of peanuts sitting on my counter." But Susan has learned how to handle her highest-temptation foods. "I have a bag of cashews in my cupboard, but I don't start because I know I won't be able to stop." She admits to an occasional urge to go on a food binge. "So I go downtown and buy an expensive candy bar. It takes care of a craving. I give in to it, and it satisfies me. Then I go on with my business. Once I allow myself to have it, I don't have to worry anymore."

If things get out of hand, it's just for a short time. Susan recently made a sumptuous strawberry-rhubarb pie and found herself eating three slices in one day. So she said to herself, "Hmmm, that's full of calories. You can't have pie three times a day."

Susan finds it critical to weigh herself daily. If the scale creeps up a few pounds (she never lets herself gain more than 5), she cuts back for a few days. "I might have grapefruit and dry toast for breakfast, a salad with apple and cheese for lunch, then a normal supper, but less of it. Within a few days, I'm back down again. I ask myself, 'Was it worth it?' No, it wasn't."

In short, Susan has been able to maintain a 100-pound-plus weight loss for many years, yet she still has a nice food life. It's not one of sacrifice and denial, but instead one involving moderation, trade-offs and pleasure in knowing what she really wants to eat and what she can forgo.

The Many Ways of Maintenance

When I asked each master, "What are the three most important things you do to keep your weight down?" I got more than 90 different answers. Here are some of their responses:

- ◆ "Make weekly menus and shop to fit the menus."
- ◆ "Monitor fat intake."
- ◆ "Eat differently — more fruit, less sugar/fat."
- ◆ "Eat nutritious meals — reasonable amounts."

- ◆ "Eat the bad things only on Saturday."
- ◆ "Avoid old 'problem' foods: excess pasta, bread, butter, sour cream. I don't eliminate, just watch quantity."
- ◆ "Portion control of foods."
- ◆ "Eat oatmeal every morning — no sausage, bacon or eggs."

It soon became obvious that there are just as many ways to maintain weight as there are to lose it in the first place. But, again, I was struck by certain "food facts" that emerged from the stories of the masters.

FOOD FACT #1
The masters stop seeing the way they eat as dieting.

I have an overweight friend who does all the "right" stuff when she's trying to lose weight. Vegetables in cream sauce make way for plain, steamed versions. She eats more chicken and fish in place of fattier meats. Diet salad dressing takes the place of chunky blue cheese. The freezer is filled with frozen yogurt. Then, after she sheds 30 pounds or so, she gets sick of the new way of eating. All of the changes are reversed, and on go the pounds — again. My friend lives in one of two states: she's either on a diet or off one.

Susan C., however, never used the word "diet" to describe how she lost weight that final time nor to describe the way she eats now, even when she cuts back for a few days to lose a few unwanted pounds. Actually, the word "diet" stems from the Greek word *diaita,* meaning "way of life." And it's quite clear that the way Susan eats has simply become just that for her. When Arizona researchers Drs. Robert Colvin and Susan Olson conducted their first interviews, they found themselves saying, "You're telling us what you eat *now.* How about when you were losing?" Their typical puzzled reply was, "*Of course* it's the same food — how could you ever go back to what you ate before?" Similarly, when I asked the masters, "How do you think your eating habits are different from those of people who lose weight and gain it back?" their most common responses had to do with lifestyle change and accepting that they cannot return to their old habits.

In an article on preventing weight regain, psychologists Brenda L. Wolfe, Ph.D., and G. Alan Marlatt, Ph.D., state, "The first essential step in *preventing relapse* is eliminating the artificial boundary between *weight loss* and *weight maintenance*." The masters recognize this: they see that the strategies to lose weight and those to maintain weight are essentially one and the same.

Diets can be useful tools to get you started on weight loss. But, as psychologist Dr. Ronna Kabatznick points out, "The difference between weight loss and maintenance is only a couple of hundred calories for many people. It's an extra sandwich or an extra dessert. You have to close the gap between the effort it takes to lose weight and to keep it off."

Here's what the masters have to say about breaking away from the diet mentality:

◆ Sam E., who lost 35 pounds 10 years ago, reiterates, "People need to realize that what they are doing now to get the weight off has to be what they are willing to do once the weight comes off." Like a number of masters, Sam lost weight when she stopped dieting and adopted a lifestyle of healthy eating.

◆ Bob W., who has lost 250 pounds and has maintained that loss for 21 years, says, "I keep the weight off by continuing to do what I did to lose it."

◆ Nancy K., who's kept off 60 pounds for 5 years: "I lost weight when I quit dieting and just watched what I ate."

◆ Linda W. lost her 39 pounds 6 years ago when she "decided to just try to cut back rather than going on an all-out starvation diet."

◆ Rose F. has lost 35 pounds and is still losing: "The secret is I never really denied myself anything that I really wanted. I just cut back a little each day and stayed with it. My original plan was to quit gaining and start losing without torturing myself."

I was impressed by the similarities in the way other masters ate "then" (when they were actively losing weight) and how they eat now.

◆ Marie D. **Then:** "Ate low-fat healthy foods (fruits, vegetables, whole grains) and ate only when hungry." **Now:** "Concentrate on eating unprocessed foods, whole grains, little meat and low-fat foods and eating only when hungry."

◆ Linda G. **Then:** "Ate smaller portions, watched fat and sugar intake." **Now:** "Modest portions, less fat, less sugar."

◆ Don C. **Then:** "Ate low-fat, low-sugar, high-fiber." **Now:** "Try to maintain low-fat, high-fiber diet and minimize between-meal snacking."

◆ Mindy B. **Then:** "I decided to cut out all fat from my diet. I ate no meat, but I did eat chicken and fish." **Now:** "I don't eat meat, and my fat intake is minimal. I eat fruit, raw vegetables, lots of yogurt, rice, potatoes and chicken and fish."

Accepting that you have to make permanent changes in the way you eat doesn't mean a lifetime of hardship but does mean some sacrifice and delay of gratification. Donna C. is one who admits it's a struggle to keep off her 108 pounds. She adds, "But it's worth it! My life has changed dramatically for the better, and I love it!"

Pat B. also feels great about her choice to adopt a new way of eating. "I'm lazy. I don't ever want to have to do it [lose weight] again. I don't ever want to be that unhappy again." She's kept off 84 pounds for 10 years.

FOOD FACT #2
The masters survive the transition from weight loss to maintenance.

Even with a change in attitude, the transition from losing weight to maintenance is not always easy. There's no question that most people do eat less while losing and get to eat more afterward. The difficulty is making the decision about what foods to add at maintenance, particularly for people who have lost pounds quickly through a more structured weight-loss plan and/or a strict diet. Kevin C. lost his 45 pounds in 5 months and admits, "Maintenance was a nightmare. You're probably better off if you lose weight slowly so you have more time to make behavioral changes." If you're a program person, you should stay with the program through the maintenance phase.

Many slimmed-down people, however, contradict the popular notion that maintaining weight loss is harder than losing it in the first place. Surprisingly, the vast majority of people in the National Weight Control Registry seem to disagree with that idea! Two-thirds of them said maintenance is "easy" or "moderately easy," while only one-third view it as "hard." Of course, as Kevin C. suggests, how you lose the weight may alter your perception of how difficult maintenance really is — the Registry members who lost weight on their own were more likely to say maintenance was easier than taking the pounds off, while those who used liquid weight-loss formulas as part of a formal program were more inclined to say just the opposite. It may be that the liquid dieters had it easier while losing because they didn't have to make food decisions, but it became more of a struggle when they reached their goals because they had to learn how to maintain weight while eating regular foods.

For numerous *Thin for Life* masters, learning what to eat at maintenance seemed to be a trial-and-error process. Of the difference between her current eating routine and the one when she was slimming down, Susan C. says, "When I was losing weight, I wouldn't eat pasta because I thought it was more fattening. I would eat my meat plainer and skipped most desserts. I was more focused then than now, but I don't recall a transition period. My maintenance eating just seems to have evolved from changing my eating habits." (The remaining Food Facts will help you establish maintenance food habits, as will the "Nondieting Weight-Control Plan" on page 128.)

Of course, it's easier to "settle in" to maintenance food habits if you discover the value of exercise as you're losing weight or shortly thereafter. Brian L. felt a need to cut out sweets as he was losing his 20 pounds (he's 5′5″) 15 years ago. But when he started running shortly after he lost the weight, he found that he could include his treats.

Another difficulty in making the transition is finding your "comfortable weight" (see page 48). Many masters initially dropped to a weight that was too low for comfort. For example, Brenda Z. says, "My goal of 135 was hard to maintain. I can maintain and not 'fight my body' at 140 to 145."

Susan C. still views herself as heavy and wishes she had been prepared for feeling this way as she was losing weight. Similarly, Jeffrey B. continues to see himself as "a fat person, even though I've had the weight off longer than I've had it on. And I still have to work to believe it when my friends say I look better at 180 than at 150." (He's 6′1″ tall and weighed 235 pounds 22 years ago.)

FOOD FACT #3
The masters see the beauty of low-fat eating.

When asked the three most important factors in keeping their weight down, the number-one food-related response from the masters was "watch my fat intake." In fact, 9 out of 10 masters answered "Yes" to the question "Do you eat a low-fat diet now?" Most of them told me they eat in the neighborhood of 20 to 30 percent of their calories from fat.

Patsy B. (73 pounds, 3 years): "I basically cut all fats from my diet. It's wonderful, and I really do eat a lot. I buy fat-free [products] and sometimes these things cost a little more, but they are worth it."

Shirley C. (26 pounds, 12½ years): "Even when eating out, which I do at least twice a week, I tell waitpersons I'm allergic to butter. I eat fish out — but seldom, if ever, meat. I'm careful but happy in my eating habits."

Marie D. (32 pounds, 3 years): "I focus on eating a low-fat diet and eating only when I'm hungry. I eat as much as I want of healthy foods."

Edith S. (56 pounds, 3 years): "I never starved myself as I had done many times before. I ate all the complex carbohydrates I wanted. I cut all the fats out of my diet that I could and only ate small amounts of chicken, turkey or fish. I used nonfat milk, yogurt and cottage cheese. I also quit frying. I never had hunger pangs or felt weak like before. I still follow the same program."

Interestingly, despite wide differences in methods National Weight Control Registry members used to lose weight, their maintenance diet appears to be almost universal. A study comparing members — those who lost on their own, those who lost with organized programs, and those who lost using liquid formula — concluded that all groups *maintained* their weight loss by consuming a low-fat, low-calorie diet as well as by exercising avidly. Average fat intake of the Registry members was about 24 percent of calories, which is well below the 30 percent figure commonly recommended for health. And about a third of them reported that their fat intake was 20 percent or less.

Not long ago, it was believed that paying close attention to fat intake would enable you to lose weight without paying much attention to calories. And, indeed, several studies suggest that when people are allowed to eat as much as they want of low-fat foods, they consume fewer calories than if they are allowed to eat unlimited amounts of higher-fat foods. However, reducing your fat intake without cutting back on calories is not likely to be sufficient.

The latest thinking is that what's most effective for weight control is watching fat intake and calories at the same time. In other words, don't think that if you cut back on fat, you can eat all you want of high-carbohydrate foods like low-fat crackers, pretzels, pasta, bread and rice and still lose weight.

Cutting back on fat can help immensely with weight control because it is the most fattening nutrient: each gram of fat (a gram is about 1/30 of an ounce) provides about 9 calories, while a gram of protein or carbohydrate each provides about 4 calories. Thus, any time fat is added to a food — a tablespoon of oil to a salad or a dollop of real mayonnaise to water-packed tuna — it markedly raises calories. Fat is, in essence, any food that's greasy to the touch: butter, oil, margarine, mayonnaise, regular salad dressing and cream cheese. Whole-milk dairy products and cheeses tend to be high in fat, as do many processed meats (like sausage and bologna), ground meats and marbled fresh meats. Thus, if you cut back on fat, you automatically cut back on calories. (For details on cutting back on fat, see "The Basics of Low-Fat Eating" on page 126.)

Conversely, some studies suggest that it's easy to eat too many calories (in a short period of time) when you consume fatty foods. That makes sense when you think about the fact that fatty foods tend have more calories in a smaller volume than do low-fat foods. (For instance, a 250-calorie portion of French fries would net you just a 3-ounce portion, while a 250-ounce portion of plain potatoes would weigh about 10 ounces.) Thus, if you eat a high-carbohydrate, low-fat meal — particularly one that's high in fiber — you should feel full on fewer calories than if you eat a high-fat, low-carbohydrate meal. Finally, although eating too much of any of the calorie-yielding nutrients can make you gain weight, excess fat calories are more readily converted to body fat than are excess carbohydrate or protein calories.

When her doctor ordered her to lose weight after her legs "gave out," Holly L. headed for the library. "The fact that I could have generous amounts of carbohydrates, fruits and veggies in exchange for fat put me on the road to a 54-pound loss of weight." She adds, "Now, at age 72, I walk at a fast clip 6 days a week, bend and stretch with not a worry in the world about ever gaining it back." She described how she follows her low-fat food plan at buffets and as she travels: "I always find something on the menu that is suitable. This has been my way of eating for the last 3 years, and I'm happy with life. It's a whole new world being normal in size and not having to worry about gaining weight again." Today, Holly weighs 160, down 97 pounds from her high of 257.

What about all the new reduced-fat versions of foods, like peanut butter, cookies, salad dressings and the like — do they help with weight loss? Many masters told me they make good use of these products. But good use means watching portion sizes because all of these reduced-fat foods still have calories in them, sometimes the same, more or not much less than their higher-fat counterparts.

FOOD FACT #4
The masters develop — and enjoy — new tastes in food.

Like Susan C., who's largely abandoned the meats and fatty foods of her past, many masters have done the same, discovering the satiety value of fruits and vegetables, which have bulk and are filling without providing many calories, as well as grains like breads, cereals, pasta and rice. In essence, the masters told me that they've figured out how to "eat large," which means getting the greatest volume of food for the least amount of calories. Edith S., who's kept off 56 pounds for 3 years, says, "I eat 5 starches a day, 4 vegetables, 3 fruits, 2 servings of nonfat dairy products, 1 serving of protein-rich foods. This is my daily goal, and I usually keep close to it. I stress high-fiber foods, as they seem to keep me from feeling hungry."

Despite the popularity of low-carbohydrate, high-protein diets, people who have overcome weight problems tend to eat foods

---

Two Recommended Books for "Eating Large":

Eating Thin for Life by Anne M. Fletcher. 1997. Boston: Houghton Mifflin Company.
  The Volumetrics Weight-Control Plan by Barbara Rolls, Ph.D., and Robert A. Barnett. 2000. New York: HarperCollins Publishers.

---

that are low in fat and that are relatively high in carbohydrate and moderate in protein. The "masters" of former weight problems tend to make high-carbohydrate foods like fruits, vegetables, breads, cereals and pasta the *mainstay* of their diets; and many told me they've cut back on meats, favoring lower-fat protein foods such as skinless poultry, fish and shellfish and reduced-fat cheese. More than half of the masters indicated that, at the most, they eat meat once or twice a week. Protein does seem to have "staying power" when it comes to appetite control. That is, having a small portion of low-fat protein food with each meal may help you feel full and hold you over from one meal to the next.

Adding to the weight-control value of low-fat eating, of course, is overwhelming evidence that the best diet for preventing problems such as heart disease and certain types of cancer is one rich in carbohydrate foods such as vegetables, fruits, legumes and whole grains — and limited in saturated fats. (Saturated fats come from whole-milk dairy products, meats — especially fattier cuts — and coconut and palm oils.)

Sadly, there is a pervasive attitude that anything good-tasting is automatically bad for you and, conversely, that all the good-for-you foods taste bad. Yet many of the masters seem to celebrate their new way of eating and have found ways to enliven foods and enjoy new taste sensations. Instead of dwelling on what they can't have, they focus on what they *can* have.

Carole C. (40 pounds, 20 years): "I learned to cook super low-fat. If it didn't taste good, my husband wouldn't eat it. I use lots of herbs and spices. I never feel deprived. Now, I just don't like the feeling of greasy, fatty foods. I'll eat a whole baked potato with low-fat cheese and chopped green onion: it's heavenly. We don't keep high-calorie foods in the house. We have other enjoyable things, like fresh strawberries."

Tom J. (75 pounds, 27 years): "I never sit down to a plate of protein. I eat lots of vegetables, fruits and legumes instead of meat. I know how to cook and can make a vegetarian meal that's better than most people's idea of a regular meal. I use lots of garlic, spices and herbs."

Holly L. (54 pounds, 3 years): "I get several health-conscious magazines now. They have recipes and tips that I use. Mostly I've changed my habits and find those to be second nature now. After 5 or 6 months, I was no longer interested in eating the way I had."

Ernie L. (45 pounds, 12½ years): "I started stir-frying and putting it on pasta. For me, it was heaven. I love to cook, and I'm very creative."

Leo P. (46 pounds, 3½ years): "What I have done is kept myself from feeling as if something was being taken away from me. I have developed a new taste for food. When I'm cooking, I will use a combination of common herbs and spices to enhance the food's flavor."

Shirley C. (26 pounds, 12½ years): "I love to cook and convert all my recipes to low-fat, nutritious selections. Low-fat, high-carbohydrate cooking is so easy. All you have to do is take a few extra minutes to read labels!"

And the payoff is worth it, as Gail O. explains of her eating habits and her 79-pound weight loss of 3 years: "I eat lots of carbohydrates, vegetables and fruits, chicken and fish, very little red meat. My food rewards are pretzels, raisins and a glass of red wine about four times a week. I went from a size 18/20 to a size 2/4 petite. Healthwise, I have normal blood sugar, blood pressure and cholesterol levels; all were high when I started." Ron K., who's been down 61 pounds for 5 years, says, "By 'eating smart,' one can live a normal life and not be an overweight recluse."

Contrary to the popular belief that "naturally thin" people get to eat whatever they want, one study suggests that they eat much the way the masters do. In the study on successful maintainers conducted at the Kaiser Permanente Medical Center (page 64), the researchers also examined eating habits of women who had never been overweight and found that these women consciously worked to stay trim and in shape. If they gained some weight — say, after a vacation — they made an effort to eat less until their weight returned to normal.

FOOD FACT #5
The masters develop consistency in their way of eating.

When I asked the masters to describe their daily eating habits, nearly half made a point of saying that they eat three meals a day. Quite a few eat several snacks in addition to their regular meals. Many of the masters could tell me exactly what they regularly eat for breakfast, lunch and dinner. Moreover, when I asked the masters, "How are your eating habits different than they were when you were heavy?" many responded that they no longer eat haphazardly and, instead, now go out of their way to eat regular meals and avoid skipping meals. Ron K. maintains that consistency is one of the keys to his 61-pound weight loss of 5 years. "By eating primarily the same foods on a daily basis, I can keep track of my caloric input."

Findings from the maintainers in the National Weight Control Registry suggest, too, that they eat regular meals — on average, they reported eating about five times per day, and only a small number said they ate less than twice a day. Another major finding of the Registry is that most of its members are big on breakfast — when about 3,000 of them were asked whether they eat breakfast, nearly 8 out of 10 said they did so every day of the week. Just 4 percent of them are complete breakfast-skippers.

Yet nationwide, breakfast eating seems to be on the decline — sometimes dieters forgo breakfast, thinking it will give them a jump-start on calorie-saving on any given day. In contrast, Registry cofounder Dr. James Hill suspects that the reason eating breakfast helps with weight control is that it helps you manage hunger throughout the day. "If you pace yourself during the day, you are probably less likely to have an urge to overindulge at lunch and in the evening," says Dr. Hill. Indeed, other studies suggest that skipping meals or having highly erratic eating patterns is more likely to lead to hunger and loss of control over food intake when you do eat than is eating regularly scheduled meals.

Not every master eats three square meals a day, though. Ernie L., the master profiled in Chapter 3, maintains his weight easily on two substantial meals a day. But like many other masters, he can tell you exactly what those meals consist of.

What's the best advice? If you are a meal-skipper, you might want to try a week or two's experiment of eating a small meal at the times you usually don't eat, particularly at breakfast; it may help you to eat less at other times. It does seem to be important to sit down and eat at least several planned, well-balanced meals, with some low-fat protein, vegetables, fruit and grain-based foods each day.

FOOD FACT #6
The masters keep track of what they eat.

Quite a few masters mentioned that keeping a food diary is one of the most important things they do to keep their weight down; more than a third indicated that they keep a diary or count calories if their weight rises. And 3 out of every 4 masters said they still record what they eat, at least occasionally. "Once a day, I write down the food items and their calories," admits Lois M. "It forces me not to kid myself about food. Some days I do better than I thought, and on others it's the opposite."

To be sure, one way to get yourself into a regular meal routine, as well as to get a handle on between-meal snacking, is to keep a diary of what you eat, listing every single food and beverage, as well as the portion size and when it's eaten. A number of studies indicate that people who consistently "self-monitor" their food intake and exercise by keeping regular written records lose more weight and keep it off longer than those who do not. In his book, *The 9 Truths About Weight Loss,* Dr. Daniel Kirschenbaum goes so far as to say, "Self-monitoring is the single most important aspect of effective weight control." Based on his research in this area, he maintains that if you keep a written record of what you eat and how much you exercise at least three-quarters of the time, you'll greatly increase the odds of becoming a master of weight control. Moreover, two studies in which Dr. Kirschenbaum was involved suggest that record-keeping can get you through some tough times, foodwise. These studies revealed that people in weight-loss programs who were most vigilant about writing down what they ate during the Thanksgiving to New Year's holiday season were actually able to lose some weight, while the least diligent record-keepers put on extra pounds.

It makes sense to keep track of what and how much you eat, at least for a while, because several studies reveal that overweight people have a tendency to underestimate the amount they eat. For instance, one study in the *New England Journal of Medicine* reported that a group of 10 overweight people who estimated their average daily intake to be just over 1,000 calories were actually consuming 2,081 daily calories. According to the researchers, the participants were not trying to be deceptive; rather, they seemed to be in a state of denial about how much they really ate.

Many masters also make an effort to control the portions of the food they eat. "I measure my portions," states Mary S., "or they tend to grow in size." Indeed, many experts believe that, as a society, we've lost sight of what a healthful serving size is — in large part because of enormous restaurant food portions, all-you-can-eat buffets, "super-sizing" and jug-size beverages that seem to be part and parcel of the American way of life. According to a 2002

American Dietetic Association nationwide opinion survey, more than half of the respondents overestimated the recommended serving sizes for cooked pasta, rice, lean meat and vegetables. In another study in which college students were asked to bring to class what they considered to be a "medium" sample of a bagel, muffin, baked potato, cookie or apple, average sizes of most items far exceeded recommended portion sizes.

In addition to writing down food items and measuring foods, you may want to keep track of calories or grams of fat (see page 144, "Fat and Calorie Content of a Sampling of Foods") for a while — at least until you feel you are more in touch with your real hunger. While this may sound tedious, the good news is that weighing and measuring as well as counting this and that in foods need not be a lifetime endeavor for everyone. Only 6 people reported that they count fat grams. Just 1 in 5 counts calories. And only 1 in 10 continues to regularly measure food, although some do so periodically — say, if weight creeps up. In the National Weight Control Registry, about half of participants reported that they still count calories, fat grams or both to maintain weight loss.

As always, you have to do it your way. Marie D. has found that counting calories or measuring portions doesn't work for her. What is effective is eating a low-fat diet and eating only when she's hungry. But she knows exactly what she eats during her three structured daily meals.

FOOD FACT #7
The masters indulge themselves but spend their calories wisely.

One of the ways the masters manage to eat healthfully over the long term is by not denying themselves favorite foods. Carole C. told me, "If I want it, I have it. On Mother's Day, I was given a huge chocolate 'turtle,' and it was wonderful." Marie D. says that one of her top three strategies for keeping her weight down is "allowing myself treats and desserts occasionally but enjoying smaller quantities." She finds that eating a little more food and a few treats on weekends helps her to maintain a healthful diet all week. Linda W. adds, "I found that when I get hungry for a high-fat food, I eat it. A slip-up every now and then is better for me than the craving." As Susan C. explains, "You eventually learn that you can occasionally eat those things [high-fat or higher-calorie foods] and still lose weight." (To learn how you can develop this no-guilt attitude, see "Don't Let Lapses Become Relapses," on page 160.)

In fact, when I asked the masters how they deal with food cravings, their number-one response was, "I have a little." Well over half indicated that they have a regular, nondiet dessert at least once or twice a month; many do so at least once or twice a week.

There are masters, however, who choose not to eat regular treats, although only 1 in 10 said they completely avoid sweets or desserts. Instead, some view more healthful foods, such as fresh fruits, as rewards. Or they develop their own low-fat recipes for "splurge" foods.

Virtually all the masters take steps to control their highest-temptation foods. For instance, about 2 out of every 3 masters said they keep problem foods out of the house or out of sight. Susan C. avoids buying aged cheeses because she can't stop herself from eating them. Ernie L. says his first line of defense is in the grocery store. "I shop very sensibly. If all that's in the fridge is apples and grapes, then that's what I'll eat. But if I know there's a half-gallon of butter-pecan ice cream [his favorite] in the house, I'll work on it 'til it's gone." Holly L. says, "There are certain things I do not have in the house, like chips and high-fat cheese. Sweets have never been a real problem for me. But when I do buy them, I get the no-fat ones."

The masters also make conscious choices about how to spend their calories. Jeffrey B. made it clear that he doesn't waste his calories on foods he doesn't really care for. "I decided that if I am going to eat something, it has to taste good. If I'm going to spend calories, it's not going to be on a bologna sandwich."

Part of the choice-making process is trade-offs. That is, if you have a higher-calorie or fatty item, you may have to forgo something else. "I'll sit down and eat half a pizza, but I won't eat dessert," says Susan C. "One day I may have butter but no jam on my bread. The next day, it's jam with no butter." Sometimes she has pie or cake for breakfast, then she eats more lightly at lunch. Kelly D., who has maintained a 55-pound weight loss for 4½ years, told me, "If I want to have a cocktail or two before dinner, I will eliminate dessert. If I want a dessert, which is a treat, I eliminate the cocktails." Cam L. "splurges" on fried oysters but has them with a plain baked potato and salad with no dressing.

The masters' newfound habits don't prevent them from treating themselves to restaurant meals. Although they're choosy about where they eat and what they order, 7 out of 10 of them eat in restaurants at least once or twice a week. Findings from the National Weight Control Registry suggest that successful maintainers don't eat much fast food: on average, participants reported eating less than one fast-food meal per week.

Steve S., one of the more disciplined masters I interviewed, once weighed 435 pounds and now tries to eat at least 35 servings of fruits and vegetables each week and tries to consume no more than 25 percent of his calories from fat. He's been able to maintain a 210-pound weight loss for 13 years. But, he adds, "I get to eat the things I really like, like ice cream and pizza. I rarely order fried food or steak. And I don't keep high-fat foods around my home or office."

Do the masters lose their love of eating? "It's an understanding that I will always love food — its preparation, fine restaurants, eating with friends, junk food — all of it," says Karen S. "Having kept my weight within 5 pounds for the last 15 years, I also know that if I eat a large quantity of a food that's not the best (like tortilla chips), I will not shoot back up to my original weight." Says Nancy R., who's kept off 55 pounds for 3 years, "My main problem, as with many overweight people, is that I love to eat — even with the diet plan, education and rethinking on what and how to cook, I still just love to eat, and I'm not sure that will ever change!"

Nor should it. For most people — heavy, thin, average and formerly heavy — food is one of life's pleasures. To be sure, when I asked the masters, "Do you enjoy food?" the overwhelming majority answered, "Yes." Master Rosetta F. says, "I never did plan to quit the thing that I enjoyed the most. That is, when I am eating a large meal with friends or family, I just enjoy the food and company and tell myself that I owe it to myself to do this because I have been so good for so long."

Connye Z., who's kept off 34 pounds for 5½ years, has accepted the limitations and admits that sweets are a weakness for both her and her husband, so she doesn't buy them often. "If it's there, we know we will eat it right away! However, there is nothing I cannot eat. I never told myself I can never have another chocolate doughnut. No food is forbidden to me, so I'm not deprived."

How can you start to learn to spend your calories wisely? Try answering the following four questions for yourself:

1. **What are my food strengths — things that can really work to my advantage in keeping weight off?** If you love fruits and vegetables, for instance, how can you capitalize on that? Perhaps you can stock up at the supermarket and make a concerted effort to eat at least two with every meal.
2. **What foods are really important to me?** Make a list of the ones you really love — whether French fries, hot fudge sundaes, rib-eye steaks or chocolate chip cookies. Ask yourself under what circumstances you can eat a controlled amount of these foods. Some people find that it's best to buy a one-portion package and savor every bite. Others find it easiest to have such items in restaurants, where portions are controlled.
3. **What foods do I really need to keep out of the house?** If at all possible, get rid of foods that you have difficulty controlling.

4. **What foods can I forgo and not miss too much?** Maybe you really don't mind bread without butter or margarine — as long as it's fresh and warm.

FOOD FACT #8
The masters try to listen to their bodies.

Some masters told me one of their major ways of controlling weight is to try to eat only when they are hungry. Kathleen H. says, "Don't eat just to eat! If you are not hungry, don't eat. If it takes more than 5 minutes to decide what to eat . . . I'm not hungry! If you need to eat but are not hungry, eat an apple and a glass of water."

Susan C. said, "I don't like the way overeating makes me feel." One of Nancy K.'s important strategies for keeping off her 60 pounds is, "I don't eat 'til I'm stuffed — even at holidays."

On the other hand, the masters find that it's important not to let themselves get too hungry. "I refuse to starve myself," states Cathy C. And Mary S. advises, "Don't ever let yourself get hungry; it leads to disaster." The problem with allowing yourself to become ravenous is that it lowers your resistance, and you're less likely to make wise choices. If, for instance, you let yourself get to the point of faintness after a long day at work, you're more likely to stop for a fast-food burger, fries and a shake than to go home and make yourself fish, baked potato and vegetables.

Many people have been on and off diets so much that they don't even know when they're really hungry and when they're full. As Janet Polivy, Ph.D., and C. Peter Herman, Ph.D., point out in *Breaking the Diet Habit,* many of us were brought up as members of "the clean-plate club," taught to finish everything set before us. Indeed, most masters suggested that they cannot rely solely on their internal sense of satisfaction to tell them how much to consume. As such, they take important steps to control the amounts of food that they eat — for instance, by making it a rule to leave some food on their plate after each meal, planning the day-to-day content of meals ahead of time, or going out of their way to limit portions by serving themselves finite amounts. Also, 2 out of 3 told me that they make a concerted effort to drink more water to control their weight. And nearly half of them find that eating slowly helps them limit the amount they eat.

To get in touch with physiological hunger, try some of the following behavior-modification techniques:

◆ Put your fork or spoon down between bites and drink water or a no-calorie beverage frequently during a meal so you have time to consider whether you're really hungry for more.

◆ Stop eating for 1 or 2 timed minutes at several points throughout your meal, and use these breaks to ask yourself if you are still hungry.

◆ Put only half to three-quarters of the food you usually eat on your plate. Have second helpings only if you are truly hungry.

◆ If you feel like having seconds, take a break from eating for about 20 minutes and return to the table only if you find you remain hungry.

More on Behavior Modification

Nearly 20 years ago, in keeping with the state-of-the-art techniques for working with overweight people, I instructed my patients to follow certain behavior-modification techniques in order to correct problem eating habits:

◆ Slow down your rate of eating. Put your fork down between bites of food; chew and swallow what's in your mouth before going for the next bite.

◆ Make eating a singular activity — that is, don't do anything else: don't watch TV, read a newspaper or do office work.

◆ Eat all of your meals at the same place and while sitting down, at a table.

◆ Serve your food on a smaller plate, so it looks like you have more to eat.

◆ Avoid shopping when you're hungry because your resistance will be low. Shop from a list and stick to it, so you don't buy a lot of extras.

◆ Plan ahead: think about what you'll eat for meals, as well as before going to social events and restaurants.

One day, however, the following thought hit me: "*I* like to read the newspaper while I eat breakfast and lunch; I *enjoy* my food *more* when I read while I eat, and it doesn't keep *me* from paying attention to my food." Not long after, a patient who had been in the habit of eating in front of the television said to me, "I ate *more* when you told me to shut off the TV!" Some patients felt these techniques were just plain silly and uncomfortable.

Just as with every other technique for weight control, you may have to experiment to see if these tips help you. Here are some that the masters found to be helpful:

◆ Nancy K.: "I don't tempt myself with any favorites (potato chips) in the house." At dinnertime, she fixes herself a lunch-size plate of whatever else she makes for the family. Sometimes, she has seconds.

◆ Rosemary O.: "I have selected my kitchen and dining room as designated places to eat. I avoid eating in the den, etc." When she knows she's going out, she plans ahead by "banking calories" — that is, by saving them up so she never feels she's on a diet.

◆ Ernie L.: "Food waste really bothers me. I know I won't leave food behind on my plate. So I buy foods in controlled portion sizes, like a 6-ounce steak."

◆ Karen S.: "I attempt to mimic my thin husband's eating habits, particularly his slow speed of eating."

◆ Julie J.: "I don't eat food when I can't sit and enjoy it."

◆ Mindy B. finds it helpful to avoid cleaning her plate of food and to "wait 15 minutes to see how full you really are after your meal."

◆ Joanna M.: "I keep cookies, candy and other goodies in the freezer so I know they'll be there a while, and I don't feel compelled to enjoy them before they get stale." After a meal, she removes "triggers," such as dishes and packaged foods that might compel her to eat more. To get the food taste out of her mouth, Joanna ends each meal or snack with a hot drink, carbonated beverage or small mint.

The masters who find these behavior-modification techniques to be beneficial did not just use them while they were losing weight, they continue them during maintenance.

It Gets Easier with Time

When I asked the masters to rate the degree to which they agreed with the statement "It is a constant struggle to keep my weight down," on a scale of 1 (agree) to 5 (disagree), slightly more than half of them gave ratings of 3, 4 and 5. This suggests to me that, for many of them, maintenance is not a huge struggle. And apparently, maintaining weight loss gets easier with passing time, as suggested by a National Weight Control Registry study involving more than 900 participants. Those who had maintained weight loss for 6 or more years reported requiring significantly less effort to diet and maintain weight than did people who had kept off weight for just 2 to 3 years. *And with time, the pleasure derived from weight maintenance — in comparison with the effort entailed — was found to increase.*

People who lose a great deal of weight may find the going a bit tougher and appear to be at greater risk of regaining lost weight. When the Registry researchers went back to the participants a year after they had enrolled in the study, they compared 420 of them who were still maintaining their weight loss with 248 who had regained an average of 15½ pounds. (To be in the Registry, participants had to have kept off at least 30 pounds for a minimum of a year.) The researchers discovered that the risk of regaining was significantly increased for those who had lost more than 30 percent of their initial weight as compared with those who had lost 25 to 30 percent.

There's also evidence from this same study suggesting that the longer you can keep extra pounds at bay, the more likely you'll be able to keep weight off for good. The Registry researchers found that the members whose weight had stayed stable had maintained their weight loss for longer before entering the Registry than had the regainers. In fact, maintaining weight loss for 2 to 5 years decreased the risk of subsequent regain by more than 50 percent.

Finally, this study also found that the regainers were less likely to maintain the behavior changes needed to keep weight off. That is, compared with maintainers, the regainers reported significantly less exercise, and they also increased the percentage of their calories that came from fat. It just goes to show, once again, that if you want to keep the weight off, you can't go back to your old ways.

None of the *Thin for Life* masters seem to regret whatever they must continue to do to keep the weight off. Doug S., who's lost more than 100 pounds twice in his life (he's kept off 108 pounds for the last 4 years), admits, "It's hard, it's really hard. But I know how much better I feel about myself. It's definitely worth it."

Master Kim W., who's kept off 27 pounds for 7 years and now works as a personal-fitness trainer, has a motto: "How bad do you want it?" She says, "I use this with clients when they complain about giving up certain foods. If you want to lose weight badly enough, you'll do what it takes."

How the Former Galloping Gourmet Converted to High-Flavor, Low-Risk Eating

As you may know from his Public Television series and healthful cookbooks, Graham Kerr, the gallant wine-drinking, cream-and-butter-sloshing Galloping Gourmet of the early '70s, is into a whole new way of cooking and eating. If the man who was "once paid $10,000 a day to recommend the addition of fat, salt and sugar to recipes" could adopt the low-fat way of life, anyone can. Moreover, Kerr's dietary changes also illustrate how switching to low-fat habits can facilitate weight loss.

At his all-time high, Kerr weighed 225, which he brought down and held at about 215 through most of his years as the Galloping Gourmet. Since he switched to low-fat eating, his weight hovers around 198. (He's 6'3" tall.) He recalls that in 1971, his blood cholesterol was a none-too-healthy 260; now it's 190, below the recommended cutoff of 200.

The turning point in eating habits occurred for Kerr when he was on a two-year boat cruise, recuperating with his wife from a car accident. He recalls the date: "It was May 18, 1971. We had just eaten a rich meal from a famous restaurant. There were probably 170 grams of fat in that one meal. Everyone on board felt sick. I said to myself, 'I've gone to bed many times before feeling greasy, awakening with my mouth feeling coated with fat.' And the room would be spinning, in part because of the wine and cognac." Kerr wondered if he'd been "subclinically sick" for many years and decided to remove fat and hard spirits from the boat's menu. "Within weeks, everyone felt better. I understood that my body didn't like what it had been doing."

Kerr admits that he soon became a "health-food extremist." He recalls his wife complaining, "There's nothing left to eat." He goes on, "She tossed the bologna across the floor and started throwing everything away. At that point, I realized I had gone too far. I had no joy left at my dinner table. I realized that the table is where we come for love and regeneration, but I had turned it into a place of 'No, you don't eat that.'"

Today, as he chooses his daily foods and designs his recipes, Kerr's guiding question is, "What is the least I can put in my body that will give me the most vitality, and P.S., can it taste good, too?" His approach means cooking with minimum risk from fat, sodium and cholesterol but with "maximum creativity by using taste, aromas, colors and textures." He and his wife, Treena, who has had to modify her diet because of a heart attack, stroke and diabetes, see their way of eating as "a joint venture. We don't focus on what we can't have but on enhancing what we do have. We *can* eat much more than we *can't* have."

What *does* Kerr have? He starts his day with homemade "care-mush," consisting of oats, a few raisins, some nuts and seeds and skim milk. Lunch is usually vegetable soup with grains and beans in it — poured over greens, plus a "great" piece of bread with some herb-seasoned yogurt cheese. A typical dinner would consist of a 3- to 4-ounce portion of chicken or fish, along with two or three vegetables. For dessert, Kerr may have plain yogurt flavored with vanilla and honey, served over fruit. Or he might have a sugar-free gelatin dessert with fresh fruit in it.

I asked Graham if he ever treats himself, indulging in occasional high-fat foods. He responded, "My memory menu could easily go to goose liver in a Madeira sauce or a rich, wonderful ice cream. There is a part of me that says, 'God, I'd love to eat that.' But I know I'd feel less than well. I'm the sort of person who could easily gain 20 pounds if I relent." Instead, his indulgences are foods like English muffins with marmalade, perfectly cooked sweet potatoes, roasted vegetables with a spritz of olive oil, or spinach with cilantro, red pepper and lemon. He also enjoys using a spread made with yogurt cheese and soft tub butter-flavored margarine without "trans" fat in it. He says, "You *can* find comfort in food that is good for you."

Kerr's advice for making the switch to low-fat eating is simple. "Whatever you know has fat in it, halve it. For instance, if you order French fries, only eat half of them. Then triple the amount of fruits, vegetables and grains that you'd have with that food. Always replace food that has fat with food you adore that doesn't."

The Basics of Low-Fat Eating — Going by the Numbers

Where do you start? How do you know what "eating low-fat" actually means when it comes to making food choices? Some people count grams of fat in everything they eat until they get a feel for various foods and how much fat they can consume on a daily basis. The table on page 144 gives you a sense of the number of grams of fat, as well as calories, in basic foods.

The following steps will help you determine how many grams of fat you can consume each day:

1. **Decide on your calorie level.** To go on a low-calorie diet on your own for any length of time, women should drop no lower than 1,200 calories a day; men no lower than 1,500 calories. Once you reach your maintenance weight, you should be able to consume more calories. (Hard-and-fast numbers are not available since calorie needs are highly individual and depend on your activity level.)

2. **Set your goal for percentage of calories from fat.** Major health organizations recommend that no more than 30 percent of calories come from fat, but a number of masters eat considerably less than that, about 20 percent. Yet it may be tough to make such a drastic jump from your current diet. Perhaps it makes sense to start at 25 or 30 percent and go lower if you think you can later. (Some people find that if they go too low in fat intake, it's hard to stick with it.)

3. **Figure out how many grams of fat you can eat each day for**

your chosen calorie and fat levels. Use the chart below to guide you.

If your calorie level is:	Your total daily fat gram allowance is: % of calories from fat		
	30%	25%	20%
1,200	40	33	27
1,300	43	36	29
1,400	47	39	31
1,500	50	42	33
1,600	53	44	36
1,700	57	47	38
1,800	60	50	40
1,900	63	53	42
2,000	67	56	44
2,100	70	58	47
2,200	73	61	49
2,300	77	64	51
2,400	80	67	53
2,500	83	69	56
2,600	87	72	58

To determine the amount of fat you can eat at any particular calorie level, multiply the calorie level times the percentage of fat you want — say 2,000 × .25 = 500, which is the total number of calories contributed by fat. Take that number and divide by 9 (since there are 9 calories in each gram of fat), and you'll have your daily quota for fat, which, in this example, is 56 grams.

By paying attention to the grams of fat in various foods, with time you'll get a sense of how to budget your fat grams. Let's say you've selected a 1,400-calorie level with 25 percent of those calories from fat. The chart indicates that your daily fat quota is 39 grams. If you see that a serving of a particular food provides 10 grams of fat, you'll know that's fairly steep since it provides about one-fourth of your allowance for the day. Should you choose to eat that higher-fat item, you'll know to watch more carefully the other items you eat that day. Remember that what's important is your *average* intake of fat over time — there's no harm in an occasional meal or even an occasional day of high-fat eating.

Nutrition labels make it easier to keep track of fat, as grams of fat per serving are listed on almost all processed foods and even some that are not processed. A point of confusion, however, on the labels is their listing of "% Daily Value," which is based on a 2,000-calorie diet with about 30 percent of the calories coming from fat. Unless that's exactly the calorie and fat level you've selected, it's best to use "% Daily Value" only to compare one food to another. What's better is to pay attention to *total grams of fat per serving* and see how that food fits into your daily fat budget.

Your best bet, if you want to cut way back on fat — and eat a nutritious, well-balanced diet at the same time — is to consult with a registered dietitian. You can ask your physician for a referral, call the outpatient dietary department of your local hospital to set up an appointment with one of its dietitians, or call the American Dietetic Association's Nutrition Information Line: 1-800-366-1655.

Making Food Shifts: A 6-Week Nondieting Weight-Control Plan

You don't *have* to count grams of fat in everything you eat. Studies suggest you can markedly lower fat intake by making some relatively painless shifts within each of the food groups in the Food Guide Pyramid (see facing page), which outlines the basics of healthful eating. Foods at the base of the pyramid are supposed to be the foundation of a good diet, while items at the tip are meant to be eaten in lesser amounts.

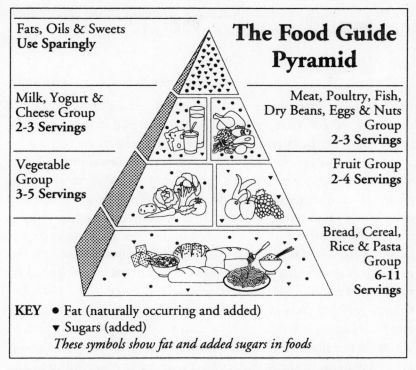

The Food Guide Pyramid

Fats, Oils & Sweets
Use Sparingly

Milk, Yogurt &
Cheese Group
2-3 Servings

Meat, Poultry, Fish,
Dry Beans, Eggs & Nuts
Group
2-3 Servings

Vegetable
Group
3-5 Servings

Fruit Group
2-4 Servings

Bread, Cereal,
Rice & Pasta
Group
6-11
Servings

KEY   • Fat (naturally occurring and added)
       ▼ Sugars (added)
       These symbols show fat and added sugars in foods

Source: U.S. Department of Agriculture/ U.S. Department of Health and Human
Services

The most important fat-saving shifts are to use less butter, margarine, oil and other fats in cooking and on foods; change from regular milk products to fat-free and reduced-fat versions; and consume less meat (most importantly hamburger, which is one of the fattiest meats, and high-fat processed meats, such as salami and sausage). At the same time, more of your calories should come from low-fat grain products, fruits and vegetables.

Many people, however, feel overwhelmed when they try to make multiple changes all at once. For this reason, the 6-Week Nondieting Plan has you take things one food group at a time, working on a single group for each one of 6 weeks. You can start with any food group, but since foods at the top of the pyramid contain the most fat, it makes sense to begin there. Each week, continue the changes from the previous week.

WEEK 1
Fats, oils and sweets

Fats include butter, margarine, vegetable oils, shortening, salad dressings, mayonnaise, cream, cream cheese and bacon. Use these items sparingly because they can markedly contribute to your fat and calorie budget. A study published in the *Journal of the American Dietetic Association* of a large group of women who were trying to restrict their fat intake to no more than 20 percent of calories revealed that avoiding fats as a flavoring — for example, on potatoes and bread — was the single most important step in maintaining low-fat intake on a long-term basis. Cut back on fats as much as possible, and experiment with fat-free and reduced-fat versions of mayonnaise, salad dressing and margarine. (Different brands vary not only in tastiness but also in fat levels.) To replace fats in cooking, try experimenting with nonstick cooking sprays, which now come in flavors like butter, olive oil, lemon and garlic. From a general health standpoint, it's wise to avoid saturated and trans fat (mainly in full-fat milk products, butter, lard, tropical oils, fatty meats, hydrogenated and partially hydrogenated vegetable oils, and fried foods). When you do use fats, stick with types that are largely polyunsaturated and monounsaturated (for instance, safflower, sesame, soy, corn, canola and olive oils, as well as liquid and tub margarine with 2 grams or less of saturated fat per tablespoon).

Sugar and low-fat sweets per se don't concern me too much as a dietitian, as long as the portions are moderate and they don't take the place of nutritious foods. Some masters treat themselves to no-fat or low-fat sweets, such as licorice, jelly beans and jelly (instead of butter). The problem is that many high-sugar foods — including regular ice cream, chocolates and cookies — also have a great deal of fat. When given a choice, it makes sense to generally favor reduced-fat or no-fat versions like frozen yogurt and reduced-fat baked goods. However, as mentioned earlier, many reduced-fat sweets don't have much of a calorie advantage. Be aware, too, that many high-sugar foods are "empty-calorie" foods, providing calories but few or no vitamins and minerals. If you consume a lot of these on a low-calorie diet, you run the risk of nutritional inadequacies. You can save sugar calories by making the shift from regular to diet soda. One of my friends lost 10 pounds just by giving up regular soda.

Alcoholic beverages are also typically considered part of this food group and can add significant calories to your daily intake. Some masters told me that they had much less trouble controlling their weight when they gave up alcohol. Master Ron K., who has kept off 61 pounds for 5 years, indicates that one of his most important weight-control strategies is to limit alcohol intake to 1 drink or beer at a sitting. Research studies suggest, too, that in nonalcoholic people, alcohol may stimulate appetite and cause them to eat more than they would without alcohol.

Goals for Week 1

◆ For 1 or 2 days, keep track of all the fats you eat, noting the exact amount. For the next several days, cut your fat intake in half. Then, if you feel you can, cut it in half once again.

◆ Take 3 foods that you would normally add fat to and try them without any fat. If that's unacceptable, try them with reduced-fat or fat-free substitutes. For instance, try a baked potato with just salt, pepper and chives. If it seems too dry, add a dollop of fat-free or reduced-fat sour cream with chives.

◆ In cooking, try cutting the amount of fat that you usually use by at least one-third to one-half. (See "The Art of Low-Fat Cooking," page 139, and "22 Ways to Shave Fat from Your Recipes," page 142.)

◆ If you have a sweet tooth, try having no more than 3 small servings of desserts or sweet snacks this week, and/or switch to some of the low-fat sweets, such as sherbet, fig bars or jelly beans, listed in the chart on pages 144–149.

WEEK 2
Meat, poultry, fish, dry beans, eggs and nuts group — the protein foods

You can save a lot on your fat budget by eating more fish and skinless chicken in place of popular meats like hamburger and steak. Note that many types of fish and shellfish, such as sole, cod, clams, shrimp and scallops, have only 1 or 2 grams of fat per 3-ounce cooked serving, provided you prepare them without added fat. (Oilier fish like salmon and mackerel are higher in fat, but much of the fat comes from omega-3 fatty acids, which are beneficial.) Skinless roasted chicken breast has just 3 grams of fat in a serving. You can substitute fish and chicken for meat in many recipes.

Although it is not necessary to cut out red meats, many masters indicated that they limit them. Says Ron K., "I eat red meat once a week and have 3 to 4 ounces at the most." Another way to cut back on fat is to switch to lean cuts, such as beef eye-of-round or top round; pork tenderloin, boneless sirloin chop or boneless loin roast; veal chops or roast. Use only low-fat cold cuts, such as roast turkey breast or very lean boiled or baked ham. Since Americans tend to eat more protein than they need — and since protein foods often come packaged with a lot of fat — it's generally recommended that you keep portion sizes of meats small. Be sure to trim meats of visible fat, and use hamburger (even the lean type) as an occasional "treat" food rather than as a staple in your diet.

Note, too, that a number of masters enjoy the dried-bean family, which has next to no fat and includes chickpeas, kidney beans, navy beans, pinto beans and lentils. As you can see from the chart on page 147, nuts and nut butters are quite high in fat and should be used sparingly. Eggs are not very high in fat, but they have about 213 milligrams of cholesterol per yolk, which needs to be taken into account in order to stick with the American Heart Association's recommended daily cholesterol limit of 300 milligrams. (You can eat as many whites as you want; they're free of cholesterol.) Of course, you can undo the advantages of any low-fat protein food by using high-fat cooking methods, such as frying or sautéing in butter. Stick with broiling, roasting, grilling, baking, sautéing in little or no fat in a nonstick skillet, steaming and poaching.

Goals for Week 2

◆ Have 2 to 3 small servings of protein foods each day. A serving is 2 to 3 ounces of cooked meat, poultry or fish (3 ounces is about the size of a deck of cards); ½ cup of cooked beans; or 2 tablespoons of peanut butter. One egg or ¼ cup reduced-fat or fat-free cottage cheese, which is not as high in calcium as other cheeses and thus is not in the milk/dairy group, counts as an ounce of meat or ⅓ of a 3-ounce serving.

◆ If you have a food scale, weigh meats after cooking to assure that portion sizes are appropriate.

◆ Have fish or skinless breast of chicken or turkey a minimum of 3 times this week. Try substituting one of them in at least one recipe in which you would normally use red meat. Since prepackaged ground turkey breast can be quite high in fat, buy skinless turkey breast and have it ground. Use it in recipes in place of hamburger.

◆ Experiment with one of the lean cuts of meat mentioned above.

◆ Have at least 1 serving of beans as in vegetarian baked beans, mixed with pasta and vegetables, or in homemade low-fat soup, such as Jordan F.'s "Thick and Hearty Bean Soup" on page 310.

WEEK 3
The milk, yogurt and cheese group

Shifting from regular to reduced-fat dairy products can make a big difference: the more you can use fat-free (skim) or 1-percent-fat versions of milk, yogurt and cheeses, the better. (Cheeses should have no more than 5 grams of fat per ounce.) It pays to experiment, since some brands are much tastier than others. With time, you can get used to a new taste, as master Rosetta F. has: "I changed from whole milk to 2 percent and then to skim milk. I drank the 2 percent until I started to like it better and then changed to skim months later." Even though they may be low in fat, some yogurts are still quite high in calories because of the added sugar. Aspartame-sweetened yogurts are much lower in calories.

Goals for Week 3

◆ Have 3 to 4 servings from this group each day. (If you consume fewer servings than this, you should check with your physician about taking a calcium supplement.) A serving is 1 cup of milk, 8 ounces of yogurt or 1½ to 2 ounces of cheese.

◆ If you haven't already switched to 1 percent fat or skim milk, try Rosetta's technique of making the change gradually. (My family refused to drink skim milk until after my father had a major heart blockage, when I decided to switch without telling. My kids and husband never noticed the difference.) You may find that skim milk is fine for cereal, but not in your coffee. (Some people like evaporated skim milk or fat-free half-and-half in coffee.)

◆ Sample 2 or 3 kinds of reduced-fat cheese to see which you prefer.

◆ Try 2 new flavors of fat-free yogurt.

WEEK 4
The fruit group

The remaining food groups are those you can fill up on so you're less tempted to eat higher-fat items. Fruits are virtually fat-free, with the exception of avocados and olives, which are considered fats. You can save yourself calories from sugar by sticking with fresh versions and avoiding those canned or frozen in syrup. Many people find it more satisfying to eat a piece of fruit than to drink juices, which go down quickly and have little bulk. Says Rosetta F., "I switched to more natural foods by telling myself that 'fat goes to fat.' So I picked out fresh fruit instead of the cinnamon pull-aparts that I used to get. I discovered I liked nectarines, which I had never eaten before."

Goals for Week 4

◆ Have at least 2 to 4 fruit servings per day. A serving is 1 medium whole fruit, 1 cup of juice or ½ cup of canned or fresh, cut-up fruit.

◆ Have at least 1 fruit serving with each meal: for instance, a banana on your cereal at breakfast, a juicy orange for lunch and a baked apple with cinnamon for a bedtime snack.

◆ Try a minimum of 2 less-familiar fruits this week, for example, an unusual type of melon, papaya or kiwi fruit.

◆ If you're in the dessert habit, have several different types of fresh, cut-up fruit instead at least 3 nights this week.

WEEK 5
The vegetable group

No fat to speak of here — again, unless you add it as butter, sour cream, mayonnaise or in frying. No shifting necessary — load up on vegetables.

Goals for Week 5

◆ Have at least 3 to 5 servings each day. A serving is considered ½ cup of cooked vegetable or 1 cup of raw vegetable. (On weight-loss diets, salad greens, such as lettuce and raw spinach, are usually considered "free foods" that can be eaten as often as you like.)

◆ Have at least 1 vegetable with lunch and 2 with supper. For example, at lunchtime have carrot sticks or cucumber coins (try them with fat-free salad dressing) to replace the crunch of chips. Supper might include a large spinach salad with mushrooms, red peppers and low-fat salad dressing, plus a cup of a cooked vegetable, such as broccoli.

◆ Try at least 2 less-familiar vegetables this week, such as okra, Brussels sprouts or winter squash.

◆ Experiment with various no-fat flavorings: dillweed on green beans, basil on zucchini, or lemon juice and nutmeg on spinach.

WEEK 6
The bread, cereal, rice and pasta group
(Low-fat crackers are usually considered part of this group as well.)

For a long time, many people labored under the misconception that breads, cereals, rice and pasta are taboo for weight control. Luckily, this has been shown to be false, and these foods are now considered to be mainstays of a healthful diet. The key is to avoid *adding* fats to them or to use reduced-fat or no-fat products on them, such as reduced-calorie margarine and fat-free mayonnaise. Shift away from higher-fat items like regular muffins, quick breads, oilier crackers and baked goods like doughnuts and cake. To boost your fiber intake, mainly use whole-grain versions of the foods in this group.

Goals for Week 6

◆ Have 6 to 11 servings from this group each day (6 servings are plenty for most women; 9 servings for most men). A serving is 1 slice of bread; ½ cup of cooked cereal, rice or pasta; 1 ounce of dry cereal (check product labels for equivalents to 1-ounce sizes since they vary from ¼ cup to more than a cup); ½ English muffin, hot dog roll or hamburger roll or small bagel; 3 graham cracker squares, 5 slices melba toast or 6 saltines; a 4- to-5-inch pancake. For portion sizes of other foods in this group, see the expanded list of complex carbohydrates in Week 2 of the Jump-Start Diet (page 369). (Make sure that refined products are "enriched.")

◆ Have 2 servings (men may want to have more) from this group with each meal. Breakfast might include an ounce of high-fiber cereal and a slice of whole-wheat toast with a teaspoon of jelly, which has no fat. Lunch is easy — a sandwich with 2 slices of oatmeal bread. For supper, have a serving or two of pasta and a slice of warm whole-grain bread.

◆ Take at least 3 grain foods that you normally have with fat and try them without any; for example, plain warm whole-wheat bread or pancakes with syrup but without the butter or margarine. (If this proves unacceptable, try them with reduced-fat products.)

◆ Have sandwiches with fancy mustard or fat-free mayonnaise instead of regular mayonnaise.

Here's how some of the masters have made food shifts:

◆ Tom J. (75 pounds, 27 years): "I eat very little meat, lots of vegetables, grains and beans and lots of fruit and pasta."

◆ Jean M. (60 pounds, 3 years): "Mine was a bad set of eating habits all my life: bacon, sausage, fried food, ice cream, candy." Now, she eats "every low-fat or fat-free food available," 3 to 4 fruits and a large salad with low-fat dressing every day, plenty of chicken and turkey, fat-free crackers and Diet Coke.

◆ Carol B. (75 pounds, 6 years): "I eat 3 meals a day that are low in fat and high in complex carbohydrates." Specifically, she says the staples of her low-fat diet are "cereal, fruits, vegetables, pasta, seafood and chicken."

◆ Teresa M. (36 pounds, 4 years): "I eat lots of fruits and vegetables, no red meat — just fish, chicken and turkey. I stay away from high-fat foods. It's just not worth it to me to eat them."

◆ Leo P. (46 pounds, 3½ years): "I eat 3 to 4 fruits a day, grains, legumes, vegetables, very little if any fried food and limited meat."

◆ Vicki B. (61 pounds, 8½ years): "I eat a lot of whole grains and fruits and vegetables and cut down on fats."

Compare the following two days to see how making food shifts can greatly lower fat and calorie intake. (Approximate grams of fat are listed after items containing more than 1 gram of fat.)

Higher-fat day	Lower-fat day
BREAKFAST	
1 oz. (1¼ cups) Cheerios (2)	1 oz. Cheerios (2)
¾ cup whole milk (6)	¾ cup skim milk
½ medium banana	½ medium banana
1 slice wheat toast with 1 teaspoon margarine (4)	1 slice wheat toast with 1 teaspoon reduced-calorie margarine (2)
COFFEE BREAK	
1 yeast doughnut (14)	English muffin with 2 teaspoons jelly
LUNCH	
3 ounces bologna (24) on 2 slices rye bread with 2 tablespoons mayonnaise (22)	3 ounces very lean baked ham (3) on 2 slices rye bread with 1 tablespoon reduced-fat mayonnaise (5)
1 ounce potato chips (10)	1 large carrot
2 chocolate chip cookies (9)	2 fig bars (3)
SUPPER	
4 ounces roast leg of lamb, lean (9)	4 ounces broiled halibut (3) in 1 teaspoon margarine (4) with lemon juice
½ cup au gratin potatoes (9)	1 medium baked potato with 2 tablespoons light sour cream (2)
large tossed salad with 2 tablespoons blue-cheese dressing (16)	large tossed salad with 2 tablespoons low-calorie blue-cheese dressing (2)

Higher-fat day	Lower-fat day
1 cup cooked spinach with 1 teaspoon margarine (4)	1 cup cooked spinach with lemon juice
1 cup vanilla ice cream (14)	½ cup low-fat frozen vanilla yogurt (1) with ¼ cantaloupe
SNACK	
3 cups microwave popcorn (7)	3 cups reduced-fat microwave popcorn (2)
8 ounces regular cola	8 ounces diet cola
Total fat = 155 grams	**34 grams**
Total calories = 2,630	**1,604**
% calories from fat = 53%	**19%**

The Art of Low-Fat Cooking

Let's face it: fat does nice things for food. It adds moisture and what chefs call "mouth feel" — that smooth, velvety sensation. How do you make up for the loss of fat? First, you can still get a lot of the goodness of fat simply by cutting back — by using one-half to two-thirds the recommended amount of butter, margarine, mayonnaise or oil in recipes. (Each tablespoon that you cut will save you about 100 calories and at least 11 grams of fat.) A number of masters leave fat out altogether and sauté in beef or chicken broth.

But many foods will surely lose their appetizing moisture and mouth feel when you remove some or all of the fat, so you have to add something back. You can substitute reduced-fat versions of the fats you take out, or add moist, nonfat ingredients like apple-sauce to baked goods. Low-fat or fat-free versions of yogurt or sour cream also work well to moisten certain dishes. In fact, many reduced-fat or fat-free dairy products make good substitutes for whole milk, sour cream and cream.

Sometimes products with just a small amount of fat work

better than those that are fat-free. Reduced-fat cheese products vary greatly in palatability, so experiment with them or try using a small amount of reduced-fat or regular cheese along with a fat-free kind.

Small amounts of flavorful fats, like butter, olive oil, bacon fat and sesame oil, can go a long way. A tablespoon may be all you need to enhance a recipe. Creative use of herbs and spices can also make up for the lack of fat. It also helps to use lemon and lime juice, as well as lots of vegetables in cooking. Aromatic vegetables like onions, garlic, peppers and celery can pick up the flavor of small amounts of fat and carry them through an entire recipe. Freshly squeezed lemon and lime juice, fresh herbs and spices and fresh garlic and onions deliver more flavor than dried and powdered forms. (Consult the list beginning on page 388 for cookbooks and magazines devoted to the subject of low-fat cooking.)

Two Before and After Recipes from Masters

A number of masters are adept at low-fat cookery. Two of them submitted the original versions of the following recipes, along with their adaptations. Don M. was able to bring about more than an 85 percent reduction in fat in Mallory's Lean Delight, while Bonnie R. shaved off virtually all of the fat from Fruit-Filled Coffee Cake. (Grams of fat follow each ingredient containing significant fat. Directions for these recipes are on pages 333 and 356 respectively.)

Mallory's Lean Delight
with Don M.'s adaptations

Original recipe	Don's version
1 large onion, chopped	1 large onion, chopped
2 tablespoons butter (23)	(No butter)
1½ pounds ground beef (84)	1½ pounds ground turkey breast* (4)
15-to-16-ounce can tomato sauce	15-to-16-ounce can tomato sauce
1 can (6 ounces drained weight) pitted black olives, drained (18)	20 medium pitted black olives, drained (7)
16-ounce can cream-style corn	16-ounce can cream-style corn
1 tablespoon chili powder	1 tablespoon chili powder
(No salt)	½ teaspoon salt
8 ounces elbow macaroni (4)	8 ounces elbow macaroni (4)
6 ounces sharp Cheddar cheese (56)	(No cheese)
1 cup unseasoned bread crumbs (6)	1 cup unseasoned bread crumbs (6)
Serves 8	Serves 8
Before:	After:
Fat = 195 grams	Fat = 25 grams
Calories = 4,229	Calories = 2,621
Per serving:	Per serving:
Fat = 24 grams	Fat = 3 grams
Calories = 529	Calories = 333

*Use skinless turkey breast, and have it ground or grind it in a food processor.
*Combine 1 cup 1% cottage cheese with several tablespoons skim milk in blender until smooth.

Fruit-Filled Coffee Cake
with Bonnie R.'s adaptations

Original recipe	Bonnie's version
1 cup oil (218)	1 cup unsweetened applesauce
1½ cups granulated sugar	1 cup granulated sugar
3 eggs (15)	1 egg, plus 4 egg whites (5)
3 cups all-purpose flour (4)	3 cups all-purpose flour (4)
1 tablespoon baking powder	1 tablespoon baking powder
2 teaspoons baking soda	2 teaspoons baking soda
1 cup sour cream (48)	1 cup fat-free sour cream
1 tablespoon vanilla	1 tablespoon vanilla
1 teaspoon almond extract	1 teaspoon almond extract
20-ounce can pie filling	20-ounce can light pie filling (any flavor)
2 teaspoons cinnamon mixed with	2 teaspoons cinnamon mixed with
2 tablespoons granulated sugar	2 tablespoons granulated sugar
Serves 12	Serves 12

Before:
Fat = 286 grams
Calories = 5,990
Per serving:
Fat = 24 grams
Calories = 500

After:
Fat = 10 grams
Calories = 3,246
Per serving:
Fat = negligible
Calories = 271

22 Ways to Shave Fat from Your Recipes

Substitute	For	Fat omitted (grams)
¼ cup butter, margarine or oil	½ cup butter, margarine or oil	46
¼ cup reduced-calorie margarine	¼ cup regular margarine or butter	24
⅓-second spray of nonstick spray	1 tablespoon oil	14
2 egg whites	1 large egg	5
3 tablespoons unsweetened cocoa	1 ounce baking chocolate	13
4 tablespoons chocolate syrup	4 tablespoons fudge topping	8

Substitute	For	Fat omitted (grams)
½ cup evaporated fat-free milk	½ cup heavy cream	44
1 cup plain low-fat yogurt	1 cup sour cream	45
1 cup "mock" sour cream*	1 cup sour cream	46
1 cup reduced-fat sour cream (2 g fat/2 tablespoons)	1 cup sour cream	32
white sauce made with 1 cup 1% milk, 2 tablespoons flour	white sauce made with 1 cup whole milk, 2 tablespoons flour, 2 tablespoons margarine	28
1 pound swordfish (raw)	1 pound pork shoulder (raw, lean only)	20
8 ounces Neufchâtel cheese	8 ounces cream cheese	32
4 ounces fat-free cream-cheese product	4 ounces cream cheese	40
⅔ cup plain low-fat yogurt	⅔ cup regular mayonnaise	113
⅔ cup light mayonnaise	⅔ cup regular mayonnaise	63
⅔ cup fat-free mayonnaise dressing	⅔ cup regular mayonnaise	116
4 ounces reduced-fat cheese slices (2 g fat/ounce)	4 ounces Cheddar cheese	30
4 ounces reduced-fat Cheddar cheese (4 g fat/ounce)	4 ounces Cheddar cheese	22
3 ounces reduced-calorie Swiss cheese slices, plus 1 ounce Swiss cheese	4 ounces Swiss cheese	18
8 ounces 1%-fat cottage cheese	8 ounces whole-milk ricotta cheese	27
1 cup applesauce	1 cup oil	218

Fat and Calorie Content of a Sampling of Foods
(Lower-fat or fat-free versions exist for many of these products. Check labels.)

Food	Amount	Calories	Fat (g)
GRAIN PRODUCTS			
Bread (French, Italian, mixed grain, raisin, pumpernickel, rye, wheat, white)	1 slice	72	1
Bagel, plain, 3½-inch	1	195	1
Biscuit, baking powder, 2-inch	1	157	3
Croissant, 2-ounce, 4-inch	1	265	16
Muffin, 2-ounce			
Blueberry	1	177	5
Bran	1	172	7
Corn	1	170	5
English muffin	1	133	1
Hamburger or hotdog bun	1	121	2
Cold cereal	1 ounce		
Unsweetened	(about 1 cup)	105	0
Sweetened	(about ¾ cup)	108	1
Granola	(about ⅓ cup)	127	4
Oatmeal, regular or instant, cooked	½ cup	73	1
Crackers	½ ounce		
Saltines	(5)	65	2
Graham, 2½-inch square	(2)	60	1
Cheese, 1-inch square	(about 14)	75	4
Oyster	(varies)	61	2
Butter-type	(about 4)	72	4
Nabisco Wheat Thins	(about 8)	67	3
Keebler Wheatables	(about 6)	68	3
Pepperidge Farm Goldfish	(about 25)	66	3
Pasta	½ cup		
Egg noodles, cooked		106	1
Spaghetti or macaroni, cooked		107	0
Rice, white, cooked	½ cup	103	0

Food	Amount	Calories	Fat (g)
Pancake, 4-inch	1	78	3
Waffle, 4-inch square	1	94	3
Tortillas			
Corn, unfried, 6-inch, ½ oz.	1	33	0
Flour, 6-inch, 1 oz.	1	91	2
Popcorn	3 cups		
Oil popped		165	9
Air popped		92	1
FRUITS AND VEGETABLES			
Fruits, fruit juices		varies	
Vegetables		varies	
Onion rings, frozen, breaded	1 ounce	88	5
French fries	1¾ ounce		
Frozen, baked		76	3
Fast food		156	8
Scalloped potatoes	½ cup	105	5
Potato salad, made with mayo	½ cup	164	9
Potato chips	1 ounce	150	10
MILK PRODUCTS			
Milk	1 cup		
Skim		86	0
1% fat		102	3
2% fat		121	5
Whole		150	8
Cheese			
American, blue, Cheddar, Swiss	1 ounce	107	9
Feta	1 ounce	75	6
Mozzarella, part-skim	1 ounce	72	5
Parmesan, grated	2 tablespoons	57	4
Cottage cheese	½ cup		
1% fat		82	1
2% fat		101	2
4% fat		130	5

Food	Amount	Calories	Fat (g)
Ricotta cheese	½ cup		
Whole milk		214	16
Part-skim		170	10
Yogurt, made with low-fat milk	½ cup		
Fruit-flavored		114	1
Plain		71	2
Frozen, vanilla		102	1
Ice cream	½ cup		
Vanilla		133	7
Fruit-flavored		128	6
Low-fat		115	2
FISH, POULTRY, MEAT			
Fish (skinless, flesh only, cooked without added fat or sauces) White-fleshed fish (cod, flounder, haddock, halibut, ocean perch, orange roughy, pollock, sole)	3 ounces	99	1
Shellfish (except oysters)	3 ounces	88	1
Oysters	about 12	101	4
Catfish	3 ounces	142	9
Rainbow trout	3 ounces	142	6
Salmon (Atlantic, coho)	3 ounces	162	7
Mackerel (Atlantic, Pacific)	3 ounces	213	13
Chicken (roasted, meat only, no skin)			
Breast	3 ounces	140	3
Leg	3 ounces	162	7
Thigh	3 ounces	178	9
Turkey (roasted, meat only, no skin)			
Breast	3 ounces	115	1
Dark meat	3 ounces	159	6
Ground turkey, broiled			
With skin	3 ounces	200	11
Without skin	3 ounces	115	1

Food	Amount	Calories	Fat (g)
Lean beef (cooked, meat only, trimmed of fat)			
Eye-of-round	3 ounces	141	4
Top round	3 ounces	153	4
Top sirloin	3 ounces	166	6
Tenderloin	3 ounces	175	8
Flank	3 ounces	176	9
Ground beef, 90% lean	3 ounces	144	8
Ground beef, 80% lean	3 ounces	231	16
Lean pork (cooked, meat only, trimmed of fat)			
Tenderloin	3 ounces	140	4
Chop (sirloin, loin, rib)	3 ounces	172	7
Boneless loin roast	3 ounces	178	8
Boneless rib roast	3 ounces	182	9
EGGS			
Whole egg, large	1	75	5
Egg white, large	1	17	0
NUTS AND LEGUMES			
Nuts: Almonds, cashews, peanuts, pistachios	1 ounce	165	14
Peanut butter	2 tablespoons	190	16
Legumes, cooked			
Lima, pinto, kidney or black beans, lentils	½ cup	113	0
Chickpeas	½ cup	135	2
FATS AND OILS			
Butter or margarine, regular stick	1 tablespoon	102	12
Reduced-calorie margarine	1 tablespoon	49	6
Oil, any type	1 tablespoon	120	14
Shortening	1 tablespoon	113	13
Salad dressing, regular, commercial	1 tablespoon		
Blue cheese, Italian, French, ranch		75	8

Food	Amount	Calories	Fat (g)
Mayonnaise	1 tablespoon	100	11
Mayonnaise, reduced-fat	1 tablespoon	50	5
Cream cheese	1 ounce	99	10
Cream cheese, Neufchâtel	1 ounce	71	6
Sour cream	1 tablespoon	31	3
Cream	1 tablespoon		
Light		29	3
Heavy		51	6
Half-and-half		20	2
Avocado	2 ounces	91	9
Olives, green or ripe	about 5	23	2
SWEETS			
Sugar	1 tablespoon		
White		48	0
Brown		52	0
Powdered		29	0
Jam, jelly, preserves	1 tablespoon	56	0
Carbonated beverage	12-ounce can	162	0
Syrup	2 tablespoons		
Maple		105	0
Chocolate		102	0
Milk chocolate candy	1 ounce	145	9
Candy corn	1 ounce	104	0
Caramels	1 ounce	108	2
Licorice	1 ounce	99	0
Marshmallows (1 ounce)	4 large	92	0
Gumdrops, jelly or gummy candy	1 ounce	108	0
Sherbet	½ cup	124	1
Coconut, sweetened, shredded	¼ cup	88	6
Pie, 9-inch	⅛ pie		
Fruit-type		330	14
Custard, cream-type		303	14

Food	Amount	Calories	Fat (g)
Cake	2-ounce piece		
Plain with frosting		212	10
Angel food		146	0
Pound		220	11
Gingerbread		221	8
Cookies	2 cookies		
Chocolate chip		156	9
Sugar		137	6
Peanut butter		190	10
Sandwich-type		102	4
Fig bars	2	120	3
Vanilla wafers	5	90	4

Note: Values are approximate. Brands vary.
Source: Primarily taken from U.S. Department of Agriculture data.

5

Key to Success #5

Nip It in the Bud: Break the Relapse Cycle

At last! You've lost the weight — you're finally at your goal. But soon you find yourself "slipping" — a few desserts here and there, a social situation that throws you, a bad day at work — and you decide a hot fudge sundae would soothe your soul. A few pounds return, then some more, and before you know it, your weight's right back where you started. A familiar scenario? It doesn't have to be. The good news is that you can break the "relapse" cycle.

Without a doubt, the most striking similarity among the masters is that they have discovered a way to *nip weight gain in the bud*. That is, they monitor their weight closely, and if they gain just a small amount, they *immediately* take it off. Nearly every single master has a game plan for getting back down when a small amount of weight comes back.

Janice C.'s Story

When I asked Janice C. the three most important things she does to keep her weight down, her first reply was, "I have a weight range — the top being 118. Once I get beyond that, I decrease snacking and/or meal portions and moderately increase exercise." This method of nipping weight gain has enabled Janice to maintain a 50-pound loss. For the past 10 years, she has weighed 116, give or take a few pounds — no small feat for someone who is 5'2" tall.

Janice's weight problem began when she was about 12 years old, after her parents divorced and the family moved. "Before that, I lived in the country. If I wanted to play with a friend, I had to ride my bike for 45 minutes. But when we moved to the city, my best friend was two or three blocks away, and I had more access to food: the 7-Eleven store was right down the street. Also, my mother started working and going to school. We stopped having regular meals." By the time she was 14, when she stopped weighing herself, she was up to about 165. "It really was a combination of a change in activity and a change in eating habits that led to my weight problem."

People always told Janice that she "carried her weight well" and that she had a "pretty face." "Boys would befriend me, but they tended to have long-term relationships with thinner girls." As a teenager, she tried various diets but didn't get serious until she was 15, when a relative paid for her to go to a clinic where she got hormone shots and was placed on a 500-calorie diet. "I stuck to it like glue, and I got myself up to running 5 miles. When I woke up in the morning, I felt like I would pass out." Within several months, Janice was down to 109 pounds.

She gradually regained some but not all of the weight; for years, she stayed around 130. But she tried various schemes to recoup her losses: Ayds weight-loss candies, the Stillman diet and "crazy" diets. "I created my own things — always something drastic that I couldn't maintain. I'd eat fruit all day, only vegetables and salads or just two sandwiches a day. I was either running marathons or doing nothing. It was all or nothing." Janice adds, "I really had the good food/bad food mentality. I was good at restraining myself for a while. Then I'd go back to the 'bad' foods, gain the weight back, and the cycle would start again."

The turning point for Janice occurred about 12 years ago when she was a college student and her car broke down. "While I was waiting for my insurance company to settle, I had to ride my bicycle to work. As a result, I started to lose weight and noticed I felt better about myself. My self-esteem increased, my clothes fit better, and I had more energy, which, in turn, spurred me to continue on. I was also more careful about what I ate. I didn't deny myself anything — I just ate smaller portions, and I started eating breakfast."

Janice feels that this last time she lost weight, her goal shifted. "In high school, it was more for the external, social reward: to get the weight off and gain popularity. When I was older, I was doing it for myself. I had a more realistic view of what I wanted and lost weight for my own level of self-confidence and to feel better." She also believes that her new, sensible approach had to do with the fact that she was seriously dating, and the two of them ate out a lot and went to many family meals together. "I realized I had to learn to eat like a normal person. I knew I couldn't live the old way, with the crazy diets and the marathons." It took Janice about two years to stabilize at her current weight.

Now Janice starts her day with a small breakfast of toast, cereal or a granola bar. Her largest meal is lunch, which she usually eats in a restaurant. "I eat anything I want, but try to make it pretty nutritious. I might have fish tacos or a teriyaki bowl. I have a tendency to choose low-fat and nonfat products and still feel like I'm treating myself. I *enjoy* reduced-fat hot fudge and frozen yogurt." In the evening, she says, "I allow myself to graze on foods like salads and rice. If I do have chips or sweets, I watch the portions."

Janice's first means of monitoring her weight is going by the fit of her clothing. She also weighs herself once or twice a week, but not if she thinks it will be "bad news"; she knows weighing at that point will distress her and be of no benefit. "If I feel like I'm up to 118, judging by the fit of my clothes, I won't weigh for a few days to see if I can make some adjustments. I basically eat the same during the day, but I'm more careful about my grazing at night. I might exercise more, reduce portions and pay more attention to fat content. I know if I spend several days watching it, I'll be back down to 115 or 116."

As for exercise, Janice tries to do something three or four times a week — say, 20 minutes on a StairMaster, biking or walking, as well as some light hand weights. "My exercise can be sporadic, and it's easy for me to get into the habit of not exercising. But it *is* one of the most important things I do to control my weight."

Janice chose 116 as her goal because she knew she could maintain it without starving herself. "I learned from the past that 109 was ridiculous." It did take some time to feel confident about being able to maintain. Like other masters, she learned through trial and error that if she gains a few pounds, she can lose them by cutting back and not doing something extreme. "As time goes by, my confidence has built up."

How does Janice think she's different from people who regain weight? "I'm obstinate. I never accepted myself as an overweight person, never perceived myself in the long run as being an overweight adult."

I asked Janice if it was difficult to continue to be motivated when there was no longer the reinforcement of watching the scale drop. "I continued to feel satisfaction because I knew where I had been. I consciously reminded myself of that. Now, I focus on how good I feel," she said. I also wondered what, after all this time, motivates her to prevent further weight gain immediately, and she replied, "I feel the reward every day when I put on my clothes. I concentrate on how good I feel about my body when I give a presentation, exercise, go to the pool and when men notice me."

Day-by-Day, Meal-by-Meal

Like Janice, *the masters nip weight gain in the bud on a day-by-day basis and on a meal-by-meal basis.* Lorraine W. says that the most important steps she takes for keeping off her 37 pounds are:

"I made a vow to myself never to let it get out of hand again," and "If I have a larger meal, I make the next one very light." (Lorraine is 5'2" tall and has kept her weight off for 5 years; she lost her weight when she was almost 60!) Lou Ann L., who's kept off 43 pounds for 15 years, says, "I try to eat until I'm full and then stop. But I'm loose in a lot of ways; for example, at a party, I'll eat whatever I want. But if I eat a lot, I'll eat less the next day or two."

The vast majority of masters stop gaining before they put on more than 5 pounds; most others allow themselves no more than 10 pounds. Indeed, more than 80 percent of the masters keep their weight within a 1-to-5-pound range; another 14 percent keep their weight within a 10-pound regain limit. According to Dr. Thomas Wadden, director of the Weight and Eating Disorders Program at the University of Pennsylvania School of Medicine, "Reversing small weight gains immediately, as they occur, is the single most important skill that patients fail to learn in conventional weight-loss programs."

Closely Monitor Your Weight

If you're going to keep small weight gains from getting out of hand, you have to have some means of monitoring your weight. Dr. Susan Ross found that of her successful patients, "most realized the need for a 'red flag' or warning system to monitor weight fluctuations and prevent the fluctuations from going beyond a certain amount." When I asked the masters, "How do you keep track of your weight?" I learned that nearly 9 out of 10 of them weigh themselves regularly. Like Janice, about a third of the masters weigh in one to three times a week. About one-quarter consult the scale at least once a day. In fact, 15 people listed daily or regular weigh-ins among their top three maintenance strategies.

What did the National Weight Control Registry find among its many maintainers? Their frequency of weighing in was much like that of the *Thin for Life* masters: about 75 percent of them weighed themselves more than once a week. Nearly 4 out of 10 of them step on the scale daily.

The high incidence of frequent weighing came as a surprise to me, since dieters are warned commonly not to weigh themselves any more often than once a week. It is likely that frequent weighing is unwise when you're trying to lose weight, because the scale doesn't always register small day-to-day losses, which can be discouraging. *But frequent weighing does seem to be an important checkpoint for many people after they've lost weight.*

As with most aspects of weight maintenance, how often you weigh yourself is up to you. Drs. Kelly Brownell and Judith Rodin point out in *The Weight Maintenance Survival Guide* that "people who have difficulty with maintenance do not have a set of guidelines . . . They weigh themselves whenever they remember or feel like it." Since weight tends to fluctuate throughout the day, it is wise not to consult the scale more than once a day. Instead, weigh yourself at one particular time of day only. Note, too, that fluid retention (from menstrual changes or from eating salty foods on a particular day) can cause daily weight fluctuations that are not cause for panic, and the amount of clothing you're wearing can cause variations.

Not every master monitors weight by a scale. Carole C. "never" weighs herself but instead gauges her weight by the fit of her clothing. She adds, "I try to look great, not keep my weight down. It's a different perspective." Similarly, Tim H. says, "I rarely step on a scale. But I can tell when I gain 5 pounds because I can feel it: my clothes get tighter." About 4 out of 10 masters go by the fit of their clothes to keep tabs on their weight, often in combination with regular weighing. Doug S., who's kept off more than 100 pounds for 4 years, states, "When my pants get tight, I start dieting. I used to allow myself to buy bigger clothes. I had a range of pant sizes from 34 to 52. But I got rid of the big pants. Now, I won't buy bigger sizes."

Some masters say they keep a handle on their weight by noting how they look in a mirror. And Larry Z. monitors his 70-pound weight loss of 15 years by noting the fit of his belt, as well as by weighing himself. Joy B., who's kept 35 pounds off her tiny 5'1" frame for more than 4 years (20 of that off for 18 years), not only weighs herself once or twice weekly and checks how her clothes fit but looks at the size and shape of her legs, since that's where she tends to gain weight. "When my thighs touch, it means things are getting out of hand (and into mouth!)."

As always, pick one (or more) monitoring systems that are right for you. Be ready to experiment, and take into consideration your past experience of what did and didn't work. If you choose weighing, decide if you'll check the scale once a day, once a week or twice a week. Maybe, like Janice, you're better off not consulting it if you suspect your weight is up a bit, or if you think you're retaining fluid. If you passionately hate to weigh yourself, then perhaps judging by your clothes is best, allowing yourself to go no higher than a certain size. You could also pick an item of clothing or two that you want to feel good in. Kim W., for instance, keeps track of her weight by how her jeans fit and how she looks in leotards. The important thing is to pick a monitoring system and use it faithfully.

Be Adamant About Establishing — and Keeping — a Weight Buffer Zone

Nearly all the masters have a maximum upper limit for weight — a sort of "buffer zone" — and they are adamant about not exceeding it. Holly L. says, "I cut back if more than a pound or two stays with me for a week." (Her plan makes sense since some weight fluctuation is normal: you need only tackle the pounds that stay on for a week or so.) And Violet Y. says, "In 19-plus years, I have never let myself get over 4 pounds past my ideal weight."

A few male masters allow themselves more leeway with their

weight, as do several women who were once extremely heavy. Larry Z. gives himself 15 pounds' grace, ranging from 185 to 200. "When I hit 200, I know it's time to stop." Tom J. fluctuates 10 to 20 pounds before he takes action. And Ann F., who once weighed close to 400 pounds, tends to fluctuate between 140 and 170 pounds.

Have a Set Plan of Action If You Hit Your Upper Limit

When the masters hit the top of their zone, they do something about it. They don't harp on it, feel sorry for themselves or stall around, and within a short time, their weight is back down to the lower end of their comfortable range.

Here are some masters' plans of action:

◆ Virginia L. (97 pounds, 3½ years): "If I gain weight, I go back to a strict low-fat program and drink lots of water."

◆ Steve S. (210 pounds, 13 years): "When my weight goes up, I do more of what I'm already doing." Specifically, he eats more fruits and vegetables and exercises more.

◆ Patsy Jean B. (73 pounds, 3 years): "I gain a few pounds at holiday time when I allow myself to eat fats and goodies. I get back on [my plan] and lose those few." She does this by following a diet, exercising more, giving up sweets and sometimes skipping meals.

◆ Tim H. (40 pounds, 6 years): When his clothes feel tighter: "I watch what I eat for a while. I won't buy peanut butter for several weeks, and I work out a little more."

◆ Larry Z. (70 pounds, 15 years): "If I feel heavy, I know what I have to do. I skip meals, quit snacking and stop drinking beer for a while."

◆ Tom J. (75 pounds, 27 years): "When my weight gets high, I balance it out with a 4-to-6-week period of stringency." He also keeps track of what he eats and exercises more.

None of this is to suggest that you have to do anything stringent if you gain a little weight. *The important thing is to be aware of small gains and do something about them right away — even if it's just returning to your normal way of eating and exercising and slowly letting that take care of the extra pounds.*

Following is a potpourri of strategies that masters use when their weight rises. (The first five were the top five responses.) Check off those that are most acceptable to you, and give them a try the next time you gain a few pounds:

__ exercise more
__ stop snacking
__ keep a food diary or count calories
__ give up or cut back on sweets
__ go on a diet
__ go back to the person or group that helped you lose weight
__ apply techniques or a food plan that helped you lose weight
__ weigh and measure food

__ eat carefully for 2 or 3 days
__ give up alcoholic beverages
__ don't allow yourself to feel guilty
__ eat smaller portions
__ skip meals
__ increase fruits and vegetables
__ decrease fat intake
__ don't eat after supper
__ try inner reflection
__ drink more water

If your weight climbs, instead of viewing whatever action you decide to take as painful and punitive, paint it in a more positive light. Focus on how good you feel when you're eating healthfully and exercising. Ernie L., the master profiled in Chapter 3, has learned to look on the bright side when he gains weight as a result of his frequent travels. "I've accepted the fact that when I go to Europe, I gain 5 to 10 pounds because I love the rich desserts and get less exercise." (He knows that he also has a tendency to gain over the winter holidays, as well as on business trips, when he's less in control of the food choices.) "The moment I have slight discomfort in the waist of my pants, I say, 'That's it.' I take a look at what got me there and try to reverse it." After Europe, for instance, he immediately returns to his four days per week of aerobics classes and cuts out desserts for a while.

If resuming his normal lifestyle doesn't get rid of the excess weight within several weeks, Ernie may step up the exercise and further decrease food consumption. (Since diets didn't work for him in the past, he does not think of himself as going on one.) Ernie is also patient with himself, giving himself time to shed the weight. "I used to want to get rid of it instantly and to punish myself. But I no longer say to myself, 'Three weeks of indulgence, now three weeks of punishment.' I realize that it may take 8 to 10 weeks."

When I asked Ernie if it was a hardship to resume his normal habits after a period of being away from them, he replied, "Oh, I suppose there's a moment of feeling sorry for myself. But I try to look at the positive rather than the negative. Since I do so much of my own cooking, I reward myself with tasty low-fat recipes — I'll think of the pasta dishes I like that are really great. Or I might buy some exotic fresh fruits or expensive leafy lettuce. Instead of spending money on a dessert, I'll spend it on a wonderful salad. And since exercise is such a part of my life, I look forward to it. Rather than dwell on the drudgery of an extra aerobics class, I might go cross-country skiing on the weekend — something that's fun."

As you experiment with the masters' tips for nipping weight gain in the bud, don't think of yourself as doing something punitive. Rather, be ecstatic that you're doing something about your weight before it gets out of hand. *Remind yourself that it's a lot less painful to deal with 5 or 10 pounds at a time than with 30, 50 or 100 pounds.*

Don't Let Lapses Become Relapses

Most of the masters have broken away from the all-or-nothing attitude of either being "on" or "off" a certain food-and-exercise plan — of either following the rules or breaking them. *The masters give themselves permission to deviate from some preconceived ideal and recognize that there are no hard-and-fast rules when it comes to weight control. When they do "slip," they don't berate themselves, but they do take immediate action so the situation doesn't get out of hand. Thus, they prevent lapses from becoming full-blown relapses.*

Lapses are single events of "slipping," doing something *unplanned* that is not ideal for weight control. A lapse might be impulsively downing a Danish from an enticing tray at work or eating a second or third piece of cake that you hadn't planned into your day's meals. It might be failing to exercise for a week when you had intended to. A lapse could also be an evening of binge eating or indulging in a rich meal. In defining a lapse, I stress the word *unplanned,* because if you plan an indulgence, it's *not* slipping. I think it's healthy for most people to allow themselves treats occasionally, as long as they can learn to enjoy them and not feel guilty.

The problem when dieters view lapses as total losses of control is that the lapses often accumulate and become **relapses,** leading to significant weight gain. Relapse might occur after a month of following a low-calorie diet, then suddenly "giving in" at a party and having several snack foods or sweets. The next day, feeling that you've blown it, you skip breakfast but succumb to a grilled reuben sandwich and fries at lunch. This chain of events may go on for a week or so, and soon you find you've gained 5 pounds. *The trick of the masters is to stop it there — don't let the gain go any further.*

Eileen B. is a master who's certainly had room for potential relapse. About four years ago, she quit smoking and at the same time started on the course of losing about 45 pounds. She adds, "In the meantime, I became pregnant, gained exactly what my doctor specified and lost every pound of the pregnancy weight gain within four weeks of giving birth. I have had a weight problem all my life, and I now know, hey, it can be done! I never quit. Everyone slips. Ignore it, and carry on."

One of the keys to preventing lapses from becoming relapses is to view occasional slips as learning experiences. Think about what went awry and how you can prevent a similar situation in the future — then pick yourself up and say, "Oh well, everyone makes mistakes."

Another key to preventing relapse is to stop viewing slips as personal signs of weakness. Instead, recognize that lapses are unique responses to individual situations. In other words, giving in to a piece of chocolate cake at an office birthday party doesn't mean you are a weak person with no willpower. (If you'd looked around you, you'd have noticed lots of other people "giving in" to indulgence.) Rather, this was one highly tempting instance — one that would tempt almost anyone, not just you — in which you had unplanned food. No big deal!

Some people have even pointed out that the overweight may have a harder struggle overcoming their problem than smokers, alcoholics or drug addicts (and may be the most prone to relapse) because they cannot entirely give up the substance. Says one master who also overcame a drinking problem, "At least with booze, you can give it up completely; not so with food."

A Plan for Preventing Relapse

In the 1980s, University of Washington psychologists Drs. G. Alan Marlatt and Judith Gordon developed a now widely used relapse prevention model for helping people with alcohol problems avoid or cope with slips in their drinking. Several studies suggest that this method may play a role in keeping off lost pounds. One of the studies, published in 2001 in the *Journal of Clinical Psychology,* examined differences between 606 people who had maintained weight loss (on average, about 40 pounds) for at least 3 years and 606 regainers. (Regainers reported having lost and regained weight and had never been able to maintain significant weight loss.) The most striking difference between the maintainers and the regainers was how they said they'd cope with a relapse. According to lead author Dr. Faith-Anne Dohm, Ph.D., from Fairfield University in Connecticut, "The maintainers were significantly more likely to respond to a gain in weight by using coping strategies such as treating it as a small mistake, losing the pounds again, increasing exercise and watching food intake more carefully. The regainers, on the other hand, were more likely to say they'd react to weight gain by feeling terrible and going off a diet."

Based on an article in the *Weight Control Digest* by Yale University psychologists Drs. Kelly Brownell and Carlos Grilo, the following adaptation of the relapse prevention model provides skills to help you avoid backsliding with your weight. *They should be used both while you're losing weight and at maintenance:*

SKILL #1
Identify your potential high-risk situations.

High-risk situations are times when you are likely to "slip" or have lapses from your weight-control plan. You can identify your areas of weakness by reflecting on your past weight-loss attempts and by using the following checklist:

I am at high risk for unplanned eating or deviating from my exercise plan when I'm . . .

__ alone	__ celebrating
__ lonely	__ frustrated
__ bored	__ feeling rejected

__ depressed	__ avoiding a task
__ very hungry	__ in my car
__ with others	__ cooking
__ at a party or social	__ around certain
gathering	tempting foods
__ at a restaurant	__ walking in my door
__ anxious	__ clearing the table
__ angry	__ other
__ in a bad mood	

Ask yourself what it is about the situations that makes them troublesome for you. For instance, it may not be parties per se that pose the problem — they may only be risky when someone pushes food on you. Or eating in the car may only be a problem if you go grocery shopping right before dinner — and place the bags on the seat next to you.

SKILL #2
Prevent high-risk situations as best you can.

It's ideal if you can prevent high-risk situations in the first place. One way, according to Drs. Grilo and Brownell, is to write down several specific things you can do to prevent each of them. It's important to do this ahead of time, because if you wait until the situation arises, it's much easier to eat than to consider other options.

So if you can't resist reaching into grocery bags after you shop, try putting them in the trunk of the car. If you tend to overeat when you allow yourself to become starved, make it a point not to let yourself go any longer than three hours without eating something. Have someone else clear the table if you can't resist nibbling leftovers. Or if you eat out of loneliness and you just ended a relationship, consider signing up for a class or planning several get-togethers with special friends.

Janice knows that evenings with nothing to do are her high-risk times. "If I feel that I'm at the upper end of my weight range, I might consciously come home from work, eat some vegetables, then make sure that I'm busy. For instance, I might plan to do some chores or, better yet, go out shopping or visit a friend."

SKILL #3
Effectively deal with high-risk situations when they do occur.

You can't eliminate all high-risk situations, but you can learn to handle them more effectively when they happen. For instance, 1 in 3 masters indicated that their "tough time" of day is after supper — they can't really avoid that time of day, so their most common way of handling that tough time is to do something other than eat.

If parties are your downfall, you probably don't want to stop going to them for the rest of your life. When you do go to a party, how can you avoid overeating? First, set a realistic goal. Is it reasonable to think that you'll eat nothing there, only drinking club soda with lime? It's more realistic to scope out the food situation when you first arrive at the party, select a few items that you'd really enjoy, load up from the vegetable and fruit platters, then station yourself some place other than next to the buffet. (For more on realistic goal-setting, see page 167.)

For me, the act of coming home or walking in the door is high-risk: I automatically think of food. (I think it stems from childhood, when I'd get home from school and head right for the refrigerator.) Of course, I can't eliminate coming home, but I can bypass the kitchen door by going through my front door, grabbing the mail, then relaxing and sorting through it. Or I can plan ahead to have a low-fat food, like a juicy apple or fresh melon, waiting for me.

Is there any evidence that using these techniques in high-risk situations works? The answer is yes, according to a study by Dr. Grilo and colleagues, in which people in weight-loss programs were asked to describe two situations: one in which they overate (a lapse) and one in which they were highly tempted but did not overeat. For each situation, the people were asked about coping strategies they used: either *behavioral strategies* involving overt action like walking away from food, doing something else instead of eating, talking to someone, waiting until the urge to eat decreased or eating low-calorie foods instead; or *cognitive (mental) strategies,* like thinking about other things, encouraging themselves or thinking about the consequences of overeating.

When the dieters used either type of coping strategy, they almost always reported overcoming temptations. Better still, when they combined both behavioral and cognitive coping, they were even more likely to avoid a lapse. Combining a helpful behavior with a motivating thought may be the best defense yet against lapses. (For more on cognitive coping, see Chapter 6.)

Drs. Grilo and Brownell stress that you have to accept the fact that you cannot fix every situation or perform perfectly all the time: your goal should be to limit how much the situations influence you. In the weeks ahead, try to anticipate them and apply the coping skills you find to be most helpful. But remember, as the masters do, that you'll still have slips.

SKILL #4
React constructively after high-risk situations.

So you were in a high-risk situation, and you wound up overeating or not handling it as you would have liked. The worst thing that you can do is to react with self-blame and guilt: both increase chances of relapse. Drs. Grilo and Brownell warn that negative emotional reactions pose a "greater threat to successful maintenance than do the few excess calories."

Here are some of the ways the masters handle high-risk situations after the fact:

◆ Tim H. (40 pounds, 6 years): "I don't berate myself when I eat less than healthily. I just eat better the next time."

- Ann Q. (49 pounds, 3 years): "One of the most important things I do to keep my weight down is to forgive myself for minor transgressions."
- Jean B. (45 pounds, 5 years): "I don't feel guilty if I overeat one day. If you let yourself feel guilty, you will eat more."
- Bob W. (250 pounds, 21 years): "When I 'goof,' I just begin again."

If you handled a situation in a way that you were not entirely happy with, ask yourself the following questions:

- What went wrong? (Think about what you were thinking, feeling and expecting and what happened immediately preceding the lapse.)

- Could I have avoided the situation altogether? If not, how could I have handled it differently — what might I have done or said to myself to avoid overeating?

- How can I handle the same situation in a more constructive way the next time around?

- What can I do, in a nonpunitive way, to make up for the lapse? For a short time, can I exercise a little more or eat a bit less? Or should I just forget about it and go back to my healthful habits, which will eventually take care of the lapse?

Then congratulate yourself for your awareness of the lapse and make a pledge not to let it lead to another immediate lapse. Be aware that each time you use any of the relapse prevention skills listed above, you are increasing your sense of self-efficacy — that is, your belief in your ability to control your weight forever. As you learn to prevent lapses and cope with them without panicking when they do occur, you will gain more confidence and likely be better able to handle the next challenging situation. Lou Ann L. has overcome enough lapses to know. "As the years have passed, I've grown more relaxed and confident about how I relate to food and how I look. I also know that if my clothes are getting tight, I can eat less for a week or two, and everything will fit again."

Learning to Set Realistic Goals

Did you ever make a pledge to yourself that you'd never eat a piece of chocolate again — or, after starting a diet in May, say that you'd be a size 10 by mid-June? Maybe you've sworn yourself to not gaining a single pound over the holidays, when in fact you've never been able to accomplish the task. What about exercise: have you vowed to start running a mile a day, when you've done no exercise for the past six months? All of these vows and pledges are examples of unrealistic goals that are impossible or extremely difficult to achieve and will set you up for lapses and possibly relapse.

People who lose weight and keep it off have a tendency to set goals that are attainable. In the Kaiser Permanente study (page 64), maintainers reported setting small goals that they could meet. A Yale University study found that the women who had regained weight were either "very much on or off"; that is, for a while they would eat well and exercise, then they would go back to their old ways. In contrast, the maintainers in the same study were more realistic: they didn't feel they had to do everything all the time. For instance, they might exercise just three times a week, but they were consistent about it.

The following guidelines will help you set realistic goals:

◆ Steer clear of "never," "always" and "every day" goals.

They're too perfectionistic and reflect all-or-nothing thinking. What, after all, are the odds you'll never eat a piece of chocolate again? Or that you'll exercise every single day? In their book, *Permanent Weight Control,* Michael J. Mahoney, Ph.D., and Kathryn Mahoney, M.S.W., M.S., point out that all-or-nothing goals encourage all-or-nothing behavior. "You are asking yourself for perfect behavior, for errorless eating habits. You are leaving yourself no room for human error, for *gradual* improvement. You are constantly living one mistake away from failure, one error away from defeat." Thus, if your downfall is chocolate desserts, rather than swearing off chocolate forever, a far more reasonable goal — one that you're likely to accomplish — would be to eat them no more than once a week or to allow yourself to have them only in controlled circumstances, such as when dining in a restaurant.

◆ Set "just for today" or "just for this week" goals.

In other words, work on short-term goals, rather than focus on your long-term desires. Ask yourself what small steps you can achieve today: Drink a cup of water before each meal? Have a serving of fruit with each meal? Use the stairs instead of the elevator at work? Master Lois M. makes this point well: "When you focus on having to lose 100 pounds, you think, 'What the hell; two more cookies isn't going to make a difference.' But you can do it if you learn to set your goals just for today or just for this meal. Then you don't have to think about having to lose 100 pounds." (Actually, an occasional "two more cookies" won't make much of a difference in the context of a day of low-calorie eating. But with a "what-the-hell" attitude, many people let those two cookies become 10 or 15 — easy to do if you feel frustrated about a seemingly gargantuan task before you.)

◆ Replace "I will be" goals with "I will do" goals.

As the Mahoneys suggest, you may want to be thinner, be in shape or be a healthful eater. But what will you do to get yourself there? Make your goals action-oriented. For example, you might say, "I will walk three or four times a week" or "I will switch from a sugar-coated cereal to a high-fiber cereal."

◆ Set specific rather than vague goals.

Nebulous goals that don't describe a specific behavior tend not to work because you never know for sure if you've met them.

So instead of vowing to "exercise more" or "not eat so many sweets," promise yourself to ride your exercise bike three times a week for 20 minutes or eat a sweet treat no more than three times a week.

◆ Base goals on where you are now, not where you want to be down the road.

The Mahoneys point out that reasonable goals are relative *only* to your past and current behavior. Thus, in setting a goal for a specific eating or exercise behavior, it's important to examine where you're coming from. If you've always gained over the holidays, it's more realistic to try to keep your weight stable than to lose weight. Maybe you're accustomed to eating a big bowl of ice cream in front of the television each night — after you've had dessert at supper. Instead of giving up the sweet bedtime snack altogether, you might try having fruit for dessert at suppertime and later having a measured cup of frozen low-fat yogurt in front of the TV.

◆ Avoid "should" and "have to" goals.

Goals like these tend to make people feel deprived and guilty. Let's say you're at a picnic, and you see a huge spread of mayonnaise-laden salads and desserts. Your tendency may be to feel you "shouldn't" have any of the high-fat items and "have to" eat only salad without dressing and a plain, broiled burger. Instead, ask yourself, "Who says I shouldn't? Who says I have to?" It's important to feel that you have the choice, and it's fine to have an item or two that's not a nutritional dream food — along with more healthful choices.

◆ Set flexible goals, and be ready to change them.

If your long-term goal is to cut your fat intake to 25 percent of your calories, but you've failed at the short-term goal of eating all bread, toast and potatoes dry, maybe you should use diet margarine instead of none. Or try cutting back on fat in some other way.

None of this is to say that your goals should not be challenging. The Mahoneys add, "You should expect some difficulty in performing *new* behaviors in *old,* familiar situations." If you fail repeatedly, they say, you should "back up a step or two and try again."

Why is realistic goal-setting so helpful for long-term weight control? In the first place, it helps you experience numerous small successes, which in turn are highly likely to heighten your sense of self-efficacy, or belief in yourself. Your confidence is also raised by the fact that one success tends to breed another, as demonstrated by a number of the masters. After Janice discovered that moderate exercise could help her lose weight, she became motivated to start making reasonable changes in her diet. Similarly, Don C. found that success at exercise spurred him to tackle more goals. "Running made me feel considerably better. I lost some weight, and that made me want to change my diet. Success at one thing made me want to do more."

Linda W. gave me a more detailed description of her many small triumphs, stemming from reasonable goals. "I decided to start very easily because drastic plans had never worked for me. At the first meal, I decided to start cutting back by not using butter (or margarine) on my bread. I found that I could very easily get by without butter and still do not use it on anything. Then I started to walk, and that was when the weight really started to come off. Then I read an article in *Reader's Digest* about fat grams, and I cut back my fat intake. I also started doing toning exercises and kept that up for about 2 years. I joined an aerobics class three summers ago and love it." Indeed, one success led to another for Linda, who lost 39 pounds "slow and steady" and has kept it off for 6 years.

Drs. Robert Colvin and Susan Olson found, too, that the maintainers in their study had accumulated many "small wins," maintaining their weight losses despite personal crises, such as divorce and the death of loved ones. "It's not because their weight is more important than such catastrophes . . . but because the habits acquired through small wins are so deeply ingrained that they persist even when stressful events take the foreground."

Look at the Big Picture

When your success at weight control is the result of meeting many small, achievable goals, it becomes more difficult for you to label any single "slip" or lapse as failure. One mistake can't undo all your positive changes.

Another way to look at it is that to lose weight — and especially to keep it off — you have to make multiple lifestyle changes. You're probably exercising, making an effort to be more active in your daily routine, developing a preference for lower-fat foods, keeping fewer tempting foods around the house, eating regular meals, making more nutritious snack choices, handling your feelings better and choosing restaurants with healthful food selections. How can one single act of overeating — or even several — undo all the other positive changes you've made? Even the worst eating binge is likely to add no more than a pound or two of body fat.

When I asked Janice what she does if she doesn't handle a food-related situation as she would have liked, she replied, "I don't berate myself, and I don't fixate on it. I get it in perspective: that one candy bar won't make me 20 pounds overweight. I look at the big picture. I remind myself that there are a multitude of things I do in a day, in a week, like eating breakfast, exercising and drinking water, that help me maintain my weight. That one candy bar is a drop in the bucket."

Experts suggest that you will be less likely to view a single instance of overeating as a catastrophe if you define success as more than reaching a goal weight. The turning point for a number of masters came when they decided to focus on *lifestyle change* and not just on weight loss. Janice, for one, feels that when she ultimately lost weight and kept it off, her perspective had shifted from the short-term goal of losing weight to a long-term vision of wanting to feel good about herself forever. So set *your* sights on the small goals that lead to positive lifestyle changes, such as healthful eating, more physical activity and feeling better about yourself, and always look at the big picture of the *many* favorable steps you've taken to control your weight.

Tim H. does just that to keep off his 40 pounds. "I love chocolate, and I believe in everything in moderation: there's nothing wrong with having one candy bar a day. But in the beginning, I was more punitive and beat myself up for having chocolate. Now, I see it as long-range planning — it's a lifetime routine. I give myself credit for my gains and try not to berate myself for my losses. Yeah, I'd like my diet to be better, but instead of saying, 'I'm doing it wrong,' I always feel I'm doing it 'more right' than I did before."

6

Key to Success #6

Learn the Art of Positive Self-Talk

Have you ever found yourself running late for an appointment, only to hit every red traffic light en route, make a wrong turn out of haste and get behind every slow-moving vehicle in town? At some level, you're probably thinking, "I'll never make it. I'm never on time for anything. Why don't these jerks get out of my way?" You find yourself tapping your foot, tailgating, driving too fast, blowing your horn and feeling like you might explode. What does it all accomplish?

What you say to yourself — your *self-talk* — about running late affects your actions and your feelings. You get yourself all worked up, run the risk of an accident and accomplish nothing other than getting to the appointment at the same time or later than if you hadn't gotten riled up.

Now, what if you had said more positive things to yourself like "Oh, well. There's nothing I can do about running late now. It's not worth risking an accident, and sometimes it's just not possible to be on time. The worst thing that can happen is that I'll be 15 minutes late, and *that's* not the end of the world." More positive self-talk can lead to more positive behavior: you don't speed, you calm yourself down, you don't take a wrong turn, and you get to your destination just five minutes late.

You may not be aware of it, but a similar process goes on with food and weight control all the time. Many people engage in negative self-talk — destructive thoughts — that trigger them to overeat or eat foods that interfere with their goals. But the masters have learned to counter negative with positive self-talk — a technique that can help both as you're losing weight and as you maintain that loss.

Joanna M.'s Story

I suspected Joanna M. was adept at positive self-talk when she wrote me that she used a number of psychological "tricks" to control her weight. She doesn't know how she learned the art; she "stumbled onto it." No matter how she learned the skills, Joanna made it clear that positive thinking is a critical part of her everyday life. But it wasn't always so. Joanna struggled with her weight for many years before she ever really believed she could be successful. Intellectually, she knew that eating less could make you thinner. But up until about 15 years ago, that knowledge never influenced her food choices. At that time, she started to lose the weight, eventually dropping from 190 to 140 over an up-and-down course of about 5 years. Now, at a height of 5'8", she feels good at her weight of 143. And she should, for she's managed to keep off more than 40 pounds for 10 years.

Like many other masters, Joanna describes her early years as overweight years. "I was heavy as an infant, toddler and child." The problem was exacerbated when she was 5 and her mother died. "I was lonely and traumatized, and the person whose job it was to feed me had died. So food became very important to me." At some level, Joanna believes she was thinking, "As long as I'm eating, I'm coping without her."

Throughout her elementary school years, she recalls her stepmother "locking up" tempting food, which she would "dole out" to Joanna's thinner sisters — but not to her. "My stepmother's intentions were good, but she only heightened my desire for those foods." So Joanna would sneak money from the house to buy candy, which she would eat secretly in her room.

"By the time I was 13, I weighed 147," Joanna recalls. Every year, her pediatrician would give her a lecture about her weight, and other children taunted her. Somehow, however, she was spared in high school when she slimmed down: "I was a little overweight, but not fat."

That period ended when Joanna went to college. "I started at a weight of 150 or 160. By the time I graduated, I weighed almost 200 pounds." She attributes the gain simply to overeating. "Those were happy years. It was just that food was constantly available in the college cafeteria, and I could have multiple helpings. Then, at night, a gang of us might order pizza, and sometimes there was drinking." Joanna wasn't a diet-hopper. "I only went on diets once or twice. I went on the Stillman diet for a week, but there were no serious attempts."

Joanna lost some weight again with her hectic graduate school schedule and stayed around 173 for a number of years. After graduating, she had problematic relationships with several men, which jogged her weight up and down because of the stress. A turning point in Joanna's weight battle came when a man with whom she had been living for two years left her for someone else. Although she describes herself as "devastated," a major goal in her life was finding a partner. "I needed to lose weight to attract someone new. So I began my first serious attempt at losing weight. I ate what I wanted, but in incredibly small amounts. If I ordered a hamburger and French fries, I would only eat part of them. I drank a lot of skim milk because it was soothing to me. For some reason, I snacked on liverwurst and crackers. And I ate a lot of vegetables." This was the first time Joanna saw that decisions she made throughout the day about whether or not to eat had a connection both with her weight *and* with her goal of having a romantic relationship. "Before that, I didn't really believe that if I ate properly, it would show up on my body."

At this point, Joanna also started to use positive self-talk. "I'd say to myself, 'I'm tempted to eat this, but it's more important to be thin.' I would think about how fleeting the enjoyment would be and remind myself of my goal, which was always a certain number of pounds or a time period. I would say, 'I'll do this for two weeks, or until I'm down to a certain weight.'" When she found herself starving for her next meal, and she still had hours to go, she would tell herself, "'I may not be able to make it for three or four hours, but I can make it for one.' I planned between-meal snacks to look forward to."

In addition, she thought about a therapist she saw who also happened to struggle with her weight. "The woman ate such meager meals. I often thought to myself, 'If *she* can get through the day on lettuce and lemon juice, I can do it, too.'" To this day, Joanna will remind herself of the therapist's statement, "You and I are not the kind of women who can forget that we have a weight problem. That's just how it is." Rather than feel sorry for herself, Joanna finds strength in this matter-of-fact approach.

Between cutting back on food and using positive self-talk, Joanna got down to the low-140s. And soon, she found the relationship she had been looking for — with the man to whom she is now married. She did gain about 25 pounds after meeting him, but lost half of it in time for her wedding. Shortly thereafter, she became interested in nutrition and started eating a very low-fat diet. (Because of the risk of breast cancer, she has been conscientious about watching her fat intake for many years.) From 1983 to 1988, Joanna maintained her weight around 150 and also had a baby during that time. "I only gained 22 pounds, which I lost soon after the baby's birth." After she had her second child in 1988, Joanna dropped from 153 to 136, a weight she maintained until just recently. She did it in the space of about 6 months by eating about 1,000 calories a day during the week and 1,200 calories on the weekends.

Joanna's story isn't one of having a marked "attitude shift," then dropping all her weight and keeping it off. Her story is one of weight fluctuation, gaining and losing over the course of many years, but never gaining it all back. She doesn't present her tale as a horrible battle, nor did she seem to berate herself for her rocky history. Instead, her story comes across more as a process — one of learning what works for her and of speaking positively to herself. When she feels tempted to overeat, she talks to herself and uses visual imagery. "I picture how my stomach looks when my weight is down. Or I think about how I'll look in a new outfit or how my face looks when I'm thinner." She also remembers her maternal grandmother, who was important to her and who was careful about what she ate. "She ate very little, and she ate nutritious foods. Sometimes I think of her when I'm tempted."

Joanna does feel that all the years of watching the scale fluctuate, along with a chronically low calorie intake, lowered her metabolism. Yet in the past few months, she has revamped her eating habits and found a new peace with food and her weight. About a year ago, she consulted a registered dietitian about her diet and was told that, in order to step up her metabolism, she should consider increasing her daily calorie intake from 1,200 to 1,500 or more. But Joanna didn't follow the advice right away: she had to do it her way, on her terms and in her own time. Then, about 3 months ago, she realized how "tremendously difficult" it was to maintain her weight at 136. "My weight started creeping up for no apparent reason, and I was very resentful. So I decided to increase my calories to 1,500 a day. I said, 'Okay, we'll see what happens. I won't get on the scale for a month.'" She did, in fact, gain 7 pounds, then leveled off at 143. She says of her new way of eating, "It's great. I'm not hungry all the time. Before, I was cranky and miserable. My quality of life is much better now."

Accepting the change wasn't easy, and Joanna once again called positive self-talk into play. "It was stressful to gain the weight. In the past, if I gained a pound, it would ruin my day. I'd feel that I'd failed, that I was unattractive, and I would have to decrease my calories even more. Now if I gain a little, I say to myself, 'I know I'm eating the same amount and have the same amount of activity.' I know the weight gain is temporary, and I'm confident I'll go back down."

Along with her change in food intake came a change in body image and sense of personal value. She told me, "I used to hinge my sense of self-worth on my weight. Above a certain level, I saw myself as a failure; below it, I was a success. I told myself that if I maintained my weight, my life would change: all the clients at work would ask for me, or I'd walk into a party and be beautiful because I was so thin. But I got fed up with the struggle to weigh less than 140. I realized that my goal of 136 was somewhat arbitrary and that it really didn't matter if I weighed 7 pounds more. No one even notices."

Now, Joanna's day begins with "two breakfasts," totaling 300 to 400 calories. She's up very early and starts out having dry toast or toast with tofu cream cheese or jelly. Then at work, she will eat more of the same or have a bowl of high-fiber cereal with milk. Lunch is typically a big salad — like a Caesar salad or a salad with chicken — often eaten in a restaurant. (Since she's upped her calorie intake, she no longer "holds" the dressing.) After work comes the "high point" of her day — "decompression time" — before going home to deal with the demands of young children. She stops on the way and treats herself to frozen yogurt. "I make it a point not to come home ravenous."

Dinners are typically made from recipes from low-calorie cookbooks or magazines. "I carefully choose recipes or modify them to a lower fat content. And we eat huge salads with nonfat dressing, plus lots of vegetables. Between my husband and me, we might eat a pound and a half of asparagus!" While she's cooking, Joanna keeps a no-calorie beverage by her side. When she finds herself "looking around for more" after finishing meals and snacks, she begins to look forward to her next meal. She also finalizes each meal and snack with a hot drink, carbonated beverage or small mint.

Joanna adds that her kitchen is "full of junk food," but she rarely craves or eats it because she keeps her own special controllable treat foods on hand, like malted milk balls and special non-fat chocolate sauce from a mail-order house. "I'll eat the sauce on Fiber One cereal for an evening treat."

Joanna's exercise consists of jogging for half an hour (about 2½ miles) three or four times a week. She also rides horseback several times weekly. When I asked her if she uses self-talk to motivate herself to exercise, she responded, "Yes, when I get bored or lack motivation, I picture fat on the back of my thighs."

Her number-one high-risk time is when her schedule is "all mixed up" or when she doesn't count calories. When I interviewed her, for instance, she had just returned from a business trip to Europe and was off her regime. "I came home and wanted to go on a 2,000-to-3,000-calorie excursion, but said to myself, 'The last thing you need when coping with jet lag is to go on a major binge.'"

I find Joanna's story to be enlightening not only because of her use of positive self-talk, but because it illustrates that maintenance is not static. When she hit a point of near intolerance for how she was eating, she made a change that enabled her to stay thin for life. She adds, "If you want to keep your weight down, you have to have fluid goals and motivations because life keeps changing."

What Is Self-Talk?

What exactly is this "self-talk" employed by masters like Joanna? It's that ongoing conversation — that mental dialogue — you constantly have with yourself. As Kelly S., who lists "positive self-talk" as one of her top strategies for keeping off 50 pounds for 6 years, puts it, "We all have these tapes running through our heads." Often, the "tapes" are recurring, and they determine how we eat in a given situation. In other words, self-talk can actually cause feelings and behavior that, if self-defeating, can lead to lapses. *But the masters have learned to make their self-talk positive, which, in turn, helps them control their eating and their weight.*

Psychologist Joyce D. Nash, Ph.D., notes in her book *Now That You've Lost It,* "People whose negative, self-defeating self-talk outweighs their positive, coping thoughts tend not to do well in their weight management efforts . . . In general, the person who has a greater chance of achieving long-term weight management success will engage in more self-talk that reflects flexible thinking, how-to-cope thoughts, pats-on-the-back thoughts, more self-confident thoughts and thoughts reflecting assertiveness and coping skills."

The "Now-I've-Blown-It" Phenomenon

In my experience, the most common example of negative self-talk is the "now-I've-blown-it" phenomenon: someone who has set an unrealistic goal, such as "I'm giving up desserts," has one cookie and decides, "I may as well eat the whole bag." *It isn't just the presence of sweets that triggers inappropriate eating — it's what an individual says to him- or herself about the sweets.*

What might happen if the person says something more positive and productive? "Oh well, one or two cookies won't make me gain weight, but eating the whole bag will. It's over and done, and I'll stop right here." The very act of changing that negative statement into this more positive self-talk can stop lapses from occurring.

Kelly S. recalls, "When I was in the ultimate hell of my weight problem, I knew that if I ate one cookie or candy, I was going to literally eat pounds of it." And so she did. But not anymore. "Now I tell myself there are no 'good' and 'bad' foods. I can eat a few bites of a dessert and be fine." By using such positive self-statements, she is now able to prevent lapses when she eats sweets.

How Negative Self-Talk Gets in the Way

Negative self-talk interferes with successful weight control in two ways. In the first place, it leads to "slips" in eating behavior. Joanna M. repeatedly struggles with negative self-talk after she's been out for the evening and anticipates coming home to leftover treats not eaten by her babysitter. She finds herself thinking, "I can't wait to get home and eat that," which can lead her to over-eat. But she tries to counter this negative thought with, "Look, it's already midnight. I may as well go to bed, and soon it will be morning. It's silly to eat all this after having had such a good day."

Secondly, negative self-talk may produce feelings of depression and hopelessness, which in turn can cause more overeating. Peppi S., who has kept off 62 pounds, points out that negative self-talk "leads to giving up and the guilt and depression that go along with it. This leads to the vicious cycle that so many of us can get into: eating, guilt, depression and negative thoughts, overeating, guilt, etc."

She goes on: "To avoid slipping, I am always trying to 'talk to myself.' I feel maintenance is all about *consciously* making choices. If I choose to have a dessert that I haven't had in a while, I don't bash myself for making that decision. I made the choice, I deal with the choice and make the necessary sacrifices for choosing it. None of this 'all-or-nothing' thinking, where you say, 'Well, I blew it by eating this, so the rest of the day doesn't count.' Not that we don't all have better days than others. You've got to see these as warning signals; if you don't stop it soon, you can very easily get back into old habits."

When Is Positive Self-Talk Helpful?

Positive self-talk *can work to your advantage at all stages of weight control: when the "attitude shift" is taking place, while you're losing weight and at maintenance.* When you're in the midst of the attitude shift — or as Stanton Peele and Archie

Brodsky put it in *The Truth About Addiction and Recovery,* "When you are moving from being 'on the fence' or 'thinking about' changing your habits to a firm determination to change" — you can use your reasons for wanting to lose weight as "internal pep talks." When Joanna M. was finally ready to lose weight permanently, she told herself, "I want to look good more than I want to eat." In making the decision to lose her 50 pounds once and for all, Kelly S. psyched herself with, "The weight is no longer going to be a barrier to feeling good about myself and pursuing my goals."

When you're losing weight and at maintenance, positive self-talk is particularly helpful in high-risk situations. *Positive self-talk can work at moments of choice.* When Joanna M. felt tempted to overeat as she was losing weight, she reminded herself about her end goal, "and that was more important than the immediate gratification of food." At maintenance, one of her high-risk situations comes when she's very tired. She talks herself out of indulging by asking herself, "How am I going to feel after I eat this? I remember how it used to feel."

As Kelly S. was losing weight, she realized that one of her difficult times was studying for college exams. Her recurring negative self-talk was, "I need the M&M's to get through this test. I'll diet tomorrow." But when she was ready to lose weight, her self-talk became, "I can get through this test without binge eating."

Positive self-talk can work after the fact. If Joanna M. winds up eating some of the food left over from the babysitter, she tells herself, "I'm usually so disciplined. I can have some momentary lapses. If it shows up tomorrow, I know I'll lose it."

Peppi S. sums up the benefits of positive self-talk with, "I listen to myself. [I ask myself] why I want a certain food, how that certain food tastes, what my expectations are and how I'm going to deal with the emotions if I choose to eat it. Then, if I choose to eat the food, I sit back and think about what I'm feeling. If the food was a letdown, I register this in my mind so the next time I get a craving or desire for that food (or any other food for that matter), I will remember that the last time I tried it, it wasn't all that great, and I might be more inclined not to want it."

Learning the Art of Positive Self-Talk

A problem many overweight people have is that the negative self-talk is so deeply ingrained that they're not even in touch with their mental dialogues with themselves. Indeed, a number of my patients used to tell me, "I don't think before I eat. I just do it." Peppi S. admits that before she lost her 62-plus pounds, "I never sat down to figure out why I overate. I just thought it was because I liked to eat too much. *Au contraire!* It was because I had lots of emotions or stressful situations bombarding me, causing me to satisfy them the easiest way I knew how. And the thing I was really good at was eating."

But there are techniques — psychologists call them "cognitive restructuring" — that you can learn to get in touch with your negative self-talk and turn it around to positive thinking, making it less likely that you'll eat in ways that interfere with weight management.

In their book *Permanent Weight Control,* Michael J. Mahoney and Kathryn Mahoney popularized the following cognitive restructuring techniques to help people struggling with their weight. These steps are based on their suggestions:

◆ Detect your self-statements.

This is the most difficult step: getting in touch with what you say to yourself. As the Mahoneys point out, "If you're like many people, you may go through an entire day without monitoring what you say to yourself. This doesn't mean that your thoughts are unconscious — only that you seldom make an effort to listen in on them." They suggest performing a "mental inventory" anytime you feel tempted, discouraged or depressed. That is, when you feel the urge to engage in behavior that is inconsistent with weight control, don't just tough it out — ask yourself what is going on inside your head. If you can't come up with anything, try completing the sentence "I am acting as if . . ." For instance, if you feel you can't resist the urge to eat a candy bar, you might say, "I'm acting as if I'll die or the world will end if I don't have a candy bar."

Some people find it helpful to keep a diary of their thoughts throughout the day, asking themselves what they are thinking before, during and after they eat or feel tempted to eat. The Mahoneys suggest placing small reminders or prompts, such as stickers (Kelly S. finds Post-its to be useful), in or on highly visible places like your watch, wallet, clock, mirror and scale. Each time you see a sticker, pause and review your thoughts for the preceding few minutes. Can you find any negative self-talk?

Judy F. is both a master at weight loss and a registered dietitian who specializes in counseling overweight people. She helps them get in touch with their negative self-talk by having them list 12 reasons they want to change their behavior. Then, when they want to eat something, she advises that they reread their list so they're forced to think about what they're doing.

◆ Evaluate your self-talk.

Is what you say to yourself in any given situation true, rational, sensible, helpful? As San Francisco–area psychologist Silas M. Wesley, Ph.D., points out, "The mind *lies* (as well as tells the truth some of the time). It's important to catch the mind in one of these all-too-frequent lies, overgeneralizations and gross exaggerations . . . The discovery needs to be made that you don't have to believe everything that your mind says!"

When evaluating self-talk, sometimes it helps to ask yourself what you'd say to someone else in the same situation. For instance, how would you respond to someone who said, "I blew it, I may as well pig out for the rest of the day?" You probably would tell him or her, "That doesn't make any sense."

◆ **Turn the negative self-talk to positive self-talk.**

After recognizing the irrational nature of notions like "I'm dying for something sweet," you might say, "No, I won't die if I don't have candy. And the short-term pleasure of eating it now is not worth it when I see how great I look in my new jeans."

Another way of challenging negative self-talk is with a technique called "thought-stopping." Dr. Joyce Nash suggests that whenever you have negative self-talk, you think to yourself "Stop!" and immediately dismiss the negative thought, focusing your attention on a counterargument or positive thought. She finds that it helps some people to refocus their attention when they wear rubber bands on their wrists and snap them at the same time they think "Stop!"

It Takes Time and Practice

It takes time to learn the art of cognitive restructuring, to actually believe in your new, positive self-talk and to be able to act in ways that are consistent with long-term weight control. As the Mahoneys put it, "Appropriate self-talk *typically* takes months, even years, to develop . . . there is frequently a lag between changed self-talk and changed feelings." Joanna M., for instance, wasn't always able to forgive herself so easily when she slipped. She admits, "It took a long time. It used to be that gaining one pound would drive me crazy. But that didn't stop me; it gave me renewed determination."

Dr. Wesley suggests that, rather than deal with the notion of having to change your whole life and way of thinking, you take things one thought at a time. In essence, that's what Joanna M. did when she was faced with the prospect of having to wait for another meal: she told herself if she could just make it through the next hour, she'd be okay.

In taking thoughts and events one at a time, concentrate on your ability to overcome unpleasant or challenging situations or feelings. Use self-statements like, "I've made it through similar situations before" or "It's only as bad as I tell myself it is. I know I can make it." *Your ability to use positive self-talk to manage individual situations will boost your belief in your weight-management abilities.*

Dr. Nash emphasizes that it is not possible to wipe out all negative self-statements: "To attain success, the objective is to get the positive self-talk to outweigh the negative, aiming for a ratio of about 2 to 1, positive to negative."

In all honesty, some masters find certain rather negative self-statements to be helpful — for example, Joanna M.'s comment about picturing fat on her thighs to motivate herself to exercise. And when she's tempted to indulge, she sometimes recalls how disgusted she felt after once stuffing herself with fruitcake. Alyce C. has "a picture of a very fat person" posted on the door of her refrigerator. In her book, *Alyce's Fat Chance,* she adds, "Some people put a skinny person on their door . . . that didn't work for me. Call it the Power of Negative Thinking."

As always, you have to find what works for you. But most psychologists would agree that positive self-talk is more productive than negative.

How the Masters Put Positive Self-Talk to Work

Following are some of the categories of self-talk that dieters commonly use. Take from the masters the positive self-talk statements that will work for you:

◆ **Self-fulfilling prophecies** — setting yourself up for something by telling yourself that it will or won't happen. Says master and registered dietitian Judy F., "If my patients are talking negatively, they are almost destined to eat negatively." In other words, if you tell yourself you'll never be able to lose weight and keep it off, you'll probably see to it that you never will. Peppi S. used to say, "I can't." *Now, she uses positive self-talk to create a produc-tive self-fulfilling prophecy:* "The greatest thing I learned from Nutri/System is to say, I can; I can do anything I set my mind to do." Similarly, Doris M., who was "desperate after 30 years of diets," became inspired when she went to Weight Watchers and saw "thin, healthy people maintaining 50-to-100-pound weight losses." She adds, "I could do, and I *did!*"

◆ **All-or-nothing self-talk** — black-and-white thinking. Unreal-istic goals that establish rigid rules set you up for failure. Low-calorie diets and rules about foods he should "never" eat used to trigger all-or-nothing thinking in Don M., who, after one small deviation, would say to himself, "I'm off it. I've been bad — I've fallen off the tightrope." The next day, he'd give up. Now, with his new low-fat way of life, he still feels he needs to stay away from certain foods, but instead of being negative, he focuses on treats he *can* have.

◆ **Body size or weight-related self-talk** — bemoaning your rate of weight loss or having an unrealistic goal for your body. This kind of negative self-talk might say, "I only lost half a pound this week. Why bother?" But instead of being impatient about weight loss, Rosetta F. says, "I tell myself that if there are 3,500 calories to a pound, I can lose about a pound a month by just not eating 100 calories a day that I am now eating. A pound a month times 12 months is 12 pounds, times 3 years is 36 pounds lost." Jennifer P., who's 5'5" and weighs 142, down 44 pounds from her maximum weight, says, "I wanted to weigh 123, but my recommended weight is higher. Also, I don't want to deprive myself and be ob-sessive about exercise in order to lose. I'm a size 10, and that's okay." Don M.'s body-related negative self-talk can be, "I'm still not normal; I weigh 20 pounds more than I ultimately want to." His positive refrain is, "The difference between what I was and where I am is so vast that I can now wear 'drop-dead' clothes! I haven't been this thin since I was 13 years old."

◆ **Catastrophic self-talk** — always thinking the worst will happen or feeling things are worse than they are. For example, I frequently heard my patients make comments like, "I'm up a pound this week. I'll probably gain all the weight back." But it helps to ask yourself, "What's the worst thing that could happen?" For example, if you overeat for a weekend, the worst that could happen is that you might gain a pound or two. As Lynn M. states, "If I gain a pound, I don't panic. If it takes a week or two to take it off, I have enough confidence in myself that I will lose it." When faced with a high-risk situation, like going to a party, Joanna M. doesn't panic, but instead "blocks out" 400 to 500 calories she can spend. She uses positive self-talk: "I think of women I have known who control their weight and imagine what they would eat in this setting." She also focuses on socializing and thinks about how good she looks when her weight is down.

◆ **Rationalizing self-talk** — making excuses in order to allow yourself to overeat. When she was heavy, Joanna M. made excuses by telling herself she "was going to go on a diet sometime." But at some level, she thought, "It won't work." When she was successful, she told herself (and believed it), "If I don't eat that, I *will* lose weight." After a lapse, Peppi S. used to rationalize by saying, "What's one more day of overeating?" Now, if she slips, she says to herself, "Okay, so I ate it!" and she stops right there. After dieting and regaining weight, Don M., who once had clothes in multiple sizes, used to say, "Oh well. I've got clothes that fit me." When he lost weight once and for all, however, he put all his big clothes in a "fat box" and donated them to the homeless. "Now, when I desire a short-term 'high' from a sundae, I remind myself that I no longer have to shop in a big men's store. I say, 'Yeah, you did it!'" Then his desire for the sundae passes. Lydia R. described her self-talk at a recent dessert buffet: "I had one thing I really wanted. I told myself that all those desserts don't really taste that good anyway. Besides, they're all sugar and fat." In the past, she would have said to herself, "'They all look so good. I may as well have what I want tonight. I won't have the chance again.' So I'd have a taste of everything and wind up with the equivalent of four pieces. I used to talk myself into it instead of out of it."

• **Self-deprecation** — putting yourself down for human tendencies or calling yourself demeaning names. People who see themselves as "bad" because they sometimes stray from their goals or who call themselves names like "fat pig" and "slob" set themselves up for relapse. Mindy B. used to say, "I'm fat. Who cares? I'm going to eat it anyway." Now, if she gains a few pounds, she thinks, "I like myself here. I don't ever want to be that fat person again," and she immediately takes the weight off.

• **Punishing self-statements** — chastising yourself for lapses. Remember Ernie L.'s past tendency to feel he had to punish himself with stringent dieting when he gained some weight after traveling? Now, his positive self-talk is, "I have come to accept the weight gain when I travel, and I no longer feel I have to get it off instantly. I realize that it may take some time, so I focus on the positive instead of on drudgery." Similarly, Dorothy C. comments, "Rather than flagellate myself and vow to fast or cut back drastically the day or week after a mini-binge, I have learned to accept setbacks and move on."

• **"Should" self-statements** — beliefs about obligations that have little or no basis in fact. Peppi S. was full of "shoulds": "You should always clean your plate. You should eat what's available before someone else does. You should not let anything go to waste, so you should finish it off. You should eat now so you won't be hungry later." She adds, "These are beliefs that you have to be willing to rethink into new ideas." *So when you feel "shoulds" about foods, ask yourself, "Who says I should? Does this make any sense?"* I used to tell my patients who couldn't bear to waste food to ask themselves, "Is the 'wasted' food better off in the trash can or as excess on my body?" When Joanna M. feels the urge to "eat it now before the kids finish it up," she takes a piece of the item and tucks it away so she doesn't feel she has to down it immediately.

◆ **Have-to-have-food thoughts** — feeling you can't delay immediate gratification for a particular food: "I'm dying for a __" or "I can't stop thinking about __; I have to have one." But the masters use positive statements to talk themselves out of certain situations and foods. Margie M. uses the popular statement "Nothing tastes as good as being thin feels!" Joanna M. asks herself, "Which means more: eating this or losing fat?" She adds, "When I'm hungry, I remind myself that it's only a short time until my next meal or snack, and I can stand anything for that amount of time." When Mindy B. was losing weight, she told herself, "Whatever I want to eat that is fattening, I can have next month. It will still be in the store." A similar statement helped some of my former patients who found themselves obsessing about a food when they were trying to lose weight: "I know what it tastes like, I've had it before, I'll eventually have it again. I'm just choosing not to have it right now." Peppi S. reflects, "So often, it's the built-up anticipation for a food. I often find that when I have it, it isn't so great."

◆ **Dealing-with-saboteurs self-talk** — telling yourself you have to give in to someone else's attempts to sabotage your weight-loss or maintenance efforts. So often, well-intentioned (and sometimes ill-intentioned) friends or relatives get in the way of weight control. Don M. occasionally hears, "You're too thin" and is sometimes offered high-fat food gifts. "In the past, I would have thought, 'Oh, they're right — it's time to stop losing weight. I can't refuse food that's given to me.'" Now he can say to himself, "I know in my heart that I'm not too thin, and they don't understand what I'm trying to accomplish." So he graciously accepts the food and then gives it away. Joanna M. is also occasionally admonished by jealous relatives that she should be eating more. "But I don't cave in; I remind myself I'm not the sort of person who can be talked into anything. It makes me more determined." (For more on social pressure and sabotage, see Chapter 10.)

◆ **Poor-me self-talk** — believing that your lot in life is horrible because you have to watch your weight or feeling that weight control should be easy. A number of masters had encouraging words about coping with such feelings. When Lydia R. gets through a high-risk situation without overeating, she tells herself, "It feels good to nurture myself with healthy food; it's not torture. I feel proud of myself." Peppi S. accepts that she is more susceptible to gaining weight than other people. But she doesn't feel sorry for herself; she sees herself as making conscious choices that she feels good about. She goes on, "I look at maintenance as a lifelong commitment and not as a self-defeating punishment. Maintenance is a way of life for me; it's all about making choices: I choose to read food labels, I choose to eat what I used to consider forbidden foods when I feel the urge to eat them. But I am also very careful to register in my mind what that food tastes like, how I'm feeling when I eat it and how I feel after eating it." In short, for Peppi, maintenance is not a plight, it's a choice. Instead of feeling that maintenance is a struggle, Doris M. defines her years of "carelessness, making poor food choices and feeling like a failure" as "struggling." Mindy B. uses positive self-talk to avoid "poor-me" thoughts about chocolate, a food she feels she cannot control. "I tell myself this is one thing you cannot have. Some people can't have milk, and this is a fact of life for me."

Focusing on Where You've Been

As I talked with the masters about their positive self-talk, a recurring theme was their focus on where they have been. *When they feel tempted to eat in ways that interfere with weight control, they habitually think about their past and compare it with the present.* "I think about my body — the way it used to be and the way it is now — and all the money I've spent on clothes," states Joanna M. "It makes me not want to eat." Similarly, Fern C. admits, "It hasn't been easy; I feel like quitting every so often. But when I remember what I looked like fat, I work harder at it."

When I asked the masters, "How do you stay motivated? How do you stick with it?" they told me that they do so by recalling the pain of their heavy pasts and never forgetting why they lost the weight. But in the next breath, they would contrast their remembrances with how wonderful their lives are now that they've lost the weight.

Peppi S. motivates herself by occasionally trying on a pair of her old, large jeans. She adds, "I have to remind myself every day by looking at my body in the mirror or weighing myself that I have come a long way and know the positive feelings far outweigh the negative feelings. And when I exercise, I remember what it was like when I was heavy, that I couldn't even walk a block, much less do a step class for one solid hour! I constantly think of how it used to be, how far I've come, and how I am a happy, healthy and energetic person."

Don M. stays on track, not only by recalling "the extraordinary moment" when he found that the clothes in the big men's shop were too big for him, but when he was able to purchase health insurance at a normal rate. "Right after I lost weight, I applied for health insurance, and they still charged me higher rates because they bet I'd gain the weight back. The next year, they dropped the rates, but not all the way. Now, I'm charged the normal rate for insurance. Thinking of that keeps me motivated when I'm tempted to overeat."

The clear message from the masters is: Challenge your negative, defeating self-talk with thoughts about your accomplishments. You'll come to believe in yourself more and more.

7

Key to Success #7

Move It to Lose It

Experts say without hesitation that a critical difference between maintainers and regainers is their commitment to exercise. As Mary Ann K., who managed an 84-pound weight loss, says of her maintenance method, "Exercise is a big part: you have to move it to lose it."

"Studies show clearly that exercise increases the likelihood of weight loss," notes Yale University's Kelly Brownell in the *International Journal of Obesity*. As for *keeping weight off*, he stresses, "Given recent studies showing its association with maintenance, it would be difficult to argue that any factor is more important than exercise." In fact, increased physical activity is probably the best single predictor of who will *keep off* weight.

What may come as a surprise is that most masters are *not* exercise fanatics — people who do triathlons or work out arduously every day or for hours at a time. *Indeed, experts suggest that what's most important about exercise is consistency and enjoyment — and less so the amount or type of activity.*

I'm not going to talk about how to get your heart rate up or tell you the best way to stoke your metabolic fire. Instead, this chapter provides information from the masters for getting hooked and staying hooked on exercise by designing your own personal fitness plan — one that you can live with and tailor to your needs as your circumstances change.

Jim V.'s Story

Jim V. is a master at weight control *and* at exercise. In fact, he considers exercise to be the most important thing that he does to keep off his 250 pounds. Jim has lost more than half of his former 475-pound self. When he was losing, he found, "It came off so much faster and I felt so much better when I exercised." But Jim is the kind of guy who doesn't believe things until he sees them. "I had to put it to the test, so I stopped walking for a month. My weight loss decreased immediately. I said to myself, *'This is going to be the key.'*"

As with so many masters, it took years before Jim was ready to take control of his weight problem. He told me, "I was over-weight as far back as I can remember. From about ages 5 to 10, I was chubby; I was obese through high school and college." Fortunately, Jim had a number of things going for him that made him feel good about himself despite his weight. He was very active in the drum and bugle corps, he ranked high in academics, and he always managed to have a group of supportive friends who accepted him as he was. He endured the "typical name-calling" by peers, particularly at the all-boys high school he attended, "where 75 percent of the guys were into sports. I had to stay away from that crowd because they mocked me."

Jim maintains he didn't really become uncomfortable about his weight until he was in college. "I felt misplaced. I couldn't get involved in activities as much as other people. I wanted to be in theater, but I couldn't because of my size." What really did Jim in when he was in college was his embarrassment at his inability to fit comfortably in the chairs. "It was the main reason I left college and got a job."

When he was about 19, with his weight in the "high-300s,"

Jim made his first and second-to-last attempt at losing weight. He went to a dietitian at an outpatient hospital clinic and lost about 90 pounds on a sensible, low-calorie diet. "I went because my parents forced me. I did it to please them. But I went right back to my old habits." Within 2 years, Jim had gained all the weight back.

For the next 7 or 8 years, Jim's weight problem got worse. He had a clerical job that was sedentary, as was his social life. "I'd go to work, go home, go out to the movies. My reason to go out with friends was to go out to eat. I always ate on the run, ate lots of fast foods and ate more than three times a day. I was never satisfied."

Jim's discomfort grew, as did his size: he hit his all-time high of 475 when he was 29. (He's 6'3" tall.) His readiness to take control of his weight increased when, as the teacher of a prominent drum and bugle corps, he had to do a lot of traveling. "I was so uncomfortable and embarrassed, squishing into airplane seats." He also found himself becoming complacent about his daytime job.

It took a critical, life-threatening incident for Jim to finally take action. "It was the Fourth of July, 1989. I was out in a boat with an inner tube tied behind it. I stepped in, and the tube flipped. I got caught under it, and my pants hooked onto the boat. My brother-in-law jumped in to save me, but he practically killed himself doing it." That was Jim's turning point. "I said to myself, 'If I can't save myself because of my weight . . .' Right away, I went to my doctor, who referred me to Dr. Blackburn [George Blackburn, M.D., is a weight-control expert at Beth Israel Deaconess Medical Center in Boston]. I went the next day and said, 'I'll do anything.'"

Jim then went on the OPTIFAST all-liquid "fasting" diet for 18 weeks. He had five specially formulated "shake" meals a day and no solid foods. When I asked him if that was difficult, he replied, "The first three weeks were torture, then it was a breeze. I didn't want to stop." Jim also went to behavior-modification group meetings and special meetings for people on the fast, while seeing a dietitian/nurse for individual counseling. "I just sucked in the information — the things to change my habits. I saw the situations I had placed myself in. Even though I was just drinking shakes, I was practicing for maintenance."

Over the 4½-month course, his weight plummeted to 350 pounds. Then it was time for a break: slow refeeding, easing him onto a low-calorie diet with real food that still allowed him to lose about 3 pounds a week. "The difficulty was the choices. I knew intellectually about fat, but I had to read labels and weigh things."

Jim began to exercise toward the end of the fast: he chose walking. "I probably pushed myself too hard in the beginning. I started with an hour, but the pace was slower [than now]. I found a place where I enjoyed walking around a pond. It was peaceful, and a lot of people were doing the same thing. There was lots of encouragement. The feeling I got from it was so wonderful, and it was something I was doing for myself."

After two months on the low-calorie plan, Jim still had a lot of weight to lose, so Dr. Blackburn offered him the opportunity to go back on the liquid fast for 16 weeks. Once again, the first three weeks were rough. "It was a shock, it was brutal, but the results were amazing. I went through four different wardrobes by the time I was done." (Jim admitted that if he had it to do over again, he would not have gone on the second fast because the choices he was allowed on the low-calorie diet made him feel empowered, and he didn't want to give that up.)

Again, there came a 6-week period of weaning off the liquid formula and onto regular food. Then came a year and a half of "maintenance," which meant eating three meals a day and no more than 30 grams of fat, as well as attending weekly group meetings with a dietitian. Jim never missed a meeting, and to this day, chooses to go back to see his dietitian about once every three months. "When I feel I'm getting lackadaisical, and I need a jump start, I go back for a shot in the arm. I need to hear, 'You've been through this before, and you've done all this work. You know how you feel when you're in control.'" (All together, it took Jim about 18 months to get down to his current weight of 225. He has done so well that he now runs some weight-loss groups for the program that helped him.)

"Now, I can identify when I hit 'that' point, like when I'm busy teaching drum and bugle corps, and there's lots of food around. Usually, I look and think before eating. But if there's too much pressure, I stop thinking. I reach and eat without thinking. But I sense when it's happening. Before, I would let it go out of control."

Jim described his longest lapse, which occurred this past winter. He gained 10 pounds (the upper limit of his "buffer zone") when he was under extreme pressure, traveling with the drum and bugle corps, on top of a full-time job. "All my thoughts were consumed by the kids [I was teaching]. But I decided not to let things like that become as important as my health. I identified the problem immediately and went to see Marty [his dietitian] and got back on the track."

When I asked Jim about the transition from the fast to maintenance, he admitted it was "scary." "Your mind-set is that you don't want to stop losing weight or that sense of accomplishment. It's a real downer for a while." How did he get his sense of accomplishment when the fast was over? He told me, "By getting through every day, doing my food and exercise plan, doing the things to take care of myself. In the past, I always took care of others. It was a day-by-day process, and it still is." Also, like most other masters, Jim now sees that he couldn't conquer his weight problem until he accepted full responsibility for it. "When I finally realized that I wasn't doing it for my parents but for me — that's when I felt successful."

Today, Jim says the process is much easier. And he has little fear of regaining the weight. However, he didn't start to see himself as a thinner person until two years ago, after he went through the painful process of having cosmetic surgery to remove the excess folds of skin on his chest, legs and stomach. "Now, I feel like a typical, normal human being." For motivation, Jim will sometimes recall his surgeon's warnings about how important it is to maintain his weight loss. "If I think of myself regaining, I think I might explode!" A somewhat punitive self-talk strategy, but it works for him.

Now, Jim religiously eats three meals a day. A typical breakfast consists of cereal with 1 percent milk and a bagel, plain or with jelly. For variety, so he doesn't get bored, Jim occasionally has an egg or low-fat frozen waffles. Lunch might be a bowl of soup, a large salad with dressing on the side (usually low-fat dressing, but once in a while regular, when he "has a taste for something"), or a "light" sandwich like turkey with mustard instead of mayonnaise. Then dinner is a "good-sized meal" — usually pasta with plenty of vegetables. "Lots of chicken" is in his repertoire; he rarely eats red meat. He tries to make it a rule not to eat anything past 7:00 P.M.; if he does, it's a handful of pretzels. He also eats three pieces of fruit, spread throughout the day. Jim has a good sense of how many calories he needs to maintain (he's had his metabolic rate measured) and figures he eats between 2,300 and 2,800 calories a day — hardly a starvation level!

Since he has quite a sweet tooth, Jim tries to stay away from sugary foods. "On special occasions, like holidays, I will allow myself a treat. I choose the one thing I like best." Although he makes it a practice to avoid fast-food restaurants, Jim has not given up eating out with his friends. "I did lose a lot of friends who felt I wasn't going to be 'the happy-go-lucky, let's-go-out-to-eat-dinner person.' But I still have a core of friends who will go to restaurants where you can make [healthful] choices."

Jim says his impetus to keep his weight down is more health-related rather than a "look" he's after. "I do it because I feel better. I'm motivated by the health benefits — better sleeping and breathing." And the exercise helps him "stand taller, feel stronger and have better endurance."

As for his exercise during maintenance, Jim says, "When I stop for a bit, my weight goes up. When I increase my activity, I go back to normal." His exercise routine now consists of 60-minute walks along a river each day on his lunch hour. (He figures he covers three to four miles.) "It re-energizes me for the afternoon. I'm ready to go for another four hours. I'm not as hungry, and it's improved my job performance drastically." Jim goes on his walk every week day, unless it's extremely cold or "very crazy" at work. If it's cold, Jim walks at a mall "without my credit cards and my wallet. I don't need another bad habit." Not long ago, Jim added working out at a health club three nights a week with a personal trainer to his exercise routine. He goes on a treadmill for 15 minutes, a rowing machine for 10 minutes, followed by 40 to 50 minutes of weight lifting.

Since the health-club routine added to the walking sounds like a rather intimidating amount of activity, I asked him how he responds when people in his weight-loss groups say they can't begin to have time for all that exercise. He replied, "I tell them there are 24 hours in a day, and you have to be able to find one hour a day for yourself. If people exercise 3 times a week for 20 to 45 minutes, that's a great start. You have to set reasonable goals. Even I would feel satisfied spending an hour 3 times a week walking." (Recall, too, that Jim lost weight quickly and maintained his losses just fine by walking 5 days a week.)

To make exercise enjoyable, he uses headphones, occasionally walks with a friend at work and purposely chooses pleasant surroundings. (Sometimes he walks along the beach.) He also thinks it's motivating to exercise at places where other people are doing so. At his health club, he finds it helpful to work out around "accomplished athletes," whom he fondly refers to as "muscle heads." He finds, "They constantly encourage you. They are the most tolerant people because they want you to feel the way they do."

Ultimately, Jim's secret to maintaining a 250-pound weight loss is "planning my meal pattern and exercise." He stays hooked on exercise by "experiencing how pleasing and stress-reducing it can be."

How the Masters Move It to Lose It — and Keep It Off

When I asked the masters to tell me how they were finally successful at *losing* weight, their most consistent response was "exercise." Although the question was open-ended, and many masters gave multiple responses, exercise was mentioned more frequently than any other *specific* method of weight loss.

When I asked them to list the three most important things they do to *maintain* weight loss, their most frequent specific response was, again, "exercise." Approximately three-quarters of them included exercise in their top three.

And when I asked the masters to tell me what they do if they *gain* weight, the most common answer was "exercise more." In fact, they're more likely to step up exercise in order to deal with small gains in weight than they are to go on a diet, omit sweets, stop snacking or keep a food diary. (Again, multiple responses were possible, and many masters did all or a number of the above, including exercise.)

The masters' commitment to exercise is striking when you consider that just 3 out of 10 American adults are physically active on a regular basis, and 4 out of 10 are not active at all. In contrast, the overwhelming majority of masters exercise from 3 to 7 times a week; a third of them say they do so 5 or 6 times weekly, while about 20 percent exercise 3 or 4 times.

At the high end, about 16 percent exercise daily. There's Steve S., who's gone from 435 pounds to 225 and has maintained that loss for 13 years; he once held the world record for marathon stair climbing. And Donna C. keeps 108 pounds at bay, in large part by walking 3 miles each morning *and* night, as well as by using a stair stepper or ski machine for 30 minutes, 4 to 5 days a week. At the other extreme, a significant minority of the masters work out very little — 0 to 2 times weekly. Larry Z., for example, maintains a 70-pound loss without any formal exercise. And Jeffrey B., master of 55 pounds for 22 years, exercises only when his weight rises. (See page 209 for more typical exercise regimes of masters.)

Most successful weight controllers *do* exercise on a regular basis, as revealed by the Kaiser Permanente Medical Center study (page 64, Chapter 3) that compared women who successfully maintained their weight loss with those who had regained. In the same study, 90 percent of the women who had lost weight and kept it off reported exercising regularly — at least 3 times a week for 30 minutes or longer — while only about a third of regainers said they exercised regularly. Moreover, regainers who did exercise said they did so less often and less vigorously than maintainers. Finally, maintainers reported more activity in their leisure and daily work time than did regainers.

Another study in which overweight people lost weight on four different diets revealed that, regardless of the diet followed, those who exercised maintained weight losses far better than did those who did not exercise. In addition, people who *stopped* exercising at the end of their diets regained, while those who *began* exercising at the end tended to keep off their lost pounds.

The weight-loss maintainers in the National Weight Control Registry report that, on average, they burn off an average of 400 calories a day through exercise. That's the equivalent of walking briskly for about an hour to an hour and a quarter — on a weekly basis, this would amount to walking about 28 miles. While this amount of exercise may sound somewhat intimidating, the Registry researchers point out that this figure may be somewhat inflated because people in general have a tendency to overestimate how active they are.

Can you lose weight through exercise alone, without dieting? Typically, weight losses this way are modest, less than 10 pounds. (But recall how starting with exercise inspired some masters to then take charge of their eating habits.) And exercise will not necessarily make you lose a lot more weight when you first start your weight-loss effort. When it comes to maintenance of weight loss, however, increased physical activity appears to be particularly valuable. It's quite clear from a number of controlled scientific studies that people who continue to exercise following weight-loss programs are more likely to maintain their weight loss over time than are those who do not continue. Finally, regular physical activity may delay or even prevent weight gain that tends to occur as we age.

A number of masters told me that they see a clear connection between periods of weight gain and lack of exercise. Suzanne T., for instance, gained 10 of her 80 lost pounds back after she was in a wedding, went on vacation and her "exercise time diminished." But, she adds, "I'm currently losing those 10 pounds." Similarly, when Nancy R. stopped exercising for a period of 6 to 8 months (she also stopped watching her diet), her weight shot up about 25 pounds. Now that she's exercising again, her weight is back down to 145 — 55 pounds shy of her one-time maximum of 200 pounds.

While some experts are adamant that exercise is mandatory for successful weight management, I did locate 15 masters (about 9 percent) who say they don't exercise at all — other than engaging in daily activities — and a number of them maintain more than 50-pound losses. (Likewise, 9 percent of the Registry participants report maintaining weight loss without regular physical activity.)

Quite frankly, I don't know how these people do it! Perhaps they are more physically active in their daily routines than when they were heavy, or perhaps they eat less food than other masters, or their metabolic rates may be higher.

Master Molly A. is living proof that weight loss can be done without exercise. She told me, "I was heavy all my life, from age 18 on; I was a size 20 for years." At her heaviest, Molly weighed

227. More than 8 years ago at the age of 55, she started to lose her 63 pounds. "All without exercise. People can't say they can't lose weight because they can't get out of a chair. I did it." (She doesn't exercise because she needs knee replacements.)

For the vast majority of people who want to lose weight and keep it off, exercise is important. But for those who refuse to or can't exercise for medical reasons, it should be reassuring to know that weight loss and maintenance are still possible.

The Wonders of Exercise

Why is exercise critical to so many of the masters? Because it combines a number of physical and psychological advantages.

◆ Exercise burns calories.

The table on the following pages illustrates how many calories various forms of exercise expend. The number of calories *you* burn for any one activity depends on how often, how intensely and how long you do it, as well as on your weight. (Generally speaking, it takes more calories to move around a 175-pound body than a 125-pound body.)

It can be discouraging to see how few calories even fairly rigorous exercise like running burns off on a day-to-day basis. If a 175-pound man, for instance, were to go out for 20 minutes and run at a rate of 5.5 miles per hour — quite a lot for most people — he'd use about 250 calories, which may not sound like much for a strenuous workout. But the critical difference with exercise is in its cumulative effects: if that same man were to run for 20 minutes 4 days a week, in a year's time he'd burn off 52,000 calories, which obviously could help a lot in his weight-control efforts.

What does it all add up to? When you're losing, you'll likely lose faster if you exercise. At maintenance, you'll be able to eat more food yet maintain your weight if you exercise: that 20-minute runner could eat two hot fudge sundaes a week without gaining. Moreover, the amount of weight people lose by exercising is generally greater than would be expected from the number of calories the exercise alone expends. One theory is that healthy behaviors come in "packages" — that is, if you exercise, you may not want to "wreck it" by overindulging *and* you become inspired to eat healthfully.

Calorie Values for 10 Minutes of Activity			
	Body Weight (in pounds)		
Activity	**125**	**175**	**250**
Sleeping	10	14	20
Sitting (watching TV)	10	14	18
Standing	12	16	24
Washing floors	38	53	75
Light gardening	30	42	59
Mowing grass (power)	34	47	67
Walking downstairs	56	78	111
Walking upstairs	146	202	288
Walking at 2 mph	29	40	58
Walking at 4 mph	52	72	102
Running at 5.5 mph	90	125	178
Running at 7 mph	118	164	232
Cycling at 5.5 mph	42	58	83
Cycling at 13 mph	89	124	178
Shoveling snow	65	89	130
Badminton	43	65	94
Baseball	39	54	78
Basketball	58	82	117
Bowling (nonstop)	56	78	111
Canoeing (4 mph)	90	128	182
Dancing (moderately)	35	48	69
Dancing (vigorously)	48	66	94
Football	69	96	137

Activity	Body Weight (in pounds)		
	125	175	250
Golfing	33	48	68
Horseback riding	56	78	112
Ping-Pong	32	45	64
Racquetball	75	104	144
Skiing (Alpine)	80	112	160
Skiing (water)	60	88	130
Skiing (cross-country)	98	138	194
Squash	75	104	144
Swimming (backstroke)	32	45	64
Swimming (crawl)	40	56	80
Tennis	56	80	115
Volleyball	43	65	94

◆ Exercise is good for your body.

Exercise has been shown to have preventive health benefits, lowering blood pressure and cholesterol and helping to decrease the risk of diseases like diabetes and osteoporosis. You don't even have to lose weight for the health benefits of exercise to kick in, as dramatically revealed by studies conducted on many thousands of men at the Cooper Clinic in Dallas, Texas. Researchers found that obese men who were fit had much lower death rates than normal-weight or lean men who were unfit. And, whether or not you lose weight, exercise can improve heart and lung fitness, as well as lower risk of heart disease.

◆ Exercise does wonders for your psyche.

Studies have shown an association between higher fitness levels and better mental health. Specifically, there is evidence that exercise improves mood and psychological well-being and enhances self-esteem, while at the same time decreasing stress, anxiety and depression. Psychologists feel that these mental boosts come to-gether to bring about greater commitment to weight control. Moreover, exercise can prevent relapse by replacing problem eating and alleviating stresses that make people want to eat. You can put exercise to work for you during high-risk times, such as when you're lonely, blue or bored. In fact, it may help to exercise at a time of day when emotional eating is likely to occur. (It's not easy to work out on a StairMaster or do "power" walking and eat at the same time!)

Exercise can also pick you back up after the fact. If you've had a "slip," you can counteract it by working out, which not only offsets some of the calories you've eaten, but helps you feel recommitted and in control. Jim V., who used to eat when under stress, is well aware of the psychological bonuses of exercise. "I do it because it makes me feel better. It's the greatest reliever of stress I've ever known."

Here's what some other masters have to say about what exercise does for them:

◆ Dorothy C. (32 pounds, 8 years): "Regular exercise helped burn calories *and* reduce stress that triggers overeating. It became its own motivation: I was able to gradually 'replace' my food 'addiction' with physical activity. Exercise has helped me feel better physically, get control over my life and feel good about myself."

◆ Kelly D. (54 pounds, 4½ years): "I think, in my life, the most important part is exercise. It has become a way to live healthier and a secret to relieving stress as well."

◆ Ernie L. (45 pounds, 12½ years): "Exercise, exercise, exercise," he wrote, when asked to list the three most important things he does to keep his weight down.

◆ Ann F. (220 pounds, 10 years): "I exercise every day, which seems to have done wonders not only for weight maintenance and toning, but also for general well-being. It's helped enormously in controlling stress and in my general health."

◆ Tim H. (40 pounds, 6 years): "It forces you to pay attention to your body and therefore take care of it."

◆ Kevin C. (45 pounds, 7 years): "Exercise allows you to eat that much more on maintenance; because of exercise, I can be a lot less concerned when I do overeat."

How Much Is Enough?

Should you work out 3 days a week or 5? Is 15 minutes long enough? Or do you have to expend 400 calories a day, as suggested by the National Weight Control Registry? How intense should your workouts be? One problem with minimum exercise "prescriptions" is that they contribute to that old "all-or-nothing" thinking: if you can't meet the goal, even for one day, you may as well not bother. The truth is that *any exercise is better than no exercise,* and even modest exercise can bring about significant psychological and health benefits.

Unfortunately, according to a recent Centers for Disease Control report on thousands of people, only one-fifth of overweight adults trying to lose weight meet basic recommended exercise goals for health. The usual recommendation has been to get at least 30 minutes of moderate-intensity activity — such as brisk walking, gardening, bowling or housework — on most days of the week. (Or, 3 times a week, you could do 20 minutes of vigorous exercise, such as biking, hiking, running or climbing stairs.)

Some experts feel that, to maintain weight loss, expending on the order of 1,500 to 2,500 calories per week through physical activity is optimal. In fact, in a recommendation intended primarily for weight control, a 2002 National Academy of Sciences report advises an hour per day of accumulated physical activity such as brisk walking. (If exercise is more intense or you have a job requiring physical activity, you can probably get away with spending less time in added exercise.) *But give yourself plenty of time to reach your goal.*

When former marathon runner Tom F., the master profiled in Chapter VIII, first started running, it took 3 to 4 months before he was able to run a continuous mile. And whatever you choose for exercise, it doesn't have to be done all at once — a number of studies suggest that intermittent exercise (say, in four 10-minute bouts per day) is as beneficial for weight loss and fitness as single 30- to 40-minute stints of exercise. In addition, there is evidence that you're more likely to stick with exercise if it's less intense: the drop-out rate for vigorous programs has been reported to be as much as twice as high as for moderate-intensity exercise programs.

The bottom line is that you don't have to run marathons, become a body builder or do daily step-aerobics classes to reap the benefits of exercise. As syndicated columnist Ellen Goodman once put it, " . . . we don't have to be fully regimented, highly aerobic and thigh-mastered athletes in order to be fit. It appears that all we have to do is put one foot in front of the other. Up the stairs. Down the block. Around the corner. In the garden. To and from work."

Finding What's Right for You

As with finding the right way to lose weight, the word from the masters when it comes to exercise is, *you have to find what's right for you.* The table below shows the many forms of activity chosen by the masters. Note that the number-one form of exercise is walking — the same as with members of the National Weight Control Registry.

Approximate numbers of masters who engage in various forms of exercise:	
Walking	72
Bicycling (regular and stationary)	34
Aerobics (includes jazzercize and step)	31

Nautilus/weight lifting	21
Step climbing	21
Running, jogging (includes treadmill)	19
Calisthenics	14
Swimming	11
Ski machine	7
Dancing	6
Racquetball	4
Horseback riding	4

Note: Many masters engage in multiple forms of exercise. Some other forms of exercise were mentioned, but fewer than four times each.

Some typical exercise routines described by the masters include:

◆ Cindy B. (38 pounds, 3 years): 4 to 5 times a week, she walks briskly (2 miles in ½ hour) at noontime. Sometimes she rides a stationary bike.

◆ Carole C. (39 pounds, 20 years): 5 to 6 times a week, she either power walks 2½ miles or bicycles. On weekends, she bicycles 15 to 30 miles.

◆ Cathy C. (38 pounds, 11 years): 3 to 4 times a week, she swims or uses a total workout bike (for arms and legs) for 30 minutes at a time.

◆ Chuck F. (62 pounds, 10 years): 1 to 3 times a week, he uses a stationary bike for 15 to 30 minutes and does mat work followed by free weights.

◆ Judy F. (40 pounds, 27 years): 5 to 6 times a week, she walks 2 miles.

◆ Don M. (111 pounds, 3 years): 3 to 4 times a week, he walks briskly for 40 to 45 minutes.

◆ Becky M. (40 pounds, 12 years): 5 times a week, she walks briskly for ½ hour.

◆ Thalia P. (32 pounds, 4 years): 3 to 4 times a week, she does an aerobics class or the step machine for 30 to 60 minutes.

Granted, all of these masters exercise far more than most Americans, but they are *not* fanatics. *My sense from most masters is that exercise is a healthy obligation — part of the routine of life — not a rigid obsession.*

How Do You Find What's Right for You?

In considering any one form of exercise, ask yourself the following:

◆ Is the form of exercise enjoyable or at least not unenjoyable? The odds are that if you hate what you're doing, you'll give it up quickly.

◆ Will you do it on a regular basis — not just today, but month after month?

◆ Is there a financial cost involved, and can you afford it? You may not be able to swing a fancy health club, but a YMCA, YWCA or community center may offer what you're looking for at a reasonable price.

◆ If you have to travel to an exercise facility, how conveniently is it located? How will you get there? The greater the effort, the less likely you are to stay with it.

◆ Does the type of exercise you're considering suit your schedule? If, for example, you work 60 hours a week, it may not be realistic to have a personal trainer plan a 90-minute exercise regime 5 days a week. If you're not a morning person, you may not relish getting up every day at 5:00 A.M. to go swimming.

◆ Is privacy important to you? If you are self-conscious about exercising in front of others, you might want to consider (at least initially) a solitary activity or joining a club or class specifically for overweight people.

◆ If you choose to go to an exercise facility, is it clean and pleasant-looking? Is the emphasis on enjoyment rather than on a "no-pain, no-gain" philosophy? Is the equipment well maintained and is there only a short wait for it? "Yes" answers to questions like these help to increase exercise adherence.

◆ Is it safe to perform the type of exercise that interests you? Perhaps your neighborhood is not safe for walking after work, so you may want to find an indoor track or do mall walking.

◆ If you need childcare, is it available, and do you feel comfortable with the arrangement?

◆ Do you prefer exercising alone or in a group? Would you be more motivated if you could find a friend or relative to exercise with you? Are you more likely to stay with it if you have a leader? If so, then a class situation may be best. But if you hate classes and the "hype" of some aerobics instructors, some form of home exercise may be ideal if you have the discipline to stick with it. (See page 304 for more on social support and exercise.)

◆ Does your climate suit the form of exercise you're considering? For example, if you live in Arizona or southern Texas — and you're not an early-morning person — perhaps jogging is not the best idea — at least for the many months of the year that the temperature soars above 90 degrees F.

The masters at weight loss went through a trial-and-error process before finding the form of exercise that was right for them. For Donna C., "It was between walking and swimming. I don't like to get wet, so I picked walking. I also had a dog to walk — he lost several pounds, too!" Sam E. goes to a 50-minute aerobics class 3 times a week, but only stays for 30 minutes. Holly L. tried exercise tapes and found she was too uncoordinated for aerobics: "This was a bit frustrating. Then I began walking. This I liked but found it hard to make time for until I decided it *had* to become part of my day. Now, on weekends, when I cannot fit it in, I quite often find myself looking forward to Mondays when I will be able to."

If you're considering buying home exercise equipment, which, if you stick with it, may wind up being cheaper than yearly membership fees at a club, make sure you're familiar with the machine before you take the plunge. You might want to try a friend's machine several times or join a club for a short time, just to familiarize yourself with various forms of equipment. At a fitness club, however, the equipment may be very upscale — don't assume that cheaper home versions will be as easy to use.

Note, too, that activities you may not think of as exercise "count," like bowling, Ping-Pong, golf, leisurely walks and gardening. *What's critical is that you start defining yourself as being physically active and that you do whatever you choose consistently.*

Weighing the Exercise Options

Should you walk, run, swim or step? The following guide gives you some of the pros and cons of a number of popular forms of aerobic exercise — that is, the type of exercise that gets your heart rate up and gets you huffing, puffing and burning fat.

◆ **Walking:** In my opinion, walking is the most doable form of exercise, particularly for individuals who need to lose 30 or more pounds. It costs no money, requires no special equipment or clothing (other than a decent pair of walking shoes), can be done alone or in a group almost anytime and anywhere and is relatively easy for people who are overweight and/or out of shape. Not only is the risk of injury lower with walking, since it is less stressful to weight-bearing joints than an exercise like running, but you may be more likely to stick with it because it is lower intensity and less likely to cause exhaustion. People who have hip, knee or back problems may want to consider walking in a pool. If interested in group walking, you can contact a local walking club through your YMCA or mall.

◆ **Jogging:** Jogging has just about all of the conveniences of walking, and it burns more calories than does walking for the time invested. However, jogging can be hard on the joints, especially in overweight people, and can lead to discomfort and injuries.

◆ **Cycling:** Either on an indoor stationary bicycle or an outdoor bike, you can get a good workout by cycling. Some people find it more enjoyable than jogging, and it is not as hard on the knees, ankles and feet. With an indoor cycle, you have the option of purchasing one with pumping handlebars for arms and shoulders, so you get both an upper- and lower-body workout.

◆ **Aerobic dancing:** A lot of people like aerobics because of the variety of exercises, music and group interaction. More vigorous types of aerobics tend to involve jumping or running in place, however, and the wear and tear on the joints can be considerable, especially for heavy people. Furthermore, step aerobics that require stepping on and off a platform can worsen knee problems. (The higher the platform, the greater the risk of injury.) As such, high-impact activities are not recommended for people who have a bad back, arthritis, osteoporosis or knee, ankle or foot problems. Low-impact workouts, in which one foot is always on the ground, eliminate most of the jumpy, jerky movements that can cause injury. It's wise to shop around for an aerobics class that suits your level of fitness. Be aware that some aerobics movements require coordination and can be difficult to perform. According to the *Tufts University Health & Nutrition Letter,* ½ hour of aerobic dancing burns roughly 183 calories for a 130-pound woman and 237 calories for a 170-pound man. If you prefer solitary exercise and going at your own pace, purchase an aerobics videotape.

◆ **Stair climbing:** If you choose stair climbing as your regular form of exercise, it's best to do it on a machine because going up and down real steps can be harder on your joints. You can get a great aerobic workout on these machines, but blood pressure and heart rate can rise very quickly, so beginners should be careful not to overdo it. In fact, stair-climbers offer a tough workout and may best be reserved for after you have a good fitness base — for instance, in walking. Be aware that you can't necessarily go by the caloric-expenditure reading on the machine, because leaning on the rails reduces expenditure: an estimated 7 percent fewer calories are burned for every 10 pounds you support by leaning. (In general, machines that don't allow you to program in your weight are likely to be far more "off" for calorie expenditure than are those that have you enter what you weigh.)

◆ **Elliptical training:** Elliptical training machines are sort of a cross between bicycling and stair climbing, as your feet move in a low-impact, oval motion with your body in an upright position. (Some machines also offer handlebars for an upper-body workout.) A study comparing a number of different brand machines showed that participants using them burned about 8 to 9 calories per minute, which is similar to calorie expenditure for intense aerobic dancing or running at an 11.5-minute-per-mile pace. (Of course, this would vary with the person's size and exercise intensity.) Compared to the latter, however, elliptical workouts are gentler on the body and may be an option for people who can't run or do aerobics. As another bonus, people tend to underestimate how hard they work out on elliptical trainers — what feels like a brisk walk can have the benefits of a run.

◆ **Rowing:** A rowing machine affects more parts of the body than most other forms of exercise mentioned thus far: it works out your arms, legs, abdomen, shoulders and back. Rowing can also be easier on joints than running or aerobic dancing. But if you have a back problem, you should definitely get your physician's okay before choosing this form of exercise.

◆ **Skiing:** Cross-country ski machines do more than tone your legs, they exercise most major muscle groups, but mainly the arms and legs. A workout on a ski machine is considered one of the best overall forms of exercise. Although it takes some practice to coordinate the arm and leg movements, skiing puts little strain on the body and affords a low risk of injury. Like stair equipment, however, ski machines are quite taxing and may be best saved for when you've achieved an initial level of fitness some easier way.

◆ **Swimming:** Swimming exercises all major muscle groups and carries a low risk of injury. Because water cushions the body, swimming is especially suitable for pregnant women, people with arthritis and those recovering from injuries. The buoyancy of water can be advantageous for obese individuals because it reduces stress on joints. Aquatic exercise — perhaps with other overweight people — is also a possibility.

Yoga and Tai Chi — for Body and Mind

Yoga and tai chi — Eastern practices that involve deep, focused breathing — are trendy, but can they help for weight control? "On the surface, someone who is overweight might think that these practices wouldn't be very helpful for weight loss because they don't burn many calories (with the exception of some vigorous forms of yoga — such as Ashtanga yoga)," says Carol Krucoff, coauthor of *Healing Moves: How to Cure, Relieve, and Prevent Common Ailments with Exercise.* She goes on, "However, yoga and tai chi can be *essential* in helping people who are struggling with weight issues because they are powerful ways to relieve stress — a significant reason for emotional eating. In addition, yoga focuses on increasing awareness, which helps people stop living only in their heads and helps them become more in touch with their bodies. Much more than merely 'exercises,' yoga and tai chi can serve as powerful methods of self-discovery."

Yoga is a spiritual practice originating in India, designed to help unify body and mind. The physical postures — called hatha yoga — are just one part of yoga. In the West, "yoga" is typically used to describe the hatha yoga postures that people learn in a yoga class, along with breathing and relaxation techniques. According to Ms. Krucoff, "Recent studies have found yoga to be helpful for people with heart disease and high blood pressure — both problems for which being overweight increases the risk."

Tai chi is actually a "soft" martial art from China involving a prescribed set of movements. Ms. Krucoff describes it as follows: "Watching someone practice tai chi looks like they are doing a slow dance — almost as if they're under water — on dry land." She adds, "Recent studies suggest it may improve balance and help older people avoid falls as well as reduce blood pressure."

Is Strength Training for You?

When I was in my twenties, I jogged 5 miles a day, 5 days a week. (Up until that point, I was a real slug: I had trouble passing the President's Physical Fitness tests they gave to kids. It literally took years for me to work up to 5 miles of jogging.) But it started to become torturous, and I began asking myself, "Am I going to be able to do this — from both a physical and mental standpoint — for the rest of my life?" Truth is, I was sick of it. Then I read an article that talked about how the ideal exercise regime is one that combines aerobic exercise with strength training — lifting weights, also called resistance training — and I made the switch to a combination of the two. Indeed, your best bet for weight control is to alternate between strength training and aerobic exercise.

Quite a few successful maintainers engage in strength training — the National Weight Control Registry reports that 24 percent of its men and 20 percent of women engage in weight lifting. Some overweight people prefer resistance training to other types of exercise requiring more skill or coordination. It's noncompetitive and easy to learn. Beginners can see results quickly, which keeps them going. You don't need to knock yourself out to get benefits: lifting light weights 2 or 3 times a week for 30 to 40 minutes per session is adequate. Be sure, however, to get some instruction from a qualified trainer because injuries can occur if you don't lift weights properly. (For instance, find out if the trainer has a college degree in exercise science and/or if he or she is certified by the American College of Sports Medicine or the National Strength and Conditioning Association.)

One advantage of strength training is that, by increasing the size of your muscles, you may be increasing your body's metabolic rate. In other words, because muscle tissue burns more calories than fat tissue, strength training may help you burn more calories. And strength training can prevent loss of muscle tissue that occurs with dieting. Another major advantage of strength training is that it can significantly slow down or reverse the loss of muscle tissue that naturally occurs as you age. Between the ages of 20 and 70, the typical sedentary American loses about 30 percent of the total number of body muscle cells, resulting in a depressing loss of about 6 to 7 pounds of muscle per decade. Not only do the remaining muscle cells begin to shrink, but the pounds lost in the form of muscle tend to be replaced by fat. Strength training can, to a large degree, reverse this trend by building up the muscle cells that remain.

Strength training, however, does not turn fat into muscle: there's no such phenomenon. Muscle and fat cells are completely different and cannot be changed from one to the other. But you may lose some fat because of increased calorie expenditure related to strength training, while at the same time you look better because you've firmed up and developed muscles. However, because muscle tissue weighs more than fat tissue of the same volume, weight loss can be less than expected for some people, at least when they first start training.

Strength training can benefit anyone, regardless of age. It can improve cardiovascular health, delay or prevent bone loss, ease back pain, help posture and reduce the risk of falls — a particular problem for people as they grow older. Take the case of master Celia G., who didn't lose her 36 pounds until she was 64. (She's maintained that loss for 5 years.) About 3 months into her dietitian-supervised weight-loss plan, she started doing "body toning" with special-resistance machines because she "didn't want flabby arms." The results? "I took off a total of 12 inches in my upper arms and thighs and enjoyed the work." (Similarly, when I started doing strength training, I found that I went down a size, even though I gained several pounds from the increase in muscle mass.)

Getting Started

Since about half of all people who begin an exercise program drop out within 6 months, it's important to get off to the right start. Before jumping in with exercise, *first and foremost, get your physician's okay,* particularly if you are overweight or have/had any of the following: heart disease or heart problems of any sort, chest pain, high blood pressure or other risk factors for heart disease (such as high cholesterol), stroke, diabetes, back problems, orthopedic or musculoskeletal problems, kidney or liver disease, arthritis, osteoporosis or metabolic problems. You should also get medical approval if you have not engaged in vigorous activity for a long time or are a 40-plus-year-old man or a woman age 50 or above. If you have medical problems, it may also be wise to consult with an exercise physiologist or physical therapist. Finally, you should talk with your physician about whether a medically supervised exercise stress test is appropriate for you.

Do away with the anti-exercise excuses.

"I've been inactive for too long." If you think you're so out of shape that you'll never be able to stay with it, take heart. Think about Ernie L., profiled in Chapter 3, who started "small" by running 1 minute a day, slowly working upward. If you're a beginner, however, be forewarned that exercise is unlikely to make you feel better right away. In fact, you're likely to experience some initial soreness and stiffness that usually goes away after a week or two. *With time, exercise will make you feel good,* but it may take as long as a few months before the fitness benefits set in; the psychological boost may be evident within 2 to 3 weeks.

"Exercise is for young, slim people." Recall the many masters who started their journey to maintenance after the age of 40. At 70, Fern C. (she has kept off 28 pounds for 21 years) exercises every day. She walks and does 20 minutes of different exercises, including some for stretching and some for muscular tone. She also square dances. August J. (47 pounds, 11 years), who is 85 years old, walks every day; he tries to cover approximately 10 blocks "on an empty stomach." Jennie C. (25 pounds, 4½ years) is 84 and walks every day, weather permitting. She also gets exercise raking leaves and gardening.

"It's too risky to exercise." Your chance of developing diseases caused by lack of exercise is much greater than the risks from exercise itself, note Drs. John Foreyt and G. Ken Goodrick in *Living Without Dieting.* The probability of injury is minimal if you use a gradual approach. Even some masters who have chronic medical problems find a way to "move it." Mary S. (71 pounds, 4 years) doesn't let arthritis stop her from walking 3 to 4 miles daily. When she can't walk, she uses her exercycle, which, she says, "I hate, but it fills in the gaps." Holly L. became motivated to lose her 97 pounds 3 years ago, when, at age 69, her "legs gave out." Now she exercises 5 to 6 times a week. Although she once could barely walk "half a block," she now does power walking — "1½ miles at a fast clip" — plus 80 "step-ups" and bend-and-stretch exercises. If the weather is bad, she uses an exercise bike.

"Exercise will make me hungry." On the contrary, for overweight people, increased physical activity may actually inhibit food intake. According to *The Volumetrics Weight-Control Plan,* by Barbara Rolls, Ph.D., and Robert Barnett, "The human body may need some physical activity for satiety and hunger regulatory systems to work properly." As revealed by the many masters who have incorporated a fair amount of exercise into their daily lives, most people do not "cancel out" the benefit of exercise by eating more calories than they burn. And, of course, exercise can help alleviate the many triggers for emotional eating.

"I'd look awful in those skimpy leotards or tank tops." Who says you have to wear them? In fact, many people I see working out at my local Y have on big, baggy T-shirts that cover all the less-than-perfect parts. You're actually better off wearing loose, comfortable clothing that you feel good in. However, it can give you a boost to buy attractive warm-up suits and colorful T-shirts and shoes. Stay away from heavy sweats for indoor or warm-weather exercise — they don't make you lose weight any faster and only serve to overheat you.

"At my size, I'm too self-conscious." Instead of focusing on the two or three beautiful bodies in a gym or exercise class, look at the many people who are far from perfect. In order to feel more comfortable, you may want to shop around to select an exercise facility catering to larger people. You could also start your exercise program at a slow time of day or year, so you feel less self-conscious. "Since the health-club business is slower during the summer months, there was time for me to get into the aerobics room relatively unnoticed," says Kim W. of the time when she hit her peak weight of 162 pounds. It was then that she started working out at the health club she managed.

Jim V. points out that slimmer people often give heavier individuals credit for exercising. "When I first started walking, people were *more* encouraging because I was overweight. I never encountered problems because of my appearance. If anything, people were more helpful."

"I don't have time." The truth is that you have to make exercise a top priority and schedule it into your life — just like dental flossing, styling your hair and putting on your seat belt. If you pre-plan your exercise a week in advance, thinking about your other commitments and when you'll fit in your exercise, you'll have a better chance of sticking with it. Bonnie R. says, "I think that with busy schedules, most people have to actually write down an appointed time in their appointment books or Palm Pilot to exercise at least 3 days a week." Although he didn't think it was possible, Jim V. found the time. He says, "I used to feel like my life was so active that I had no time to do it, but it's not the truth." Now he tells himself that he "works all day for someone else," and that hour and a half at night is for him alone. No one's schedule could be busier than that of Stephan P., a chef, author, consultant and frequent traveler, who was, until recently, involved in running four restaurants. He's managed to keep off 25 pounds (he's 5'7" tall) in large part by exercising for an hour, 5 or 6 times a week.

Finally, try asking yourself, "If U.S. presidents can find time to exercise, why can't I?" Once you get past the point of discomfort and into the routine, you will likely find you really miss exercise on your days off, as does master Tim H. "Exercise is number one. You have to develop it as a habit. It's so much a part of my life that I don't feel right without it."

"My family and friends are not supportive." There's no question that a commitment to exercise changes your lifestyle, which can pose threats to your inactive partner, make friends jealous or frustrate children who aren't accustomed to your taking time for yourself. Awareness of the issue can help, as can your sensitivity to their feelings. But sometimes you just have to state, "This is how it is." It may be of value to try to get the nonsupportive person to exercise with you. (For more on support, see Chapter 10.)

"I don't have the money." Several forms of exercise cost little or nothing. There's no reason to invest in fancy equipment or clothing unless you want to. Walking is free. In fact, several studies suggest that people assigned to a home-based exercise program are more likely to stick with it than those who are part of a supervised group exercise program. However, some people who spend money on exercise equipment or a health-club membership may find that the financial investment makes them more committed. You also have to think about priorities: how much do you spend each year on restaurant meals, compact discs and going to movies?

"I'm too tired." Actually, you'll likely find that regular exercise gives you more — not less — energy. Many people who feel "beat" at certain times of the day feel refreshed after exercising. Jim V.'s noontime exercise "re-energizes" him for an afternoon of productivity.

"It's too hot/it's too cold." Once you get hooked on exercise, weather will not deter you. It's important to dress comfortably and go at the time of day when the temperature is most favorable. (Or find an indoor, temperature-controlled place to walk, like a mall or indoor track.)

Whatever form of exercise you choose, start small and set realistic goals. Your short-term goal should be to start doing something — anything — to get yourself moving. If you decide to walk for 15 minutes every other day and find you can do more, you'll feel very accomplished. But if you decide to exercise every day for an hour and end up doing it only 2 days for 20 minutes, you may feel like a failure. After you have accomplished your minimum goal, then you can add on another day of exercise and/or another 5 minutes to your routine. Lynda C. affirms, "Many years ago, I used to set myself up by saying to myself that I was going to the gym every day and compound it with a 1,000-calorie diet. If I failed at dieting or inevitably didn't go to the gym every day, I didn't meet my expectations for myself and would give myself permission to overeat. Then the cycle would start all over again. Now, I do not attempt to work out more than 4 days per week, which is realistic with all the other demands in my life — kids, husband, part-time job."

It's important that your goals have some flexibility, not rigidity. For instance, if your normal walk takes 45 minutes, but you have a slight headache or an extremely busy day ahead of you, figure it's better to walk for 20 minutes than not at all.

In the beginning, keep your exercise plan simple. Even if you have professional guidance, you should play a major role in developing your program so, like your weight-loss plan, it becomes your own. No matter what form of exercise you choose, cut back if you feel tired or overly taxed. You're better off staying at a lower level of intensity than risking discouragement and giving up. With time, you should be able to move on.

Little Things Mean a Lot

In your daily routine, you can perform many little activities that add up: like taking stairs instead of elevators and parking your car way out in a parking lot, rather than right next to a store. Indeed, walking up and down two flights of stairs a day instead of using an elevator could allow a 176-pound man to lose about 6 pounds each year.

Unfortunately, as a society, we've gotten lazier and lazier physically. From 1965 to 1977 alone, estimated average calorie expenditure in individuals declined by 200 calories a day, thanks in part to labor-saving devices from electric juice squeezers to sit-down lawn mowers to remote-control garage-door openers.

Moreover, a study conducted by Yale University's Dr. Kelly Brownell and colleagues in several public places where stairs and escalators were next to each other found that only 5 percent of

223

40,000 people used the stairs. For every 5 normal-weight people who used them, only 1 overweight person did. Can these little things really make a difference? Several studies in which certain people were assigned to structured exercise programs, while others worked on incorporating more activity into their daily routines, revealed that the latter was at least as effective for improving health, losing weight and maintaining weight loss.

The trick to increasing "routine activity" is to undo our sedentary habits. Here are some ways masters "move it" in their day-to-day lives:

◆ Jim V.: "When I go to a mall, I park my car far away from the entrance. I always take the stairs at work."

◆ Graham Kerr: "I get up every hour and move around. I think it's good to have an alarm or an hourglass as a reminder."

◆ Lou Ann L.: "I always do stairs rather than elevators."

◆ Ernie L.: "I'm not a jittery person; I'm a sitter, a leaner. So I force myself to expend energy. I walk at work and take stairs."

To reverse the nonmovement trend, try to come up with as many ways as possible to increase your exercise in your day-to-day activities, starting with the morning:

◆ Use a bathroom on a different floor to brush your teeth before leaving for work.

◆ Get off the bus or have the cab drop you off two blocks before your destination.

◆ Upon arrival at your place of work, take stairs at least part of the way to your floor.

◆ Move your wastebasket to a side of your office that forces you to get up when something has to be discarded. (No shooting baskets!)

- When in airports, don't use moving walkways.

- Take the steps to use the water fountain on a different floor.

- Walk to coworkers' offices to give them messages rather than calling them on the phone or using an intercom.

- Walk your dog instead of letting him run in the back yard.

- Get up to switch TV channels rather than use a remote control.

- Walk across the room rather than ask the nearest person to hand an item to you.

- Sit in a rocking chair and rock as you watch TV.

- Get a pedometer and see if you can increase the number of steps you routinely take each day. (One study showed that, on average, inactive people take 2,000 to 4,000 steps each day, while active people take at least 10,000.)

Sticking with It

How do the masters stick with it? How do they make a lifetime commitment to exercise? As always, their approaches vary, but many of them use techniques suggested by experts.

- **Make it fun.** Ann B., who switches from rollerblading to cross-country skiing to stair stepping, says, "I found things to do that I enjoyed, so exercise wasn't a chore." Tami B. does a similar array of exercises and states, "I try to play at exercise. It makes it more like fun than drudgery." Kim W., a master who now teaches aerobics classes, told me, "I try to bring the playfulness back [to the people in my classes]. If they enjoy what they're doing, they'll stick with it and be successful." Ernie L. has fun with aerobic dance. "My mother was a dance teacher, and I have always loved dance. I find it relaxing, almost spiritual." But, unlike running, which he could do alone, Ernie finds he needs the camaraderie of group members for aerobics. He adds, "At first, I was the only man; now I have three friends with me."

In addition to finding enjoyable forms of exercise, it helps to have pleasurable accompaniments for exercise, like watching soaps or the news on TV, exercising with a partner, reading a good book or listening to music. (There is evidence that people tend to perceive exercising with music as being easier than without.) Cindy P. says, "Whether the exercise I'm doing is aerobics, swimming, stationary bike riding or lifting weights — I HAVE to have dance music. Without that, I have little or no motivation."

◆ **Make changes.** A number of masters have switched from their initial exercise routines — either for physical or mental reasons. Ernie L. gave up running when he developed knee problems. Then, for a long time, he did aerobic circuit training (a combination of weight lifting, running in place, bicycling and treadmill running), but got bored with it. "I'll probably change again in the future," he says. "You have to keep looking at what's right for you." In the words of Dorothy C., "One of the keys to sticking with exercise is to vary the routine. It helps that I enjoy aerobics, but after 11 years, I do need to use all kinds of 'tricks' to stay motivated: special music tapes; new classes, gyms and machines; new clothing; running with my husband." It apparently helps if you vary your activities — 3 out of 5 people told me they engage in at least two different forms of exercise, such as walking and cycling. This likely prevents boredom. Some vary their exercise day by day; others do it within a workout session or by the season. Wendy M. runs in the summer and does the stair stepper and bike in the wintertime. And Ann Q. walks more in summer and spring and uses a NordicTrack and bike in the winter.

◆ **Give yourself a break.** Most masters take days off from exercise. As much as he exercises during the week, Jim V. relaxes every weekend and does "fun things" like traveling and going to the beach.

◆ **Use positive mind games.** Instead of dwelling on how much more you have to do, how far you have to go and how much a stitch in your side hurts, focus on the beautiful day, the nice neighborhood and landscaping and the smell of spring. Like some masters, you can also use inspirational thoughts to spur you on. Dorothy C. fantasizes about being an Olympic athlete. While Kim W. was getting hooked on exercise, she fantasized about being a dancer: "The movie *Flashdance* had been really popular around that period of time, and I knew that I wanted to move like her."

Jim V. uses positive self-talk to overcome his distaste for working out when it's hot. He says to himself, "Okay, so it's hot. It's no different than a cool night. Go out and work out. You'll feel all the better for it." He adds, "When it's over, I'm glad I did."

◆ **Focus on the payoff.** As Donna C. puts it, "The payoff is so great. Walking is a good mind-clearer. I feel great. I have stamina. I'm rarely sick. I have two grown daughters who marvel at me. They always used to find me at home in front of the TV. Now they may call and not find me there." Since exercise doesn't necessarily show up on the scale right away, try, as Jim V. does, to focus on other measures of success, like sleeping and breathing better, standing taller and feeling stronger. Also take note of lower blood pressure and pulse rate, as well as stress reduction. Some people find it motivating to keep records of how much they exercise, along with related improvements.

◆ **Be realistic about what exercise will and won't do for you.** Let's face it: walking for ½ hour 5 times a week is not going to turn you into a Cindy Crawford look-alike. Even Tim H., who both lifts weights and works out on a ski machine, states, "I could spend my whole life never being satisfied with my body. When I was more overweight, I'd look in the mirror and think about how I wanted to be. Now, I look at how I am." Realize, too, that not everyone falls in love with exercise. "I *hate* to work out, but it feels so great after," confesses Sam E., who has kept off 35 pounds for 10 years. Even people who like to exercise sometimes go through periods when they seem to lose interest: that may be the signal that it's time for a change.

◆ **Don't make it a catastrophe when you fall short of your goal.** As with eating, relapse-prevention strategies can help with exercise. Start by setting realistic exercise goals. Since all people fall short at times, try to anticipate potential high-risk situations that increase the odds you'll skip out on exercise. Is it when you're overtired, stressed out or when you have waited until too late in the day? Develop some sort of plan for coping.

If you do miss a day of planned exercise, don't let it throw you. When Jim V. can't get out to exercise, he doesn't feel guilty, as he did in the beginning. "I say, 'There are seven days in a week — I can make up the time elsewhere.' So I may go dancing that night." Similarly, Tami B. says, "I try to do some form of exercise daily, but I don't fret if I don't." A day of missed exercise here and there doesn't even amount to a pound of weight gain.

◆ **Give yourself time to get to the point of pleasure.** Jim V. agrees that one reason why so many people give up on exercise is that they don't stick with it long enough to be able to enjoy it. For him, it took nearly a year. "You have to try it — suffer it through at first. You get there faster than most people think. You have to set that time aside for yourself. It's not being selfish, it's being wise."

Some Recommended Exercise Resources

The American College of Sports Medicine's ACSM Fitness Book, Second Edition, 1998. Available from Human Kinetics (1-800-747-4457 or www.humankinetics.com).
Biomarkers: The 10 Keys to Prolonging Vitality by William Evans and Irwin Rosenberg. 1992. New York: Fireside.
The Exercise Habit by James Gavin. 1992. Champaign, Illinois: Human Kinetics.*

---

*Out-of-print, but may be found through an online bookstore.

Getting Active and Staying Active 10 Years Later

A decade after I first contacted the masters, many of them are as active and fit as ever. Here's what some of them do to stay in shape, along with some words of motivation:

Liane F. "It has been 15 years since I lost 28 pounds. I go to the gym 4 times a week, spending 30 minutes in aerobics and 20 minutes doing weights. I also walk 5 to 7 times a week with friends. I would not do this without my buddies. The buddy system is a wonderful way to exercise. I feel really good about myself, and when I'm with my grandchildren, I'm very often asked if I am their mother! I am 60 years old, weigh 130 pounds and am a size 8."

Connye Z. "I exercise for about 2 hours a day, which I know is not realistic for most people. But I really enjoy the exercise. I do it after work, and this keeps me from crashing. [She uses her own elliptical trainer and a recumbent bike, plus has several exercise tapes she likes.] I work out at home, so the weather does not keep me from exercising. Each person has to find something that appeals to him or her. I tried running, and it is not for me. I don't play tennis or bowl because of my back. So you have to try several things before you find what's good for you."

Dennis H. To keep his weight at 202 pounds, down from his all-time high of 238, Dennis H. has become an avid runner. He also lifts weights 3 times a week, "but only for 30 minutes at a time." His advice? "What gets written down gets done! I log everything I do. Drag your body, and your mind will follow. After a short while, you'll see results, and you will be hooked. The addiction will be greater than any drug!"

Patsy B. "I alternate between a treadmill and an elliptical runner, 45 to 60 minutes a day. I love the elliptical machine. My suggestion to get started on exercise is to find a partner, which I did, and to always start easy so you won't fail. I started walking when I was 242 pounds and couldn't walk a block. Make it convenient, find something you can do at home and find a time you can do it. To inspire you and keep you focused, have someone who exercises every day as a role model. I just turned 50, and people are kind to say I don't look a day over 40!"

Doris M. "When I'm going walking early in the morning, the night before, I lay out every stitch of clothing, shoes, watch, tape player (I like Sousa marches) right beside my bed so there is no hesitation looking for anything, and my brain is right on course. I keep a calendar beside my treadmill and record daily times and attitudes. Sometimes, I think I'm too tired to exercise, but once I've begun, that fatigue fades away."

Vicki B. "Going through a divorce was very hard, and I did gain some weight. But I never quit exercising, running all the while, about 15 to 20 miles a week. And I've lost most of what I gained." Vicki still runs, lifts weights and plays racquetball with her sister — and she just started doing yoga. "My advice is to pick something you like. I'm always looking for new 'passions.' Sometime, I'm going to take up fencing." She adds, "Everybody goes through tough periods when it's important to not get too down on yourself because you aren't eating quite right. But it's also important to keep up your health. Exercise has literally kept me alive the last several years!"

Fitness for Travelers: The Ultimate Workout Guide for the Road by Suzanne Schlosberg with the American Council on Exercise. 2002. Boston: Houghton Mifflin.

Great Shape: The First Fitness Guide for Large Women by Pat Lyons and Debby Burgard. 2000. iUniverse.com.

Healing Moves: How to Cure, Relieve, and Prevent Common Ailments with Exercise by Carol Krucoff and Mitchell Krucoff, M.D. 2000. New York: Three Rivers Press.

Just the Weigh You Are: How to Be Fit and Healthy, Whatever Your Size by Steven Jonas and Linda Konner. 1998. Boston: Houghton Mifflin.

Strong Women Stay Young by Miriam Nelson. 2000. New York: Bantam Books.

Thin for Life Daybook by Anne M. Fletcher. 1998. Boston: Houghton Mifflin.

ACE Fitness Matters, magazine of the American Council on Exercise, Web site: www.acefitness.org or call 800-825-3636.

The Choose to Move program from the American Heart Association — a program for women that gradually builds up to 30 minutes of physical activity on most days of the week. Web site: www.choosetomove.org. Or call the American Heart Association at 800-242-8721.

8

Key to Success #8

Face Life Head-On

Let's be honest. For most people — whether they are slim or overweight — food provides great enjoyment. From day one, food is associated with affection and nurturing. Many of us have learned that food is at least temporarily comforting when problems arise. But for some adults, food becomes life's *only* pleasure.

A number of masters reported that, in the past, they had used food to obliterate their emotions rather than confront their feelings. And research does show that some overweight people are likely to eat in response to emotions, be they positive or negative. This does not mean that most obese people have psychological problems that, in turn, are responsible for their heaviness. However, as the masters observe, learning how to cope with life's everyday ups and downs without turning to food can make a big difference in overcoming a weight problem.

There's little question that the short-term effect of stuffing yourself with food can be anesthetizing, bringing temporary relief from anxiety and frustration. Food provides immediate gratification, and overeating can lead to feelings of sluggishness, drowsiness and calmness. In the long run, however, the payoff diminishes, and the person who overeats is left with feelings of guilt and remorse, a worsening weight problem and the unresolved problems that precipitated the eating in the first place.

The masters have put an end to this vicious cycle: they've learned to face life head-on. They've learned to deal with life's problems in constructive ways, without turning to food.

Tom F.'s Story

Tom used to do all the "wrong" things: he smoked, drank too much and was too heavy. When his physicians called him to task at the age of 28, Tom decided to quit smoking and lose weight. He has been successful for 17 years. At a height of 6', he now holds his weight at about 185, down 50 pounds from his all-time high.

Tom's weight problem didn't begin until he was in his mid-twenties. "Up until that time I was trim, and weight was not an issue. I weighed about 160 when I graduated from high school. My first inkling of a problem was when I was getting out of the Navy, and none of my dress uniforms fit." After he left the service, Tom dropped the excess weight because he was more physically active, playing tennis and swimming.

But that was temporary. When Tom started his career as a field engineer, he began to gain weight once again. "I'm the kind of person who tends to have a singular focus; if I'm going to work, I really work." He threw himself into his career. As an escape, he sought refuge in alcohol. "My eating habits were atrocious. Dinner might be a 12-pack of beer, a pizza, and then I would keep on working. Exercise was completely out. Eventually, my weight shot up to 230." Tom was also smoking two to three packs of cigarettes a day.

Within a few years, there were physical and psychological manifestations of Tom's lifestyle: he had lower-back problems and many frustrations with work. After seeking the counsel of several physicians, he was told that nothing was wrong — that is, nothing that losing his "gut" and cleaning up his lifestyle wouldn't cure. "I decided either to prove the doctors wrong or find out if they were right." All at once, he quit smoking and joined the local YMCA.

"I experimented with various forms of exercise, but nothing seemed too exciting." Then Tom discovered running: "I liked the challenge and the way it made me feel. It took me three to four months to be able to run a continuous mile. When I did, I became motivated, so I started to run more." With time, Tom worked his way up to running 70 miles a week. He even ran 10 marathons.

As he got into running, Tom became more interested in diet. He went back to basics: whole grains, more vegetables, less meat and less food. Within 2 years' time, he was down to 150, too scanty for his 6' frame. He finally leveled off at a weight of 160 to 165. Eventually, Tom also swore off alcohol.

Then, 6 years ago, Tom developed a heel spur and couldn't run for about a year. That's when emotional eating set in. "I had become addicted to the running, and it was an escape from my problems. When I had to give up running, I had no substitute, and I felt sorry for myself. So I reacted by turning to 'eats.' In the middle of the day, I would make myself a sandwich and say, 'That tasted good, I'll have another.' Then I might make a batch of chocolate chip cookies and eat half of them."

Tom eventually came to the realization that he had been avoiding many issues in his life related to past family relationships. "I had been using running, then it became food." He came to grips with his problems — and his eating — and his weight settled in at 175 to 185.

Today, Tom's exercise consists of about five hours a week of some combination of running, stretching, step-machine workouts and weight training. He is excited about his decision to start competitive running once again. "Exercise is one of the greatest joys in life, particularly running," he says.

In his eating habits, Tom tries to avoid caffeine, most white flour, salt and fat. He tries to keep tempting items out of the house. He loves to bake and prides himself on his homemade breads. Typically, breakfast is his largest meal of the day, consisting of foods like fruit, yogurt, cereal and bagels. (He may eat all of these in one meal.) Tom usually skips lunch, then eats a light supper of, for example, baked potato, soup or spaghetti.

Of his relationship with food, Tom says, "For me, concern about diet comes and goes. When I'm stressed, diet is the first thing to go: I 'pick' more and buy more high-calorie foods at the grocery store. I might stop at the store, buy a box of cookies and eat the whole thing. Food is easy: I can do it alone, and it works in a hurry. But when I accept whatever the problem is and do something about it, the overeating disappears."

Tom is well aware that his main emotional trigger for eating is fear: for example, if he is worried that he may lose a major business client. "At first, I think, 'I'm inferior; I'm no good,'" he says. "So I have to fight that. I've started to write down my problems, write about the fear and anguish that can build. With brutal honesty, I list the fears as well as the bright side. The fear doesn't go away, but I can then make a decision to do something, to take action. This prevents my turning to food. As things come up, I'm able to deal with them."

Tom continues about his problem-solving philosophy: "My problems are all within, and that's where the solution lies. I used to delude myself by saying things were outside of me, so they weren't my problems. Now, I feel the key is accepting responsibility — once I accept the problem *and* the responsibility, it eases. I say to myself, 'What can I do about that?' Then I'm working on a solution so it doesn't happen again. That way, I'm building my personal integrity, instead of getting out of my worries by eating. I'm looking the problem right in the eye." He adds, "You know, life is full of obstacles. You have to take the deaths and disappointments and move on. The solution to all of life's problems is within you. It's simply a matter of self-talk to do something."

Tom is not a "touchy-feely" kind of guy. It's not always easy for him to identify his feelings, let alone express them. I mention this because some studies suggest that overweight men are less prone to emotional eating than women. Perhaps the truth is that, in addition to having trouble admitting difficulty in handling their problems, men are less aware of the emotional side of eating.

Like so many of the masters, Tom has identified the connection between eating and his emotions. He uses problem-solving skills to put an end to temporary lapses in eating habits, and his positive self-talk allows him to manage life's stresses without turning to food: *he's learned how to face life head-on.*

Maintainers vs. Regainers: How They Cope

Stress, which can come in many shapes and forms, is one of the primary causes of relapse and overeating. It makes sense, then, that several studies suggest that positive coping skills contribute to weight control. Masters at weight loss appear to handle stressful events in their lives very differently from people who regain weight.

In the Kaiser Permanente study comparing women who successfully maintained weight loss with those who regained (page 64), researchers found that "maintainers believed themselves capable of handling their problems and used problem-solving skills to cope with their difficulties. In contrast, relapsers did not deal with their problems directly (perhaps because they lacked effective problem-solving skills) and reported that they used food to make themselves feel better when upset."

When asked "How are you dealing with this?" concerning a troubling issue, few regainers in the study used "confrontive" ways of coping. Compared with maintainers, regainers were more likely to try to escape from or avoid their problems by eating, sleeping, drinking or wishing the problem would go away. Maintainers were more inclined to "talk out their feelings" or seek professional help than were regainers.

A striking 95 percent of maintainers used "planful problem-solving" skills or confronted issues; in contrast, just 10 percent of the regainers used these skills. And the difference wasn't that the relapsers had more serious problems; aside from weight-related and health issues, there were no significant differences in their types of difficulties, which included those related to relationships, self-fulfillment and job or career.

Most of the masters I interviewed were once regainers themselves, who at that time handled problems and emotions ineffectually. Before she lost her 43 pounds, master Lou Ann L. recalls, "When I was fat, food was a kind of 'forbidden fruit.' I always felt guilty about eating sweets. But they were also a reward and a way to push down negative feelings." And Peppi S. states, "I never realized that [difficult] emotions or situations were causing me to fall back on eating blindly, without any thought. Then I would feel guilty and guess what? Overeat some more. I never got in touch with my emotions." (That was before she lost 62 pounds.)

But the masters have shifted their behavior from that of the regainers to that of the maintainers. They have not only learned to identify emotional situations that make them want to eat, but to deal with their feelings *and* problems more constructively.

Bob W. recognizes that, starting in grade school, he used food to comfort himself, "to make a difficult family situation more bearable." He goes on, "I heard voices in my head [saying], 'Ah, have some food — it will make it all better.' I used to use food to 'fix' my life and emotions." By the time he was in eighth grade, Bob's "voices" had spurred him all the way up to 400 pounds. Now, having been at a weight of about 150 for 21 years, Bob says, "I have changed my life and found other ways to cope with emotions. I finally arrived at a place where I no longer wanted to hide my feelings with excess food."

Quite a few thin-for-life masters, like Tom F., still find themselves slipping into emotional eating from time to time. As he aptly puts it, "Just because you know how to do something doesn't mean you're going to do it all the time." Doug S., who keeps more than 100 pounds at bay, admits, "If I have a bad day at work, I will come home and eat constantly. Sometimes I have good command of it, and sometimes I don't." Still, Doug has made progress in recognizing the connection between tension and overeating.

Similarly, Ann F. finds, "During periods of stress or fatigue, I still struggle with overeating and will go back to my comfort foods, such as potato chips and candy (in lesser amounts)." But like Tom F., Ann has gone one step further in dealing with emotional eating. She adds, "When I want to overeat, I try to figure out if it's fatigue, anxiety or if I need comfort; I try to figure out what I really need. Then I might go out for a swim."

Alisa S. notes that she sees a link between periods of depression and weight gain. But like many masters, she finds strength in adversity: after 7 years of keeping off 64 pounds, Alisa finds, "I do struggle at times with feeling fat and defeated, but I feel the gratification of regaining control over my emotions and my weight."

"The key to successful living is to figure out what emotions trigger you to want to overeat, find an effective strategy [for coping] and recognize the satisfaction gained by your strategies and, last, a sense that YOU are in control," says Peppi S.

Labeling Your Emotions

How can *you* learn to handle your emotions more effectively, so you turn to food with less frequency? As Peppi states, *the critical first step is getting in touch with what you're feeling — labeling your emotions.* When you have a burning desire to eat or to continue eating and eating — but you know in your heart of hearts that you're not even hungry — ask yourself what's going on. Are you angry, lonely, bored, depressed, anxious or using food to relax or celebrate?

Some people find it helpful to make themselves wait for a set amount of time — say, 20 minutes — when they have a desire to eat or find themselves craving a particular food. Indeed, in the University of Iowa study on 82 people who had kept off more than 50 pounds for an average of 4½ years (page 12), the most commonly mentioned strategy for dealing with cravings was to wait them out. The delay provides an opportunity to focus on what you're really feeling and to talk yourself out of eating.

Sometimes, however, emotional eating has gone on for so long that it's become automatic: you're so used to stuffing yourself when you're upset or bored that, like a robot, you turn to food and feel you *can't* sort out your emotions. Says Ann B., "My feelings were vague — I didn't know what I felt." Wendy M. had her "heart broken" as a teenager, so she used food as a shield to protect herself from being hurt again by men. "I was afraid to look at the hurt, so I turned to food. It helped for a while. Then I said, 'I've got a long life ahead of me; I'm gonna get hurt a lot.'" Now, Wendy sees that she held on to her weight because she wanted people to like her for her personality, not her appearance. "I realized that I didn't need to be heavy to have people like me for me." Wendy is now 40 pounds lighter and has maintained the loss for 8 years.

Similarly, Ann B. used to hide behind her weight. Then, in her weight-loss program, she tried to confront and visualize her fears of becoming thin. "I had to deal with being more sexually attractive to men. Realizing that helped me move on."

How can you get in touch with emotions that trigger eating? If your emotional eating has become automatic, you may find there are signals that the problem is about to occur. All through college, for example, whenever I was under tension, I had a habit of wandering into the kitchen and searching through the cupboards or refrigerator. It almost always happened in the evening after supper, so I wasn't really hungry. I have since come to realize that when the uncontrollable urge to snoop through the kitchen comes over me, it usually means that I'm tense or that something is bothering me. For you, the signals may be different: perhaps craving something salty or sweet or simply thinking about food when you know you're not hungry.

Another way of tuning in to your feelings is to write them down, as Tom F. does. Or like Aileen Y., who says, "When I feel a lot bombarding me, I write how I feel; it's stream-of-consciousness writing." Just the act of putting it down on paper helps Aileen get in touch with her emotions. Recently, for instance, within the space of three weeks, her grandmother, father and dog died. "Writing saved me because I wasn't keeping it bottled up. If I hadn't dealt with those feelings, I believe I would have gained a whole lot of weight." Writing her feelings out has been a major tool for Aileen in keeping off 115 pounds for more than 11 years.

Putting a Lid on Emotional Eating

Once you've labeled the emotions that trigger you to overeat, and when you're ready to stop dealing with your problems by eating and come to terms with your feelings, the next step is to find another way to cope. Claudia B. says of her final effort to lose 115 pounds, "I was ready to deal with the feelings that came up when I put the food down."

You need to ask yourself if emotional eating actually accomplishes anything. Does it truly cure your boredom? Does it make the loneliness go away? Does it cheer you up in the long run? Most masters would agree that the answer to each of these questions is "No."

Master Bob W. has developed a "problem checklist" for the people he now counsels at Kaiser Permanente's "Freedom from Fat" weight-management program. He suggests first asking yourself, "Am I really hungry? Why am I in this place with this food in my hand? Do I need it?" He advises gently reminding yourself that food is not a "cure-all" for life's problems, then thinking,

"What do I need right now? To talk to someone? Rest? A hug? A pleasant activity? A cup of tea shared with a friend? Will food help me out? Has it ever really made me feel better? Maybe food isn't the solution."

Mindy B., who has lost and kept off 84 pounds for 7 years, is aware that she has a tendency to rummage through the cupboards when she's upset with her husband or herself. Her self-talk is, "Look, you're just hurting yourself." Then, if it's nice outside, she goes and works in the yard, which "mellows" her out.

Ann B. states, "Exercise helps — it's empowering." Tami B., who finds boredom to be a sore spot in her struggle to maintain her 38-pound loss, says, "I find other things to do when I'm bored, like exercising."

Some masters find that interpersonal communication helps them deal with their issues more constructively. Compared with when she was heavy, Ann B. finds, "I talk to people more about my emotions." Tom F. sometimes works out his problems by talking them over with another person. "If I keep that problem to myself, it just goes around in my mind — say, at a rate of 800 words per minute. But when I verbalize the problem, it comes out at a rate of 150 words a minute and helps me see what the issue is. It shines an honesty spotlight on the situation, and I become more rational about dealing with it."

Certainly, positive self-talk has an important place in learning to face life head-on. As you read through this chapter on how masters cope with emotional eating, you'll find example after example of positive self-talk. When Ann B. coped with loneliness by eating, she used to say to herself, "Oh well, it doesn't matter what my body looks like anyway. It's inevitable to be heavy." In the next breath, she shared her new self-talk (at her weight of 115), "I really, really like having a healthy, strong body and the way people react to me. Having this body outweighs whatever comfort I got from food. It's not worth sedating myself with food."

Finally, since food is often used to release tension, just learning to relax may help prevent emotional eating. The psychology section of a good bookstore is filled with guides for relaxation. Some people take courses in yoga or transcendental meditation. Another technique, called "progressive muscle relaxation," involves tensing and relaxing certain muscle groups, paying close attention to the relaxation phase. Or you might choose a simple home remedy like reading, going for a bike ride or having sex — the "grab-your-mate-instead-of-your-plate" solution!

"The quickest relaxation technique is deep breathing," according to *The Truth About Addiction and Recovery,* by Stanton Peele and Archie Brodsky. They suggest leaning back, closing your eyes, picturing a pleasant scene in great detail, taking as much air as you comfortably can into your lungs, then breathing out slowly. Repeat at least several times. The idea is to practice the technique so you can call it quickly into play at tense moments.

Dealing with Specific Emotions

Special words are in order about the emotions overweight people are likely to "stifle" with food: anger, loneliness, boredom and depression. (See page 257 to determine if professional counseling is in order.)

◆ **Anger.** Says master Aileen Y.: "I used anger and angry behavior as a buffer to keep me from having an honest relationship with people. If I was angry, I didn't have to be intimate. I could keep people at a distance. Instead of being honest with myself, I used food to sate my feelings." Now, Aileen, who is an active Overeaters Anonymous member, deals with her anger by sharing it — either with her OA sponsor (support person) or by writing about it. "Now, I look at my part of the situation and am honest about my feelings. I make peace, accept the situation and move forward."

Of course, the way you deal with anger depends on the circumstance and the individual. You may find it useful to make a list of appropriate ways to handle anger, as well as other emotions that trigger overeating. For anger, your list might include:

- Talk to myself to see if it's really worth being angry.
- Walk away from the person or situation.
- Tell the person how I feel.
- Use relaxation techniques.
- Go for a walk or bike ride.
- Buy a book on dealing with anger and assertiveness.

- **Loneliness.** "I started to gain weight when I was a senior in high school," recalls Kelly S. "A lot of my friends had steady boyfriends, and I didn't. So on weekends, I'd volunteer to work at a homemade ice cream shop. I learned to pacify how hurt I was with food . . . [and tell myself] that an ice cream sundae at the moment would make me feel better. I would wake up in a 'drugged' state. I was dulling the pain. In a short period of time, I gained 30 to 40 pounds." But at some level, she recognized what she was doing. "I knew it made me feel worse. I gained weight, couldn't fit in my clothes; it was self-imposed isolation. I realized that I had to start reaching out." As Kelly saw more clearly the connection between her emotions and overeating, she was able to channel her energy into her career goal: becoming a registered dietitian. Now, 50 pounds lighter for 6 years, she specializes in counseling people with weight problems.

Your list of appropriate ways to cope with day-to-day loneliness might include:

- Call a friend or relative.
- Go shopping.
- Join an adult-education class.
- Go to a support group or club.
- Rent a movie.
- Get a pet.

◆ **Boredom.** In the process of losing her 62 pounds, Peppi S. figured out that she is likely to overeat when she first comes home from work and is bored. Now, when she finds herself searching through the cabinets, she asks herself, "What am I doing? Am I bored, hungry? I try to figure out why I'm doing what I'm doing. In the past, when I came home from work, I wouldn't know if I was hungry or bored. Now I might try some other activity or drink water."

◆ **Depression.** Before Ann B. lost her 35 pounds, she was in the habit of "anesthetizing" her feelings of vague depression and loneliness by eating. After going through a Shaklee group weight-loss program that helped participants identify the triggers for eating, she stopped using food "as a drug." Ann said to herself, "Whatever is going on with me, it isn't worth being overweight." In fact, Ann's number-one strategy for keeping her weight down is, "Don't eat for emotional reasons . . . I think it's most important to find out why you're using food." Now, Ann sorts out her emotions on paper. "I keep a personal journal of my thoughts and feelings to identify them. When I write it down, I can figure out what's bugging me."

Some ways to cheer yourself up when feeling blue:

- ◆ Get a new haircut or a facial.
- ◆ Exercise.
- ◆ Buy yourself something special.
- ◆ Get together with a friend.
- ◆ Take a day off from work just for you.
- ◆ Forget the chores and play with your kids.
- ◆ Go to a play, movie or sports event.

Unpleasant emotions and problems are part of life. They will be there whether or not you turn to food. Sometimes, you just have to accept what you are feeling. Master and weight-control counselor Kelly S. says, "I think sometimes people need to be

For stress management, check out this book: <u>Mastering Stress 2001</u> by Drs. David H. Barlow, Ronald M. Rapee and Leslie Reisner. 2001. Dallas: The LifeStyle Company. (800-LEARN-41 or www.thelifestylecompany.com)

'there' for that feeling — or just to feel something and do nothing. You can choose to use food one more time, but you know what the consequences will be."

A Primer on Problem Solving

Psychologists have developed some strategies for helping people cope with life's stresses more effectively, and the techniques can be applied to weight-related problems, as well as to day-to-day issues. I've combined several strategies for problem solving in the following six-step process:

STEP #1
Define the problem.

What is getting in the way of losing weight? Look for patterns: the time of day that your problem occurs, what precedes it, what follows it, whether it happens when you're alone or with certain people. It's important to be honest with yourself. As psychologists Daniel Wheeler and Irving Janis advise, if the problem is genuine, do not ignore it, rationalize, procrastinate, bypass or panic.

Weight-related example: You have no trouble sticking to your low-fat food plan all day long, but you find yourself thinking about food and picking all evening. What precedes the problem? You've finished supper and are full. At about 8:00, your skinny husband starts getting out chips and sweets, leaves them on the counter and marches in and out to munch on them as you both watch TV. You tell yourself,

"I'm not going to have any snacks after supper." What happens? You always give in, and once you start snacking, you have trouble stopping. What's the upshot? You go to bed feeling fat, defeated and guilty.

Nonweight example: You feel overwhelmed because, once again, your babysitter has canceled at the last minute, forcing you to take another vacation day from work to care for your kids. The problem is that you have an unreliable babysitter and may have to find a new one.

STEP #2
Come up with alternatives.

What can you do about the problem? Psychologists believe that by coming up with many alternatives, you increase the odds of finding effective solutions. Think about your past experiences with similar problems and evaluate what worked and what didn't. Ask yourself how a friend who is a good problem-solver might handle the situation. Or, as Tom F. does, talk with a friend about the problem. Use the information to generate additional strategies for yourself.

Weight-related example: What are other possibilities for handling the nighttime snacking problem? Get out of the house: go shopping or join an exercise class. Ask your husband to snack on more healthful foods or to stop eating in front of you. Ask him to put open packages of food away. Buy snack foods you're not particularly fond of. Watch television in a different part of the house. Try to engage your husband romantically. Plan your own after-dinner snack and wait until a specific time to have it. Start a new hobby to take your mind off food. Go to bed early.

Nonweight example: What to do about the unreliable babysitter? Have a long talk to find out what's going on. Confront the sitter, saying that if she cancels again, you'll fire her. Quit your job and stay home with the kids. Place your children in a daycare facility. Ask a relative or friend to care for the children.

STEP #3
Evaluate the alternatives, listing pros and cons for each.

In essence, Tom F. does this when he writes down his fears as well as "the bright side" of a problem. Mentally picture yourself engaging in each possible solution for the problem. Think about how feasible each option is: consider time and effort, financial implications, your likelihood of succeeding in the short run *and* long run, emotional costs and gains, consistency with your values and possible impact on others in your life.

Weight-related example: Evaluate whether it's realistic to think you'll go out every night: what would the impact be on your marriage? Are you likely to engage in nighttime exercise on a long-term basis? (On the plus side, it would get you out of the house and make you come home feeling refreshed; on the downside, you may be a morning person who knows that you've never been able to stick with evening exercise.) Is it reasonable to expect your thin spouse to switch to healthful snacks? Is he likely to put food away if you ask nicely? Is it realistic to think you'll go to bed early each night? If you're more romantic, will it change the snacking? Can you envision yourself looking forward to a treat that you've saved for an evening snack?

Nonweight example: You know that talking to your sitter will have little impact because you've tried it before. Are you prepared to follow through if you have to fire her? Can you afford to stay home with the kids? What are the pros and cons of group daycare versus having a sitter in your home? If you ask your relative or friend to help, are their views of child rearing consistent with yours?

STEP #4
Make a decision and a commitment.

Choose the alternatives that give you the greatest benefits at the least cost.

Weight-related example: You decide that the most viable options are to ask your husband to put packages away and to save a snack for yourself for later in the evening. And although evening exercise is not realistic for you, you decide that you can go out with a friend or go shopping one or two nights a week.

Nonweight example: You decide to try childcare outside of the home since it will give your children exposure to other kids their age and is less expensive than having a sitter.

STEP #5
Implement the strategy.

Develop a plan to actually carry out your decision(s).

Weight-related example: Buy some low-calorie treat foods for yourself and plan what, when and how much you'll have each night. Put out some individual bowls for your husband to serve himself, and remind him to put packages away after he has a helping. Call a friend and "make a date."

Nonweight example: Call friends and neighbors for daycare recommendations, prepare interview questions, do some preliminary phone screening, then check out the best ones in person. After you make a choice, give your current sitter notice and prepare your children for the change.

STEP #6
Evaluate the plan and switch gears if necessary.

Compare the actual outcome with the desired outcome. "Your problem behavior doesn't have to be totally eliminated for your experiment to be a success," point out Michael J. Mahoney and Kathryn Mahoney in *Permanent Weight Control*. If the plan was partially successful, how could it be improved? If it didn't work, consider the possible reasons. Did you give it your best effort? Did you try the plan for a long enough period of time? Were your goals realistic? Was your strategy too ambitious? What other tactic can you try? (Go back to your list of alternatives, or come up with some new strategies.) Finally, if the plan didn't work, ask yourself what you can learn from it.

Weight-related example: Are you snacking less at night than you did before? Are you able to avoid free-for-all snacking by saving a low-fat treat for later? Do you go to bed feeling better about yourself? If your husband refuses to put packages away, perhaps *you* can do it so they're not constantly staring at you. You also might try buying treat foods for him that are not your favorites or engage in some new evening activities that remove you from television and food.

Nonweight example: Is your new daycare provider more reliable? Do you like her/him, and are your philosophies compatible? If your children still cry every morning when you drop them off, have you given the situation enough time? If the daycare is not working out, do you want to consider your second choice of having a relative provide childcare?

Do You Have Binge Eating Disorder?

There's a difference between occasional emotional overeating and "binge eating disorder," or BED, which is often called "compulsive overeating." In *Now That You've Lost It,* Dr. Joyce Nash points out, "All binges are episodes of overeating, but not all overeating episodes qualify as binges." When overeating happens only occasionally and "is accompanied by few or mild emotional reactions, it falls into the category of simple overeating," which may or may not be triggered by emotional stress. Dr. Nash emphasizes that all people, both heavy and thin, overeat from time to time, but those who engage in simple overeating do not feel out of control, while a true binge eater does.

You are at risk of having binge eating disorder if you answer yes to all or most of the following questions — and the behavior has gone on regularly for some time, say 6 months or so:

- Do you often consume unusually large amounts of food, larger than most people would eat during the same time period, under the same circumstances — for instance, a quart of ice cream, 6 brownies and 16 chocolate chip cookies — within 2 hours?
- Do you feel your eating is out of control during these times — that is, that you cannot stop eating or control what or how much you eat?
- Do you eat much more quickly than usual during such episodes?
- Do you often keep on eating, even though you are full to the point of being uncomfortable?
- Do you commonly eat alone because you're ashamed of how much you eat?
- Are such periods of overeating followed by intense feelings of disgust, depression or guilt?

How common is BED? According to the Weight-control Information Network, about 10 to 15 percent of people who are mildly obese and who try to lose weight on their own or through commercial weight-loss programs have BED. The problem is more common in women and in severely obese people. (Although most people with BED are overweight, even normal-weight people can have the problem.) If you have BED, it can be psychologically and medically devastating.

Note that binge eating also takes place in the context of another eating disorder called bulimia nervosa. But with this problem, binges are usually followed by efforts to "get rid of" the food by such practices as fasting, purposeful vomiting, strenuous exercising or abusing laxatives or diuretics. (This is in contrast to BED, where the person makes no deliberate, sustained effort to compensate for the food.) If you engage in these practices, you should be evaluated by a mental health professional who specializes in the diagnosis and treatment of eating disorders. (See page 257 for advice on finding a reliable counselor.) Because of possible serious health consequences, it would be wise to consult with your physician as well.

People with BED frequently have major depression, low self-esteem and other problems such as substance abuse that need to be treated in conjunction with the bingeing. It is not known whether their psychological problems contribute to the abnormal eating or result from it. Whatever the case, binges often occur in response to feelings such as anger, sadness, boredom and worry. Fortunately, there is evidence that depression lessens when binge eating declines.

Overcoming Binge Eating

If you think you have BED, your best bet is to see a mental health professional who's an expert in this area. Since a number of studies have shown that both cognitive-behavioral therapy and interpersonal therapy can markedly reduce binge eating in people with BED, many of the positive self-talk and behavioral techniques used by the masters are likely to be of value to binge eaters. Antidepressant drugs may also help some individuals with BED.

According to Dr. Susan Bartlett, a psychologist and specialist in

BED at Johns Hopkins University School of Medicine, "If some-one really does have binge eating disorder, simply going on a strenuous diet to quickly lose weight is unlikely to work in the long run. This may, in fact, make the problem much worse." She advises that binge eaters focus first on regaining control by re-turning to the basics of sensible eating, such as structured meals and mealtimes, menu planning and portion control. Since many binge eaters tend to consume little or nothing, then overeat all at once, having scheduled meals and snacks may help prevent exces-sive hunger by spreading the calories throughout the day. She also recommends limiting the amount of "binge" foods brought into the home.

Dr. Nash suggests that if you decide to binge, you should wait 15 minutes then "go ahead and binge, but do it in a particular way: Give yourself permission to eat without guilt. Eat slowly and savor each bite." She also stresses the value of exercise be-cause it can help with feelings of calmness and relaxation. She cautions, however, that exercise should be reasonable and not become a compulsive habit in itself. Dr. Bartlett adds that it's im-portant to not allow yourself unlimited access to food during a "planned binge"; rather, determine in advance how much you'll eat, then make sure only that much food is available.

Binge eaters tend to have rigid rules about dieting, weight goals and how they should perform. Thus they are likely to benefit from learning how to set realistic goals, as well as from relapse-prevention strategies (see Chapter 5). In addition, problem-solv-ing techniques may help binge eaters. Indeed, the masters who said they had problems with binge eating in the past indicated that their top technique for stopping bingeing is talking to them-selves and trying to figure out why they feel like going on a binge.

Whatever time of day a binge is most likely to occur is a good time to get away from areas that provide easy access to food. Since evening is often a high-risk time for bingeing, Dr. Bartlett helps her clients avoid the temptation to binge by encouraging them to plan evening activities with family or friends or go to exercise classes. A telephone buddy may also be helpful for difficult moments.

Five masters were helped by Overeaters Anonymous (OA), a free, nonprofit self-help group for compulsive overeaters based on the 12 Steps and spiritual underpinnings of Alcoholics Anonymous. The steps involve admitting that you are powerless over food and turning your life over to a "higher power." (OA does not espouse any particular diet; the goal is not weight loss per se, but to break free from compulsive overeating.) However, Dr. Bartlett points out that the approach, methods and members' philosophy in OA vary widely from group to group, even within the same city. She says that some individuals in her studies and clinics have reported they did find the daily support offered at OA helpful. However, others have received inappropriate or inaccurate advice and delayed seeking the medical and psychological treatment they really needed.

To date, there is little research evidence to support the safety and efficacy of OA, and some of its principles contradict those of most behavioral weight-loss programs that have been shown to help compulsive overeaters. If you do want to give OA a try, attend several different groups to get a feel for the leader's and participants' approach. Trust your instincts; if some of what you observe doesn't sit well with you, try another OA meeting. Whether or not you try OA, if your problems with binge eating are severe, long-standing or continue, be sure to see a psychologist, social worker or psychiatrist who has experience with eating problems.

How Some Masters Conquered Binge Eating

◆ Ann F., who once weighed 380 pounds and has kept her weight in a range of 135 to 170 pounds for 10 years, overcame her problem in large part by telling herself that there are no "good" and "bad" foods and by recognizing the value of exercise. (She tried

Overeaters Anonymous but found the approach to be too restrictive.) She states, "Probably the biggest changes in my eating behavior are that I basically eat what I want (in moderation), do not go on stringent diets or fasts (I had a long history of this), and rarely 'binge' since I eat what I want. In other words, I might have a piece of cake or two but never the whole cake anymore (thank goodness)! I may overeat at a party on Saturday night, but rarely wake up Sunday wanting to overeat. I usually feel lousy from the excess and will make it a point to exercise and eat really well the following day." It's worth noting that Ann had gastric bypass surgery, which puts a mechanical limit on the volume of food she can eat. But if she hadn't overcome her habit of binge eating, she could have undone the benefits of the procedure.

◆ Aileen Y., who has kept off 115 pounds for more than 11 years, once "had to be eating all the time. There were times when I didn't know what I wanted — [it was] that 'insatiable hunger.'" She recalls "going through boxes of cereal, loaves of bread, quarts of milk, half gallons of ice cream" — all in one day and in secret. Of the time when she lost weight once and for all, she told me, "I recognized that my eating — of any kind of foods — was out of control. I felt suicidal and depressed. I was desperate. When I started [going to] OA, it was such a relief to find support and a solution!" She gained control of her binge eating by "living and working my OA recovery program, which includes prayer, meditation, calling a sponsor [OA member], attending meetings, writing my feelings out, using the OA Steps and tools." She also plans — in writing — the foods that she will eat each day, which include "three moderate, nutritionally balanced meals with a snack of fruit." She "chooses not to include" sugar or red meat, alcoholic beverages or caffeine. Aileen has become more realistic about what she "should" weigh. "I thought 125 to 130 was to be my weight." Now, with age and after some health problems, she accepts herself at 145 (she's 5′5″). "I'm being reasonable now!"

◆ Dorothy C., who has weighed 123 for 8 years (down 32 pounds from her all-time high), remembers eating an entire frozen Sara Lee pie after a large quantity of granola cookies. "At my worst, I did it every day." She also used to make herself vomit. When I asked her how she solved her problem, she told me, "One day I decided to leave two cookies in the box. I thought, 'This feels like I'm more in control, like a normal person.' Before, it was always all or nothing: eat everything in sight so it doesn't torment me until it is gone." She adds that in conquering binge eating, "There was no one epiphany; it was gradual. For a number of years, I channeled my compulsive energy into exercise, which provides structure: psychologically, it gives a sense of control. Now I'm less compulsive." Since she realized that she did a lot of binge eating out of boredom, stress and depression, Dorothy learned to fill her time with other activities, like reading, calling friends, shopping and using delay techniques (waiting out her urges to eat), as well as exercising. Dorothy admits that she occasionally has lapses. "I still turn to my favorite foods out of boredom or stress, but less frequently. And now my definition of a binge is gobbling a bagel with butter or five or six cookies — before it was the whole bag. It's a victory to learn that you can cut it off." She also tries to satisfy sweet cravings with no-fat hard candy or jelly beans (rather than with chocolate) and usually eats some kind of dessert with meals, such as yogurt, a Weight Watchers brownie or fruit, "so as not to feel deprived."

◆ Nancy K. has conquered binge eating for 12 years, which has enabled her to maintain a 60-pound weight loss. When her problem was at its worst, she might have eaten "a dozen doughnuts and three Hostess fruit pies" secretly within the space of an hour. Then she'd feel guilty, so she'd go and buy a salad because she felt she needed "something good." She'd go through this routine at least once a week, then say to herself, "What a jerk. How stupid. You're fat and ugly, and now you make it worse." That commonly led to another day of binge eating, followed by several days of starvation: "just Tab and salads." Nancy attributes her triumph over binge eating to her becoming a born-again Christian. "I decided I couldn't continue life eating the way I was. I believed that faith in Jesus would give me the strength to overcome it." From then on, she told me, "I quit dieting, quit saying 'I cannot have this, this and this. I tried eating in a more reasonable, consistent manner: three meals and a snack. I never said, 'No, this is not allowed.' There were no weight-loss goals and no rules. My goal was to quit bingeing and be a better eater." She lost her weight very slowly, at a rate of about 10 pounds a year. She said to herself, "Hey, it's better than gaining." Now, at a weight of 135 (she's 5'7"), Nancy says she still struggles to be a "good eater. If I eat four cookies, that's a lot for me." Sometimes, she finds herself skipping meals and grabbing snack foods. But when she hits her upper weight limit of 139, she says, "Okay, start back to healthy eating." She adds, "Sure, I wish I could eat whatever I want, but I've accepted that I can't. This is something that I'm going to deal with for the rest of my life; I'm thankful for where I am."

Recommended Reading

Overcoming Binge Eating by Dr. Christopher Fairburn. New York: Guilford Press, 1995.

Some Organizations for Help with Binge Eating Disorder

National Eating Disorders Association
603 Stewart Street, Suite 803
Seattle, WA 98101
Phone: 206-382-3587 or 800-931-2237
Web site: www.nationaleatingdisorders.org

Academy for Eating Disorders
6728 Old McLean Village Drive
McLean, VA 22101-3906
Phone: 703-556-9222
Web site: www.aedweb.org

Is Professional Counseling a Good Idea?

If your weight serves as a shield or a way to hide from psychological issues, you may need professional help, both in uncovering the issues as well as in dealing with them. For instance, some women who are seriously overweight may have backgrounds of sexual, emotional and/or physical abuse that require counseling. And, as indicated earlier, some overweight people — particularly those with binge eating disorder — suffer from depression and anxiety, as well as low self-esteem. According to University of Pennsylvania psychologist Dr. Thomas Wadden and colleagues, about 10 percent of obese patients have clinically significant depression and should receive professional counseling before undertaking weight loss.

Professional counseling not only can help you deal with these issues, but it can also help you anticipate how life will be when you slim down. As master Nancy K. states, "People blame all their problems on their weight, but the problems don't go away when you're thin." (Contrary to what some think, weight loss will not "cure" major depression. However, for people who are mildly depressed, weight loss may improve mood.) Sometimes, without the weight to hide behind, the problems become magnified. A number of masters told me that new issues arose because they had never been of normal weight before. Some, for instance, had problems in relationships, while others had (and still have) a difficult time seeing themselves as thin.

How do you go about finding professional help? Start by making sure that the person is a licensed mental health professional such as a psychologist, social worker or psychiatrist. Each state has its own laws regulating the practice of psychologists and social workers. In some states, there are strict laws about who can call him- or herself a "counselor" or a "therapist"; in others, there is little or no regulation. It is wise to seek out someone who has met certification criteria from a long-standing professional organization with licensing requirements that have been established and are monitored by a state board. While this is not an exhaustive list, the degrees one should look for in a counselor would be "Ph.D.," "Psy.D.," "M.D." or "M.S.W." — any one of which should have been granted by an accredited institution of higher education.

Dr. Joyce Nash advises that the best way to choose a counselor is to ask for a referral from someone you trust, such as a physician, other counselors, religious leader or nurse. It's best if the counselor you choose is not someone whom you know socially or whose personal life you know a great deal about.

There is no guarantee that working through your problems will lead you to become thin for life, but it may increase your odds of becoming a master. Indeed, one study on overweight people in a professional weight-loss program revealed that those with the fewest psychological problems lost about twice as much weight as those who had the most problems. The more resources you have, the more likely you are to succeed at permanent weight control.

9

Key to Success #9

Get More Out of Life

How's the balance in your life? Are your days filled with "shoulds" as opposed to desires? In other words, how much time do you spend doing things you feel you *have* to do versus things you *want* to do? Do you put everyone else's needs first, always leaving your own concerns for last? Do you ever reward yourself with anything other than food? Are you happy in life? Does your weight keep you from activities you'd really like to take part in? Are you satisfied with the way you spend your time? How about your relationships: are they what you want them to be?

En route to becoming successful maintainers, many masters sorted through these questions and found they weren't satisfied with the answers. Somewhere along the way, they decided they weren't getting enough out of life and were spurred to develop more fulfilled, balanced and happy lives. Many also made positive changes in relationships and found ways to get their own needs met. They learned to feel better about themselves as well. *In short, these masters found a way to get more out of life.*

Jennifer P.'s Story

After struggling with her weight most of her life, food and weight control are now "almost nonissues," Jennifer P. told me. Why? "A stable environment and a healthy family life" are among her major keys to success. After sorting through some serious emotional traumas of childhood, Jennifer has developed a rich and rewarding life — one that doesn't revolve around food or force her to hide behind her weight anymore. At a height of 5'5", she feels happy with herself at 142 pounds. She's stabilized at around that weight for the better part of 7 years — down more than 40 pounds from her maximum of 186. "I've had two children since losing and still maintain this 140-ish weight."

Jennifer remembers herself as a "chubby" child, whose weight first became an issue around second grade, when she heard her parents comment, "We have to watch Jennifer." By the time she was in sixth grade, her weight was up to 115 (her height was 5'3") — certainly not obese, but heavier than most other children her age. She attributes her weight gain around this time to two incidents of sexual molestation, one by a relative, the other by a boy at a party. She recalls saying to herself, "If I just get fat, then boys will leave me alone." The abuse by the relative occurred for about two years, every two to three months at family gatherings. Years later, Jennifer realized, "The real issue was hiding my sexuality behind my weight."

Jennifer steadily got heavier, gaining 10 pounds each year around the time of the holidays, which marked the anniversary of the first incident of sexual abuse. "In seventh grade, I went from 115 to 125, in eighth grade from 125 to 135. At the same time, I would roller-coaster: diet and eat, diet and eat. I was an all-or-nothing kind of person. By the time I graduated from high school, I weighed 175." She continued to gain weight until the end of her freshman year in college.

Her weight-loss efforts included the usual methods: most often calorie-counting, but sometimes liquid diets, over-the-counter diet pills and fasting. She also went to Weight Watchers as a teenager, which she found to be helpful. Her typical "reward" for her dieting efforts was a 5- to 10-pound loss, which she would quickly regain. She attributes her weight problem to the diet-binge cycle: "I'd do 1,000 calories [a day] for weeks, then I'd lose control and go for it. After having three meals, I might eat a Dairy Queen parfait, then two or three doughnuts. A few hours later, my friends and I might go to a 7-Eleven store and get some candy bars. I'd say to myself, 'I'll start over tomorrow.' But it always took me a few weeks to get back on track."

Jennifer's triumph over her weight problem was a long, slow process that began the summer after her freshman year of college. That June, she started dating a man who told her she'd be a "10" if only she lost some weight. Angry at his lack of acceptance, she refused to do anything about her weight until he was out of the picture. After he went away that August, she somewhat sheepishly admits, she fasted for 7 days and lost 15 pounds. That started her pattern of losing weight during the summer and gaining some — but not all — back during the school year when she was around the boyfriend. "After the first summer, I gained back 5 pounds. The next summer I lost 22 and regained about 10 pounds. The summer of my junior year, I lost another 12."

Jennifer certainly did it her way. How? "I got addicted to exercise. I would run about 30 miles a week." (She is no longer an exercise "addict.") When I asked her about how she ate, Jennifer replied, "I figured out the low-fat thing. But I didn't know what to call it back then. My plan was semimodeled after Weight Watchers'. I always liked healthful eating and found new treats like frozen yogurt and diet ice cream." (She figures she consumed about 1,500 calories per day.) During the school year, she was able to maintain some of her losses by continuing running. She refused to diet, although she continued to watch her fat intake. "I just ate a lot, so I would gain some weight back."

When I asked Jennifer how, without therapy, she was able to stop hiding behind her weight, she replied, "I got distracted from the need to keep men at bay by my anger at my boyfriend. My need to show him I was okay overpowered my need to hide behind the weight. Otherwise, I might have kept the weight on." She added, "Somewhere along the way, I also learned to like myself: all of me, my body included, as I was. I felt my weight was mine, and I was going to do it my way." (Jennifer did undergo therapy about two years ago. She told me, "I had to deal with why I put the weight on, and I had to learn to deal with the way men look at me, now that I'm thinner.")

During the summer of her junior year, Jennifer met another man, one who loved her unconditionally. "He was someone who liked me for me. It was healing. Then the weight really became *my* issue." At first she regained 10 pounds, but she took it off in time for her wedding the following year. At that point, Jennifer was down to 152.

Jennifer made the break from the "all-or-nothing attitude" during the first two years of her marriage after deciding, "I'm just going to be normal. I asked myself, 'What would a normal person without a weight problem eat?' One bowl of cereal. One sandwich. One or two cookies. And that's what I would eat. I let the weight thing be whatever it was." Slowly, over the course of the next 5 years, Jennifer lost the last 10 pounds. Toward the end of that time, she learned a great deal from a registered dietitian. "I wanted to make sure my weight was down before I started a family because I was afraid of ballooning. The dietitian taught me about low-fat eating. I learned you can eat a lot and stay full." The dietitian also taught Jennifer to stop depriving herself. "Sometimes, I'd eat everything but the food I really wanted. So once a day, if I had an urge, I'd eat the food that I wanted.

"The long, drawn-out process of losing and maintaining taught me that sometimes my body is ready to lose weight, and sometimes it's not." She learned that, for her, a good time to lose weight was when stress was low and she could focus on losing. When she hit a plateau, she would accept it and slowly increase her calorie intake until she "felt comfortable again."

Jennifer believes that in order to lose weight permanently, she had to put herself first. Her parents were missionaries, and Jennifer had been taught that her own desires were secondary to those of others. "I was always trying to meet everyone else's needs, please everyone else. The message was that I should always be perfect, nice, godly and unselfish — that I shouldn't feel better than others. When I was trying to meet everyone else's needs, there was a big hole inside me. And I filled it up with food. We had a family rule that no one should be better than anyone else. But I knew I was my dad's favorite and that I was the prettiest of my three sisters. My sisters' boyfriends were attracted to me. I had to play myself down so I wouldn't be hated by my sisters. My weight equalized things."

Eventually, Jennifer was "able to push others' needs aside and let weight loss happen." Today, one of Jennifer's "shoulds" is, "Be selfish when you need to." When I interviewed her, for instance, she had just had a birthday. "My family and I were at a lake, and my husband was taking care of the kids. I told myself, 'It's okay to sit here selfishly, relax, read a book and let him take care of them.'"

Another important part of her success, Jennifer believes, is developing a calmer lifestyle. "I think a lot of my eating was because of family stress and chaos. Having a calm husband has helped me. I also do some meditation and journal writing to let out anger and anxiety and to explore my emotions. And I enjoy quietness." Jennifer admits that for the first 5 years after losing the weight, maintenance was "really tough, but now it's easier. I think it's emotional. My life is more peaceful. I think about food less."

Jennifer also makes a conscious effort to stay "internally aware" of why she's eating. "I try not to eat because of emotions. When I want to eat for reasons other than hunger, I stop and think, 'What is really going on here? What's the real issue creating this anxiety?' Sometimes I figure it out and choose to eat anyway. But I try, instead, to take time out and be by myself to determine what's going on. I write in my journal or go jogging. When I run, I can obsess in my own space. Then I tend to be okay." Jennifer is pleased to say she is no longer a compulsive exerciser. Her exercise frequency varies from "not at all" to three or four times a week, depending on the season and her schedule. When she does exercise, she either jogs for three miles, does a circuit-training program for ½ hour or does aerobics for 30 to 45 minutes.

Jennifer's maintenance food plan consists mainly of low-fat healthful foods. "It's habit to me to find fun things that are low-fat." A bowl of cereal (low-fat granola) with skim milk constitutes breakfast. Lunch is usually a yogurt, wheat muffin or plain bagel, fruit and diet soda. Supper might be chicken, tuna or other fish with pasta or rice, a vegetable and a roll; sometimes it's beans and rice or soup. She treats herself to sweets once a day: a handful of chocolate chips, several cookies, licorice or some low-fat treat. Her other snacks include fruit, unbuttered bread, pretzels or diet soda. Jennifer doesn't feel deprived. "I eat what I want. If everyone else is eating nachos with cheese, I have them too. Sometimes when people see me eating like this, they ask, 'Do you eat like this all the time?' They don't realize that I then watch what I eat for the rest of the day."

Jennifer weighs herself about once a week. She used to do so every day until recently. But after her scale broke, she realized she was "addicted" to weighing herself and decided to change. If she gains between 1 and 5 pounds, she cuts back on sweets and makes an effort to stop and think about what she's eating. She also consciously lowers her fat intake.

What, for Jennifer, is the secret to long-term weight control? "Determine what eating does for you. You need to start figuring out what your weight keeps you from. Consider getting some therapy. You need to sort out your issues and your eating."

What's "Getting More Out of Life" Got to Do with Maintenance?

Jennifer's past history of putting her own needs last fits with a pattern observed by G. Alan Marlatt, Ph.D., a relapse-prevention expert and director of the Addictive Behaviors Research Center at the University of Washington. He believes that a number of over-weight people have unbalanced lifestyles bogged down with a multitude of "shoulds." Their lives have little room for pleasure. If your life is unbalanced in this fashion, he says, you may feel de-prived and seek immediate gratification from food as a payoff for your martyrdom. I often saw this behavior in my overweight cli-ents who gave to others so much that the only "nice" thing they did for themselves was to indulge in food.

To remedy the situation, Dr. Marlatt advises, "Balance your lifestyle, and your sense of craving and deprivation likely will be less." In a review article on long-term weight loss, obesity experts Kelly Brownell and Robert Jeffery note that people who succeed at weight control tend to develop new hobbies, interests, friend-ships and job skills.

Jennifer P.'s story illustrates how strongly her ability to main-tain weight loss is connected with establishing a stable environ-ment, sorting through personal issues, taking care of her own needs and finding career satisfaction. Many of the other masters I spoke with also donned protective armor against weight regain by developing more fulfilled and interesting lives and, at some point, starting to feel better about themselves. Losing weight was just part of an unfolding process including many positive changes that seemingly had little or nothing to do with food and eating. *For some masters, the changes happened beforehand.* It was as if certain aspects of their lives had to be in place before they could be ready to take on permanent weight loss. Ann F. told me, "Some people make changes in crisis, but I needed to feel good about myself outside of my weight before I lost it. At that point, I had a good job, stable friendships, and I liked myself, despite my weight."

For other masters, lifestyle changes happened along the way, as they gained confidence because of their initial weight loss. For instance, as Charlotte O. was losing her 96 pounds, she started to branch out by becoming more involved in community organizations. *For a third group of masters, certain aspects of their lives changed and motivated them to begin losing weight, and their newfound confidence helped them make more changes that, in turn, reinforced their weight loss.* Take the case of Vicki B., who wasn't ready to lose her 60-plus pounds until her three sons were in school, when she had time to herself. "I went to work and started to lose." After she lost the weight (nearly 9 years ago), Vicki achieved her dream of becoming an actress: she's landed parts in local productions, TV shows and commercials. She admits that the "frequent scrutiny" she's under is a powerful incentive to keep her weight down and creates high stress levels. "But," she adds, "I'd rather be 139 pounds with high stress than 200 pounds with high stress from being overweight."

When her weight approached 200 pounds, Peppi S. says she did not want to go out, felt sorry for herself, stayed at home and ate. Now, her 62-pound weight loss has given her the confidence to become "a happy, healthy and energetic person. That's who I always dreamed of being and now that I am here, I will never go back. If I can be an example of how one can go from being depressed, overweight and a bitter person to one who is willing to take risks, try new things, get the most out of life and be happy and comfortable with myself, then I am truly successful."

Tom F., the master featured in Chapter VIII, got more out of life by making a career change. When he first decided to do something about his weight, he was "fundamentally dissatisfied with life." He was no longer happy in his work as a field engineer, so he had a talk with "the little boy inside. One of the things that I always wanted to be was a fireman." That's what Tom became for 14 years. He's moved on now and owns a software engineering business.

Dr. Ross found in about half of her maintainers a connection between being in control of losing weight and how they felt about the rest of their lives. She stated, "It appears that food intake could be the result of being in control in general or that it can be the means of getting control."

The Self-Esteem Connection

Not only does having a healthy lifestyle appear to be related to long-term weight control, but some studies suggest that having a good concept of self and a positive attitude are associated with losing and maintaining weight. It makes sense that improved self-esteem and developing a more fulfilled life go hand-in-hand. If you feel better about yourself, you are likely to have confidence to make other changes in your life.

For some masters, their improved self-image came *before* the weight loss, while for others it took place *as a result* of becoming thinner. Before Vicki B. began losing weight, she decided, "If I'm going to be this way, I'm going to look nice. I finally started buying some nice 'fat' clothes for myself and began to accept and like myself; then the changes began." Within a year, she started to lose weight. Similarly, Ann B. stated, "I accepted that I could like my body even if it never changed. There was a tremendous power for me in simply accepting myself as I was. Not 'I'll like myself when I lose weight,' which is what I said to myself for *years,* but 'I like myself, period.'" (Ironically, for some masters, accepting themselves as heavy was the precipitant for losing weight!)

Self-esteem played a role in weight loss for Tami B., too. "As I was gaining weight, I wouldn't go out because someone might see me," she says. "So I stayed home and ate and felt sorry for myself. I was in a failure cycle. Once I figured out what was happening, I decided to break out. Having fun and feeling good was more important!"

As for the boost in self-esteem that often takes place *as a result* of losing weight, Charlotte O. says, "I finished losing the weight [96 pounds] and gained enough self-esteem to get a job, leave an unhappy marriage and raise my two children alone. That happened 13 years ago; now at age 39, I feel better, and I look better than ever." Glenda L. told me, "After losing [45 pounds], I had a better sense of myself and self-esteem. I was the same person, just a better one." And Irene S. says of her 77-pound loss, "It has changed my life with high self-esteem and confidence."

Similarly, Dr. Ross's maintainers all mentioned positive changes in self-esteem, which, in turn, enabled them to project a more self-confident image. Some people then felt they could take on more responsibility at work or make job changes, while others reported they no longer felt they had to give in to or be dependent on others. "They could now be more self-directed and 'lean and mean.' There was no more need to do things that would compensate for being fat." Likewise, Drs. Colvin and Olson found that 18 months after the initial interviews with their successful maintainers, "The most important personal change, as perceived by 68 percent of the subjects, was a powerful positive increase in self-image, self-esteem and confidence." Losing weight won't automatically cure a long-standing self-esteem problem. That's why you have to develop other incentives and reinforcements in your life to protect against weight regain.

So how can *you* start feeling better about yourself? Psychological counseling can be of great help. Like Jennifer P., quite a few of the masters mentioned in this chapter told me they had counseling at some point in their lives. But there are also some steps you can take on your own.

Start Living Now

For starters, a number of psychologists suggest that you *stop living your life for the day when you will be thin.* Don't wait until you're thin to start looking nice, buying new clothes and exercising. Buy some great clothes that fit you as you are right now. Get a new hairstyle, a facial, a beauty makeover. Start thinking of yourself as an attractive person.

If you begin seeing yourself in a more positive light, it can enable you to be treated in ways that reinforce feeling good about yourself, which, in turn, may ready you for weight loss. Ann F. recalls, "About two years before I lost the weight, I spent a lot of money on nice clothes, and I let my nails grow. (I had always taken care of my hair and my face.) Before that, I went through a period of only wearing black slacks and overblouses. But I changed that completely. People started reacting to me differently. They didn't look down on me. It made me feel that it was possible to lose weight."

Drs. Zafra Cooper and Christopher Fairburn point out in an article in the journal *Behavior Research and Therapy* that people don't try to lose weight solely to watch the numbers on the scale drop. They also hope to improve their appearance, feel more attractive (or at least less unattractive), be able to wear more flattering and fashionable clothes, as well as improve self-confidence and self-respect. Some see weight loss as the only means to these ends. And, sadly, some people avoid social and professional situations because of their weight — they feel that until they lose weight, they cannot function normally in life. Then, if they don't achieve their weight-loss goals, they feel they've failed at all their other goals. Sometimes, people put off important plans until a certain weight loss is reached. *It's important to recognize that all of these objectives can be achieved whether or not you reach your weight goal.*

Dr. Joyce Nash told me that another way to improve self-esteem is to close the gap between the person you are and the person you think you should be, your ideal. (The greater the gap, she points out, the lower your self-esteem.) The problem for many people is that the ideal is unrealistic, based on perfectionistic goals. Dr. Nash recommends closing the gap by reevaluating your goals and working on day-to-day behavior and successes. She states, "We've learned to evaluate ourselves in negative ways. We tend to look for where we've failed instead of how we've improved. You need to acknowledge little positive steps, day by day." She suggests that, at the beginning of each day, you make a pledge to be successful at one small task. Then, in the evening, focus on the small things that went right that day.

Psychologists Stanton Peele and Archie Brodsky advise making a list of your personal resources. Itemize the things you like about yourself, what you're good at, your accomplishments, what others like or respect about you. You might list your conversational ability or friendliness, skill at playing an instrument or fixing broken household items, graduating as a top student in your high school class, or your parenting skills. The authors stress that by doing this, you focus on your assets and are reminded of your own worth. They add, "Being the first to recognize your own successes will help provide you with the strength to do better." The idea is to focus on your positive attributes, all of which are tools to fight your weight problem.

I must stress that there is no guarantee that boosting your self-esteem will ensure permanent weight loss. When interviewing experts, I found a number who said that, all by itself, developing a positive self-image is not likely to lead to losing weight for good. It's my hunch that, in order for it to be helpful, improved self-esteem must be coupled with a number of the Keys to Success, such as "taking the reins," "doing it your way," "accepting the food facts" and "facing life head-on."

Beyond Weight Loss

After studying successful maintainers, Drs. Colvin and Olson drew the following conclusion: "Weight loss is not an end in itself; it is the means to an end . . . It is a means to more important goals." In fact, they suggest that weight loss as a goal in itself is a guarantee for failure.

The masters have, indeed, found far more success than simple weight loss. Their newfound lifestyles and improved self-esteem now extend to other areas of their lives:

◆ Peppi S. (62 pounds): "The how-to's of maintaining my weight spilled over into other aspects of my life. I've become a more assertive person and am willing to take risks now — be it speaking up for myself or trying things I would never try before. Losing weight has not only rid me of my fat shell, but it also stripped me of some of my inhibitions and fears. I can handle almost anything now because of all the things I've learned."

◆ Charlotte O. (96 pounds, 13 years): "I'm not afraid to stand up for myself. When I was heavy, I took what people handed me. Now, I figure if I could take enough control of my life to lose weight, I can take enough control not to let people treat me badly anymore." She adds that another big step for her is getting on an airplane by herself. "When I was heavy, I would not have done that. I was always so self-conscious about my appearance. Now, I know I can walk in anywhere."

◆ Glenda L. (45 pounds, 4 years): "Part of it is physical: I look good and have more confidence. But part of it is mental: you know you can overcome a problem and translate that to other problems. If I can do this, I can do something else. You want to do more things." When I asked Glenda what weight loss enabled her to accomplish, she replied, "Get a divorce. Things that were bad became less tolerable. I felt better about myself and felt I didn't have to put up with it anymore. I knew I could make it. I also got back into opera, which I had neglected. I knew I could do it because of the discipline of weight loss."

◆ Thalia P. (32 pounds, 4 years): "I started waking up. I had more confidence to tell others where my limits were. I began to get more respect by taking risks to be assertive. This has come very hard to me, but with continual practice, I've become more free." She admits that her career as a research and development scientist at a chocolate company presents somewhat of a problem in her struggle to maintain her weight, but adds that it is "very, very minor compared to the other changes I had to make and struggles I had to overcome in my personal growth to achieve permanent weight loss."

Once weight loss is started or completed, people gain new confidence, like themselves better and tackle new challenges. These, in turn, become powerful reinforcements for keeping the weight off.

Developing a More Fulfilled Life

Two of the studies on successful maintainers have made a similar observation: the women who lost weight and kept it off were more likely to have developed lives outside of their families. In the Kaiser Permanente study comparing female maintainers with regainers (page 64), the researchers found that significantly more maintainers had salaried positions in addition to their jobs as homemakers.

Researchers Drs. Robert Colvin and Susan Olson found that well over half of their female maintainers, while heavy, had been full-time homemakers. "The years between the ages of 18 and 35 were characterized by marriage, childbearing and rearing, semireclusion in the home . . . and weight gain." After mastering weight loss, however, Drs. Colvin and Olson reported the women had "moved out of the home into the outside world." After losing weight, more than 60 percent were full-time business and professional women. And many of the maintainers who didn't work had substantially increased the amount of time they spent outside the home.

None of this is to say that being a traditional homemaker leads to obesity or that, if you choose to remain one, you can't reduce your weight. It suggests, however, that some individuals predisposed to a weight problem may find more success in losing and maintaining weight loss if they cultivate a life outside of the home. Here's what some of the masters have to say:

◆ Vicki B. was primarily a homemaker and a mother when she was heavy. "I was happy being a stay-at-home mom, but I wasn't fulfilled. It wasn't a horrible life, but I didn't have the courage to do things because of my weight. I didn't have confidence." Now, Vicki does a lot of volunteer work and public speaking in addition to acting and professional writing. She also finds herself doing more physical activities, now that she feels "good enough to wear Levi's."

◆ Jennifer P., who established her career before starting a family, attributes her ability to make food and weight "nonissues" in part to career satisfaction: "I love my job. I'm too busy to think about food." Jennifer hasn't gained weight during the summers she's been off from her college job. She's enjoyed having that time with her two young sons. (Jennifer got a master's degree in psychology and works as a counselor.)

◆ Tami B. gained weight when she was in college and raising a small child by herself. "I couldn't get out of the house. I'd come home, watch TV and eat. I was bored. I didn't want to do anything that would put me in the public eye. Then, once I started to lose weight, I developed interests in physical activities I never would have done before, like rollerblading and aerobics. Now, I keep busy; I have an active lifestyle." (Tami completed college and is now a registered dietitian.)

◆ Charlotte O. says the biggest change in her life since losing weight has been getting a job. "When I was heavy, I was a homemaker. I baked bread, cooked for the kids and ate it all. I was happy staying at home and taking care of the kids. But I wouldn't have had the confidence to get a job. When you're heavy, you sit back and envy people who do what you want to do." Not only has Charlotte gone to work, but she has made major changes in her outside activities. "I go camping, hiking, boating, swimming. But when I was heavy, I didn't do even minor things, like play games at a family picnic. I didn't want to make a fool of myself. Now [my attitude] is, 'Okay, let's go.'"

◆ Lorene N. became very involved in a food and clothing bank as she was first losing her 61 pounds. By keeping busy, she has less time to dwell on herself and food. "I also got reinvolved with church so I have less time think about poor little me."

◆ Cindy P., the master profiled in Chapter 2, lists "staying social" as one of her top three maintenance strategies. "Being with people makes me want to stay thin." She adds, "Now, I go dancing or horseback riding instead of going out to dinner."

By now, you may have noticed the near-absence of men in this chapter. I found that few men divulged information about "getting more out of life." It may be that men are less likely to share their feelings about this subject. *Whatever the case, the techniques and advice suggested in this chapter are meant for women and men alike.*

Developing a more fulfilled life doesn't mean you have to go out and get a master's degree or have a full-time career. It simply means finding new interests, hobbies, pleasures and activities, some of which take you outside of your home. Irene S. says, "I used to play tennis, but I quit because I was fat. (I'm thinking about going back.) Now I hit golf balls with my husband, jump off the diving board and slide down a slide at the pool." Mary Ann K. is "into physical, fun activities like volleyball and bike riding. Before, I would come home, watch TV or go to the mall."

Here are some activities you can try in order to help yourself develop a more fulfilled lifestyle:

◆ **20 Small Pleasures.** Make a list of 20 things you enjoy doing and post it in a prominent place. (Think about activities that you used to like to do, perhaps before you had a family.) My patients used to find it helpful to consult their lists when they had an urge for "nonhunger" eating. Master Bob W.'s list of "simple things" that make him happy includes sharing a cup of tea with a friend, singing songs, sitting looking at the stars, watching his garden grow and playing with a neighborhood cat or dog.

◆ **The Three-List Strategy.** Each day, make three separate lists: things I *absolutely* have to do, things I want to do for me and things that can wait. The idea is to cull out the necessities and get them done promptly. Then be certain to move on to at least one or two activities that you want to do for yourself, and postpone the other stuff.

◆ **Things I've Always Wanted to Do.** Make a list of activities that you've thought about doing. Then rate their feasibility on a scale of 1 to 5, with 1 being "possible" and 5 being "impossible." (My list might include running in a marathon and taking singing lessons. I'd have to rate the marathon as "4," in part because I don't think my knees could take it, in part because I wouldn't want to take the time to train away from my family and my career. Singing lessons would be a "1": I could find a way to work them into my life.) After you develop your list and ratings, choose one or two activities that received a "1" or "2" and make a step-by-step plan of action.

Learning to Reward Yourself — Without Food

Many of the items on your lists can be used as rewards — bonuses you can give yourself for meeting certain goals when you feel good about yourself, or to boost yourself when you're feeling down. Finding ways to reward yourself is important long after you've reached your weight goal, when you no longer have the reinforcement of watching the scale go down and attention from others has waned.

As Jennifer P. was losing, she allowed herself to do anything but eat as a reward. "I'd get a haircut or new clothes. Today, I treat myself with movies, clothes, activities with the kids, going to a women's group once a month. I also see exercise as my time, my treat." When Charlotte O. went down several sizes en route to her 96-pound loss, she would go out and buy herself several dresses. She also sent herself flowers.

As seems to be the case with the masters, Dr. Ross found that a common reward used by her maintainers was clothing. She also found that getting rid of clothes that were too large was "an almost universal behavior. It was as if the commitment was being made to never again gain the weight." Master Maxine D. advises, "Give your old clothes away. If you keep them, you are saying to yourself, 'I plan to gain again.'" When Don M. reached his weight goal, he rewarded himself with new all-cotton sweaters — 27 of them! "It reminds me of accomplishing my goal, so I don't overeat."

Don also developed a reward system for himself as he was losing weight. "It used to be that I'd lose 10 pounds and reward myself with homemade ice cream or a hot fudge sundae. I was sabotaging my own efforts. Then I'd be off the diet. But when I started OPTIFAST, my wife said, 'Don't reward yourself with food.' She planted the seed, and it sprouted into music, my one vice. For each 10-pound loss, I bought myself a compact disc or a tape."

Similarly, when Donna C. was losing her 108 pounds, if she

went down a size, she might buy herself new clothing, "not a hot fudge sundae." When getting together with a friend, she might suggest going for a walk or to a movie. Vicki B. also gave herself new treats as she was losing. "At a certain point, I planned a professional [beauty] makeover; at another point, I got my nails done — I have ever since. Now, I try to base my rewards less on pounds lost and more on my level of exercise and keeping my fat intake down. I might treat myself to a massage, a hairstyle or new perfume."

Irene S. says that when she first started losing weight (she also gave up alcohol at the same time), she went through a period of feeling, "This is no fun." Then she decided, "I have to face things with a clearer head. Now, I will take a nap, a bubble bath, do a facial mask, listen to a relaxation tape or elevate my legs and read. I may take a whole day and pamper myself, do whatever I want to do."

She periodically rewards herself by looking at three photos of herself: before, during and after her 77-pound loss. She admits, "I have to constantly remind myself of my success." Similarly, Peppi S. keeps a picture from when she was heavy and glances at it when she feels dissatisfied with her body. "I need to accept that there is always room for improvement, but I've come a long way."

Taking Care of Your Own Needs

Drs. Colvin and Olson found that their female success stories had become "selfish," meaning they had learned to act in their own self-interest. (The psychologists also state that most men in their study didn't see this issue "as a big deal.")

A number of masters confirmed the psychologists' findings:

◆ Jennifer P. told me, "It's important for me to know my own needs, wants and desires in addition to helping others. But when I help others, it's a choice. I try to be human, not perfect."

◆ Vicki B.: Her philosophy is, "You can't fill others' needs unless your own are met. Like a lot of women, I spent a lot of time doing things for everyone else and feeling put upon and hating it. I started taking care of my own needs. When I started running, my 5-year-old son wanted to come with me. I felt bad, but I knew if he did, it would have thrown off my plan for myself." It was hard, but Vicki had to say no.

◆ Mary Ann K.: Shortly before her decision to lose weight, her father died. "I was always taking care of him, always taking care of others." Then she read a book about codependency. "I learned I had been a second-class family member. It took about six months to say, 'Hey, I'm as important as everyone else.' If you're not number one physically and mentally, you're not good for anyone else."

◆ Irene S.: As she approached readiness to lose weight, she said to herself, "I am important, so why aren't I doing something about it?" She added, "I needed to be selfish and prioritize. I think a lot of fat people don't give themselves time and attention because they don't feel good about themselves."

◆ Charlotte O.: She still feels her children come first. "But," she stated, "instead of it being the kids, my husband, the dog, then me — I've moved myself up to second."

◆ Ann F.: One of her top priorities is to take good physical care of herself. "I have to exercise, eat well and sleep. I can give more to others when I'm less worried about what I'm not doing. Today, [before work] it took me 20 minutes to put together my breakfast and lunch. I have no qualms about it."

Changing Relationships

When you start to feel better about yourself, cultivate new interests, get involved in a career or other outside activities, take care of your own needs more, become more active and look better because of your weight loss, these changes can affect your relationships. *For some masters, the impact was painful, but apparently best for them in the long run.* Susan C., the master profiled in Chapter IV, stated that when she lost her weight, she also lost her first husband. "My husband had been happy with me the way I was. But when I lost weight, I wanted to go dancing, go to parties, wear nice clothes. Men started looking at me. I got a sports car. My head started spinning. I went out a lot with friends and did things I'd never done before. My husband and I grew apart, and the marriage ended."

Jeffrey B. thinks, too, that his weight loss of 55 pounds had something to do with his marital split. "I started to fool around. I never had the confidence to do that before." About a year after Charlotte O. lost 96 pounds, her then-husband told her he would have left her if she hadn't lost weight. She decided, "'If that's all there is [to our marriage] . . .' so I went out and got a job. I changed everything. He couldn't understand the changes. We drifted apart, and about two to three years later, we got a divorce." Finally, Thalia P. stated that the changes she had to make to keep her weight off led to her recent separation from her husband. "I am sad about this, but ultimately I'm becoming more and more myself and not living by someone else's rules."

The conclusion to be drawn is not that losing weight and losing your spouse go hand in hand. Rather, it's important to realize that all change entails risk.

There are masters who note positive changes in relationships since their weight loss. Lorene N. and her husband decided to work through their marital problems by getting counseling. Vicki B. found, "The sparkle came back into my marriage. My husband started sending me flowers. He wanted to show me off." Irene S. notes that, when she first started losing, her husband would encourage her to eat fattening things. "When he really noticed the changes, he got kind of ugly. I think he thought I had a boyfriend. Then he started walking with me. Now, he's proud of me and tries to emulate me. Our relationship is better." Mary Ann K.'s husband also became her partner in exercise. "At my halfway point, he decided to lose 40 pounds." Now, they work out at a gym together.

Some people noted positive changes in relationships outside of their marriages. Jennifer P. states, "People treat you differently. I feel that, jobwise, people see me as a more disciplined, professional person." As for friendships, she adds, "When I was in college, I used to pick a friend and hide behind her. Now I have a greater variety of friends. Having more self-esteem because of the weight loss has allowed me to branch out more." Vicki B. finds that she, too, has more friends since her weight loss. "It's not because people didn't like me, but because I have the confidence to make friends. It has opened up avenues because I feel good about myself."

When people lose weight, another part of changing relationships can be others' reactions to the "new you." Some of the people in Dr. Ross's study found that certain of their friends were supportive until their success became obvious. Then they became jealous and almost mean. "It took adjustment and sometimes loss of a friendship before the issue was resolved." Master Liz D. found after she first lost her 55 pounds, "I really got tired of everybody noticing and talking about it, seemingly constantly. I just wanted to be normal, to be just an average person instead of having to talk about it to everyone. I guess I was putting so much pressure on myself to succeed that I felt anyone who talked about my weight loss was just adding pressure. But now I have come to enjoy talking about it and try to encourage others who are dealing with weight."

You Are Much More Than Your Weight

Reaching your goal weight isn't all there is to life. Jennifer P., for instance, sometimes thinks she could stand to lose another 10 pounds. So she talks to herself, saying, "Life is not a beauty contest. Who cares if I weigh 130 or 140? I'm fine the way I am, and it isn't worth giving up other things to focus on that."

Likewise, Connie M. feels that it's important to enjoy life and not worry about being a size 10. "I'm satisfied with myself at a size 12. Life's too short to struggle with your weight. Goal weight is important, but not to the extent that it's the most important thing in your life. The emphasis is on the thin body, but let's be healthy and happy too." Similarly, Dr. Joyce Nash states, "Life is not about weight control. When you find yourself at the pearly gates, God forbid that you should say to St. Peter when he asks what you did with your life, 'I watched my weight.'"

It may help to de-emphasize the importance of appearance, as you find other sources of satisfaction. Consider the things happy people have in common, according to psychologists John Foreyt and G. Ken Goodrick in their book, *Living Without Dieting:* they are active and busy, spend more time socializing, are organized, are productive at meaningful work, are realistic in their goals, have close relationships and focus on the positive. Nowhere do you see mention of appearance. Placing too much value on attractiveness thwarts personal development and can prevent you from feeling good about yourself and going out and getting more out of life. As master Ann B. states, "Part of my feeling good is that I'm not caught up in how society says you have to look."

Paradoxically, this acceptance that life is about more than weight control and appearance leads to weight loss — at least for some people. Kelly S. states that her motivation to lose weight once and for all came when she realized that her "entire life and self-worth" were tied up in her weight. "Very draining and unempowering," she says. Likewise, Becky M. attributes her success to being able to look beyond her appearance. "There's so much more to life than weight!" She says this acceptance enabled her to lose 40 pounds, which she's kept off for 12 years — minus the periods when she had her five children.

*   *   *

If you stop allowing your weight to get in the way of a more fulfilling life, as well as feeling good about yourself, the need to use food to enrich your existence will diminish. Then you can get on with more important aspects of life — those things that make it worthwhile to maintain whatever weight you choose.

10

Key to Success #10

Don't Go It Alone

Now that you've accepted responsibility for your weight, you should be able to go it alone. Right? Not necessarily. Taking the reins, making exercise a way of life and getting more out of life may seem like overwhelming propositions. *The good news is: you don't have to go it alone.* Many masters turn to others for support, some on a regular basis, others as needed.

Weight-control experts have determined that support from family and friends is associated with long-term success at weight control. Conversely, lack of encouragement and interpersonal conflict can lead to relapse. So how can you use support from others to work for you? Whom should you turn to — a professional, a group or an individual who's close to you? How can you deal with people who are not supportive of your weight-control efforts? Examples from the masters will show that you can find strength from others in your effort to take personal control of your weight.

Muriel and Jordan F.'s Stories

They lost weight together, they keep it off together. Combined, they've lost more than 100 pounds and have maintained that loss for 3 years. I knew Muriel and Jordan F. would have a lot to say about "Don't Go It Alone" when she wrote me, "My husband and I did our program together, and we support each other strongly." He told me, "We do it together; I have to watch her, and she watches me." Yet they don't have a watchdog relationship: they maintain a strong sense of independence along with the sharing that characterizes their lives together.

After a lifetime of struggling with weight, it took both of them until they were in their fifties to finally find success. Years ago, Muriel was inspired by Oprah Winfrey's weight loss, so she decided to try Health Management Resources' liquid diet. Jordan joined the program, too, but only to support Muriel. "I didn't think it would be successful beyond the diet. It was just another attempt. I figured we'd lose and regain the weight." Muriel did the liquid "fast" for 16 weeks and went from 207 to 150 pounds. (She's 5′5″ tall.) Jordan could only take the fast for about two weeks. "It bothered me. So they told me to add a 4-ounce potato to the liquid meals each day. That worked for me." Within 12 weeks, Jordan dropped from 242 pounds to 205. (He's 6′2″.)

What led Muriel and Jordan to this point? Muriel's battle with weight began when she was a teenager. At the age of 19, when she was about 30 pounds overweight, her doctor gave her diet pills. But she never lost much weight, and her pharmacist eventually refused to refill the prescription. As she got older and had two children, her weight steadily increased and tended to stay around 185 — that is, when she wasn't trying some new weight-loss scheme. "I tried every one of them — TOPS, Weight Watchers, Overeaters Anonymous, Weight Loss Clinic and Diet Workshop." With most programs, she had very little success.

When I asked her what she thought was the main cause of her weight problem, she responded, "Being home with my kids, not working, boredom, not thinking about what I ate and watching TV." She added that socializing played a role as well. "Any time we got together with friends, food was involved. We would play cards, but the snacks were very important."

Muriel went back to work in the 1970s, when her children were teenagers. Around 1980, she had her greatest success until that time with Diet Center; she lost 60 pounds, but slowly regained the weight.

Then several important events came together. Muriel was working as the administrator of a synagogue when the rabbi, who was also a health-conscious friend, said to her, "Muriel, please, for your own sake do something about your weight." She felt that his comment came from caring, not meanness. At the same time, it really sunk in that her mother had died when she was 65. Muriel was 50 when the rabbi spoke to her, and she realized that she was "getting older and wanted to live longer. I knew I had to do something."

In retrospect, Muriel now sees as well that her father's death had an impact on her readiness to lose weight. I asked her if it had been difficult to lose weight during that stressful time. "I loved my dad, but there are certain things from childhood that I don't forget," she replied. "When he died, I was finally free. He always wanted me to be a blonde: I was the fat blonde. Now, I'm the slim brunette." Today, Muriel can see what her weight may have been doing for her. "My father wasn't pleased about my weight. I may have kept it on in anger. It was the only way I could show my disapproval of him. As long as he was around, I had one thing over him: the weight. When my father died, I grew up."

When did Jordan's weight problem start? "I was always overweight, always the biggest baby, always fat. My parents were both heavy." Jordan's father owned a bakery, and pastry and baked goods were always in the home. "If we were good, pastry was the reward." Jordan also recalls "coming home from school, throwing a steak under the broiler, eating it as a snack, then eating dinner shortly thereafter. There was always lots of food around, and I always indulged in it." By the time he graduated from high school, he weighed 262 pounds.

Like Muriel's, Jordan's first serious attempt at weight loss, when he was in his late twenties, involved diet pills. "I lost 40 or

50 pounds but gained it back when I went off the pills." From there he "tried the gamut": Weight Loss Clinic, Diet Workshop and Weight Watchers, to name a few. But the most he would lose was about 20 pounds.

Jordan doesn't recall any critical event or change in motivation that led to his readiness to lose even more weight four years ago. He merely did it for Muriel. The difference for him from all the other times was "education from a dietitian." Specifically, he related to HMR's intense education about calorie intake and expenditure. "I learned that if I exercised to this level and ate this food, I should lose weight. I believed it because they proved it to me. I'm an engineer, and I identified with the facts and figures. It was purely educational." As an example, Jordan remembers the time the dietitian demonstrated how the calories can add up in a typical tuna sandwich: "She showed us the tuna, the bread and all the mayonnaise." Muriel concurs, "The key was working with a registered dietitian. The most important things we learned were about fat, calories and portions. We just never knew about it." And of course, the support from each other played an important role.

Neither Muriel nor Jordan had a difficult time making the transition from the liquid diet to "real" food, primarily because they stuck with the HMR program and retrained their eating habits. Muriel states, "We were weaned onto good foods, so there was no problem." For Jordan, the transition to low-fat "real" foods was exciting but somewhat scary. "But I continued to lose weight, so I was encouraged." Muriel and Jordan stayed in HMR's maintenance group and saw the dietitian regularly for about a year. Had they not had this follow-up, they both feel they probably would have gained the weight back. Muriel states, "The learning process continued that year."

What about now? Jordan has elected not to continue with any support system other than Muriel but admits he could use help: his weight is up some, in part because he hasn't been able to exercise. Muriel has found it difficult to exercise as well. They both have long commutes and are in the process of moving but plan to get back into exercise when they relocate. Jordan admits, "It makes me feel good, and it's good for me."

Muriel now goes to a Jenny Craig facility, which she decided to join the summer of her second year of maintenance after she regained 18 pounds. That was when she discovered she is not the type of person who can "have a little. I love sweets. If I have one little piece, the next time it's bigger." She also attributes the weight rebound to giving in to friends who wanted to go to restaurants with poor food choices. "I realized I couldn't make everyone else happy. I had to either back off or stand my ground." She stood her ground, and friends now "ask her permission" before selecting restaurants.

She chose Jenny Craig because it was local, and she found it to be a good program. Although she does not consider herself a group person, she enjoyed the classes. Muriel continues to go back once a month to weigh in. That way, if she ever gains weight, she says she can go back to the program at no charge.

Currently Muriel weighs 152, down 55 pounds from her all-time high. At a weight of 196, Jordan is 69 pounds down from his maximum weight. They both feel it was critical that they achieved their success together. Says Jordan, "I probably wouldn't have done it without her." Although they go their separate ways during the day, their maintenance eating patterns are similar: three low-fat meals a day with several snacks in between. (Muriel can tell you exactly when she eats them.) Unlike Muriel, Jordan allows himself occasional treats like a piece of pizza, a drink or candy. Most evenings they both treat themselves to a "measured" cup of low-fat ice cream.

When it comes to planning and cooking meals, they work as a team. Jordan states, "We both work, so it's unfair for me to come home and say, 'Make me supper.' So we share the responsibility. We plan ahead and make sure someone has purchased the food for supper." Muriel adds, "He loves to cook, and I like to clean up." Jordan has become "a fanatic about oil and butter and the way they're used in food." Yet he has learned creative alternative ways to make food tasty. For instance, he talked about making broccoli with peppers, scallions, lemon juice and a little Parmesan cheese.

It's quite clear that the main source of support for Muriel and Jordan is each other. She maintains, "We talk about what we're doing all the time. We catch each other. One of us might say, 'I think you're losing it.' It's not critical or mean, just caring."

Support for the Support Theory

Like Muriel and Jordan, a number of masters told me they find support for their maintenance efforts from significant people in their lives — spouses, friends, relatives, counselors or groups.

◆ Michael and Cindy F. are another couple who control their weight together. Combined, they've lost 288 pounds, and each has kept weight off for at least 7 years. In addition to their joint efforts, both say that one of their keys to success is continued involvement with Weight Watchers.

◆ Linda Sue S. (78 pounds, 6 years) continues to see her counselor at Diet Center if she gains some weight.

◆ Mary B. (90 pounds, 11½ years) goes to a weekly Take Off Pounds Sensibly (TOPS) meeting.

◆ Cindy B. (38 pounds, 3 years) weighs in once a month at Weight Watchers.

◆ Bob W. (250 pounds, 21 years) initially lost weight by going to Weight Watchers but now goes to Overeaters Anonymous for support.

◆ Steve S. (210 pounds, 13 years) has gone back to the HMR program (where he lost his weight) four times in the last 13 years for "professional coaching" when he began to gain.

◆ Mary Ann K. (84 pounds, 3 years) returns to Jenny Craig classes when "I feel like I'm slipping."

◆ Connye Z. (34 pounds, 5½ years) gets support from her husband. "To this day, he still comments on my size, like 'Let me see those skinny legs!'" Connye also goes to Weight Watchers once a month.

◆ Jim J. (181 pounds, 5 years) goes to a weekly class with fellow long-term maintainers and talks on the phone with a professional weight-control counselor once a week. He also finds support from his wife, who makes an effort to cook low-fat foods.

A number of studies involving individuals who were enrolled in research-based weight-loss programs lend strong credence to the notion that getting support is important for maintenance, at least for certain people. Some of the most important work was conducted by Michael G. Perri, Ph.D., currently at the University of Florida, and coworkers. They completed a series of studies suggesting that support — from therapists or peers — is associated with the ability to maintain weight loss. All people in their studies were mildly to moderately obese when first treated with a comprehensive behavioral program that included a 1,000-to-1,500-calorie diet, behavior-modification techniques and positive-thinking strategies. Afterward, some of the patients received no further treatment. Others were assigned to various combinations of maintenance strategies, including the following: an aerobic exercise program; relapse-prevention training; ongoing therapist contact by mail and telephone; and peer support groups that met regularly to monitor weight, to praise and encourage each other and to use problem-solving strategies. (The therapists in most of these studies were either psychologists or graduate psychology students.)

The studies consistently indicated that people who received therapist and/or peer support kept off more weight than did those without such support. Moreover, people who took part in multiple maintenance strategies tended to do better than did those who simply went through the behavioral program or who were involved in one maintenance strategy. For instance, one of Dr. Perri's studies revealed that the group receiving three different maintenance strategies, as opposed to one or two, was the only group that showed significant *additional* weight loss during the 18-month follow-up period. People in this group maintained almost all of their initial weight loss. Dr. Perri and his coworkers concluded that the combination of therapist contact, frequent exercise and peer support holds promise for improving weight maintenance.

In another study, Dr. Perri examined the value of weight-maintenance programs involving peer support, therapist support or neither in 3 different groups of people. The groups involving either form of support maintained their weight loss significantly better than did those without such support.

What conclusions should you draw from these studies? First, support has something to do with maintenance. Second, multifaceted approaches to maintenance are best. In other words, finding support alone may not sustain weight loss. But when support is coupled with such Keys to Success as exercise, problem solving and facing the food facts, the prospect of losing weight and keeping it off is enhanced.

Support can also come from a commercial weight-loss group such as Weight Watchers or a self-help group like TOPS or Overeaters Anonymous. One study revealed that Weight Watchers members who continued to attend meetings in the same location and with the same leader after reaching their goal weights were more likely to keep their weight off than were members who did not.

Finally, support can come from family and friends. Robert

Jeffery and colleagues at the University of Minnesota studied a group of overweight men who had taken part in a 15-week behavior-modification program. The men were later contacted to see what factors had contributed to successful maintenance. One factor was support of family and friends. (Support was defined as family cooperation in weight-loss efforts or as having friends who had changed eating or exercise behavior in response to the study participants' involvement in the weight-loss program.) Two years after the initial program, men who reported high family cooperation kept off about 21 pounds; those with low cooperation from families kept off an average of about 6 pounds. The men who reported that friends had changed their diets kept 19 pounds off; those who reported no changes on the part of friends had maintained only about a 10-pound loss. This study also found that men who used a variety of different techniques to keep their weight off were the most successful.

What Can a Support System Do for You?

Whether you elect to seek the help of a professional counselor, formal group, friend or family member, having a support person or persons can do a lot to keep you at your new weight. What can you get from others?

◆ **Advice and new ideas.** Sometimes it helps to have input — say, when you're having a rough time with food intake, struggling with a personal problem that makes you want to overeat, slacking off on exercise or anticipating a social situation. Jim J. admits that, in the past, he'd use any excuse to "blow it all off. I would gain 5, then 10 pounds and throw up my hands. Now, if I gain 5 pounds, the group helps head me off. It talks openly and helps you come up with a plan." He particularly benefits from the last 15 minutes of his weekly maintenance group, when members pair off to come up with a plan or "tricks" for the week ahead.

"Sometimes, it helps to hear someone say, 'Why don't you try this again?' The broader your repertoire of tricks, the better off you are."

◆ **Empathy, encouragement and commendation.** After having kept off 71 pounds for 4 years, Mary S. has found, "The general public doesn't want to hear about my problems or my diet. My family is tired of hearing about it." But when she goes to her maintenance group, she can "let my hair down."

◆ **Education.** As Muriel and Jordan stated, the knowledge they gained from a dietitian about calories, fat and energy expenditure was invaluable. Likewise, Connye Z. gained new ideas from Weight Watchers, "like steaming vegetables." She added, "I really internalized which foods were better for me or lower in calories. I changed my eating habits, and I haven't changed them back."

◆ **Assurance that you are not alone.** Nick R., who once weighed 288 pounds and now holds his own at 210 (he's 6'2" tall), finds that going to OA allows sharing of common experiences, "like when I used to eat on my way home, but didn't tell my wife, then I'd eat dinner. [At OA] when you see the nods, you know they understand, so you don't feel like you're so different."

◆ **Help with getting your problems in perspective.** After Jim J. took a recent 3-week vacation from work and his maintenance group, he worried that he had regained weight and became "a little panicky. After all the years of being heavy, I thought, 'Maybe I really am slipping.'" But talking with his counselor and returning to group meetings helped him get things in perspective and reassured him.

◆ **Heightened accountability to yourself.** Connye Z. has been at her goal of 118 pounds for nearly 6 years, yet she goes to Weight Watchers once a month to weigh in and sometimes stays for the meetings. "They record your weight in a book that you keep. It motivates me to see the stability once a month."

◆ **Constructive criticism from others.** Muriel and Jim "catch" each other in a caring way. Jim V. gets his feedback from his dietitian who, as noted in Chapter 7, reminds him of all his hard work and how far he's come. Steve S. makes the following analogy: "Just as any professional athlete needs a coach, sometimes you need someone with an objective eye outside of you."

◆ **Reminders of where you've come from and what you need to do to stay there.** Joy B., who's kept off 35 pounds for more than 4 years, finds, "I just slide a bit, get lazy or space out every once in a while and find that I've put on 3 to 5 pounds without even knowing it. If I do gain a few pounds, I find going back to Weight Watchers meetings really helps me. It reminds me of why I want to be at a certain weight [115; she's 5'1"], and the process of going 'on-program' makes me recheck portion sizes and reeducate myself."

Support or No Support?

Before discussing the best type of support system for you, let's address the question "How do you know when you need support?" Does everyone who wants to be thin for life have to undergo intense long-term treatment and maintenance programs? Obviously not — as demonstrated by the many masters who lost weight and keep it off on their own. It's really a question of how frequently and how intensely you need support and from whom.

For certain formerly overweight people, long-term help is required. The same applies to other problems, such as alcohol dependence: while some individuals quit drinking on their own, others get aid from a self-help group for the rest of their lives. They need that reinforcement all the time, whether they're doing well or struggling. Master Jim J. feels he needs intense support. He maintains his 181-pound loss by going to weekly meetings with other maintainers at the HMR facility where he lost weight more than 5 years ago, and he also checks in with his behavioral counselor by phone once a week. He states, "I'm a lifer, if that's what it's going to take."

Others, like Jordan F., get professional support for a while, then go it alone, knowing they can return for help if they need it. Some people use support only for crisis intervention — if, for instance, they've been maintaining their weight for years and suddenly gain 5 or 10 pounds. Master Ed G., for example, has kept off at least 30 pounds for 17 years. When his weight creeps up, he returns to Weight Watchers. "I've gone back twice now; I need to do it again." (At a height of 5′10″, he's up about 10 pounds above his desired weight of 170.)

Many people, like Muriel and Jordan, need more support in the beginning, within the first year or two of reaching their goal weights. Franca Alphin, R.D., former nutrition director at Duke University's Diet and Fitness Center (a residential weight-loss facility), notes that a number of their successful patients come back for a "refresher" three to four times the first year. Within a few years, they return just once a year.

The trick is to not let your weight get out of hand before you take action. And having some place to turn, particularly right after you've reached your goal, may be critical to your success. *Like many people, you've probably had some success with weight loss but very little with weight maintenance, and it's critical to get support before matters feel out of control.*

It's not always easy to seek help when you've gained, admits Teresa M., who has gone through HMR's "restart" program twice, after she gained back some weight. "I felt like a failure, but I wanted to be thin more than anything. They made me see the positive." After initially losing about 60 pounds, she's never crept back up to her all-time high of 196, but she has regained as much as 30 pounds. Unlike her first attempt with HMR, however, she currently goes to weekly classes with fellow maintainers. (She's now down to 140.)

Time and time again, I had patients who would stop coming for appointments when they regained some weight. Some would refuse to come in until they were "doing better." *They didn't realize that they needed help most when they were struggling.* As the University of Pennsylvania's Dr. Thomas Wadden points out, avoiding help when you're having a hard time with your food intake is analogous to avoiding your physician when you have the flu!

The masters, on the other hand, recognize when they need outside aid. Paul A., for example, found his weight creeping up when he stopped his involvement with Weight Watchers. "I realized it was because I didn't have my support group, and that within a year, I'd be back up 60 pounds." Paul returned to Weight Watchers and is now one of their leaders. Likewise, Peppi S. lost 65 pounds in 1986, which she maintained until 1½ years later when she had a debilitating back injury. She regained about 40 pounds, but went back to Nutri/System to lose the extra weight and now maintains at about 138, down 62 pounds from her all-time high.

What Are Some Warning Signs That You Need Support?

♦ You are 5 to 10 pounds over your goal weight and cannot seem to lose it. Says Ed G., who goes back to Weight Watchers, "Every once in a while, I think I can do it on my own, but I don't."

♦ Your "thin" clothes are getting tight, and you find yourself buying new, bigger clothes. Teresa M. told me, "When my clothes didn't fit, I knew I had to do something, or I'd be right back where I started."

♦ You find the "tricks" that used to help you control your weight are no longer effective. Muriel F. knows she needs help when "I find myself falling off, eating high-fat foods."

◆ You find yourself turning to food to handle stress or problems. When Jim V. finds himself eating without thinking when he's under pressure, he visits his dietitian.

◆ Your mental attitude has changed. Jordan F. realizes he has a problem when he finds himself not being as careful with food, succumbing to pressure to eat in social situations.

◆ You find yourself getting lazy. Mary Ann K. says she goes back to Jenny Craig when she starts buying high-fat foods again — like ice cream instead of yogurt — and when she slacks off on exercise.

◆ You are feeling somewhat hopeless about your weight, wondering if the effort is worth it, or you feel out of control. After losing more than 25 pounds with TOPS, Maxine D. found herself regaining when she no longer had transportation to get to meetings. (She does not drive.) "I was actually only 5 pounds over, but out of control." Then her husband agreed to take her each week and wait for her. Now, she faithfully attends meetings and has kept off 38 pounds for 9 years.

Finding Support That's Right for You

The most effective way to head off trouble is to have a support system in place before the "warning signs" hit, as does Muriel F., who maintains her relationship with Jenny Craig so she can return if she needs to. If you're a private person, you may prefer to get support from an individual counselor, close friend or family member. If, however, you're more of a social, self-disclosing, outgoing person, a group situation may be more to your liking. Here are some factors to consider when making your selection:

◆ **Individual counseling.** If you're a loner, you may feel more comfortable finding a support person with expertise in weight control: a psychologist, physician, registered dietitian, social worker or trained employee of a weight-loss organization. (This is for counseling for weight-related issues, not for psychological problems.) You may want to go for a few in-depth visits, then go back on an "as-needed" basis. Or you may start out with more frequent visits, then taper off. For the first several years after she lost her 50-plus pounds, Susan D. saw a dietitian "religiously" every week. "I'm the type of person who needs to be monitored. It helps me to focus." Now, she's on her own but plans to join the YMCA and possibly go back to a dietitian.

You can also get one-on-one support from a peer at a group like Overeaters Anonymous. Attendees are encouraged to form a relationship with another OA member whom they call a "sponsor." These people are not trained weight-control counselors; they're fellow group members who are experienced with the OA program. Some masters find great support from their sponsors. Nick R. says of his, "That person understands me. With a sponsor, you can also share personal stuff that you couldn't share at a meeting." In return, if you become a sponsor, as Bob says, "you have to live it. It's an incentive to be honest. It makes you appreciate what you have and where you've been."

◆ **Group support.** Many people like groups because they find it helpful to be with others who have the same problem. "We're in it together," says Jim J. of his group of fellow maintainers. Connye Z., who lost 34 pounds with the help of Weight Watchers, found, "To hear people say that they had a similar success or similar problem was encouraging — to know they had gone through it too. They're encouraging. Once I gained 2 pounds, and they said, 'Oh, you're still way under your goal.'" And you may want to join a group with a few friends. A study by Drs. Rena Wing of Brown University and Robert Jeffery of the University of Minnesota found that people who participated in a behavioral weight-loss program with a group of four friends were better able to maintain weight loss 6 months afterward than were people who were loners in a similar program.

Another advantage of groups is the motivation you can get

from being around others who have found success. When Nick R. first went to OA and saw thin people there, it gave him hope. "I saw people who were losing weight, and their lives were getting better." After having kept off 78 pounds for 5 years, Nick points out that there can also be great satisfaction in helping someone else.

Groups can also provide a way to "get more out of life." Maxine D., for instance, says she has "an enlarged social life with all the TOPS family." Mary S. says of her maintenance group, "We shared hints. We discussed upcoming events and how to cope." Finally, some maintainers, like Paul A., choose to lead weight-control groups because, "For me, it isn't enough to go to meetings. I need to stand before the group. It's a watchdog for me; I can't be in front of the group and not keep my weight down."

If you go the group route, it pays to shop around. Muriel F. found self-help groups to be discouraging because of members who could eat more than she, yet still lose weight. Yet she liked the professionally run group at HMR because, "It was only learning. There were no comparisons of weight gain or loss."

Shopping around entails checking out umbrella groups, as well as individual chapters. For example, don't rule out TOPS, OA or Weight Watchers on the basis of one meeting and one group. If you investigate several different meetings or chapters, you may find that you like the personality of one group or leader better than another. The size of the group may enter into your decision: some individual groups of any one organization are larger than others. (TOPS and OA are self-help groups, while Weight Watchers meetings have a leader who lost weight on the program. Another option chosen by certain masters is a weight-loss group run by a local hospital.)

Instead of attending a formal weight-loss group, you may want to start one of your own. It could be a group of friends, or you could start a low-fat cooking class. Another possibility would be to approach a local dietitian or psychologist to lead a group of fellow maintainers. (Of course, you'd have to pay him or her.) It's probably wise for the group to set up certain ground rules for attendance and for calling each other between meetings or if someone doesn't show up. The group could also have a particular focus, such as a helpful weight-loss book or a weekly predetermined topic.

◆ **Support from family and friends.** Many maintainers get their support from an individual. Like Muriel and Jordan F., Cindy and Michael F. attribute much of their success to their "team approach." Cindy states, "We plan meals and work together to keep our motivation high." Connye Z.'s husband is willing to eat low-fat cooking and keep tempting foods out of the house. She says of her husband, "Since he won't cook, he eats whatever I prepare. None of this preparing two different meals. We do not keep candy and potato chips in the house. He did not try to sabotage my efforts by cooking or offering foods I needed to stay away from."

Mary Ann K. involves her whole family in the process of maintenance. Not only do she and her husband help each other in the kitchen, they share their knowledge about low-fat cooking with their kids. She exclaims, "All four of us support each other!"

Rosemary O. turns to her sister. Nearly six years ago, they joined a weight-loss program at a medical center, and they continue to work on maintenance as a team. "We live together, work together, play together, walk together. We talk about it. I ask [my sister] to keep reminding me how to eat. It's a togetherness issue."

Interestingly, studies on the effectiveness of involving spouses in weight-control efforts have yielded conflicting results, probably because some people are better off with group support, while others prefer to go it alone, and still others simply have unsupportive spouses. In the Kaiser Permanente study comparing maintainers with regainers, more than half of both groups of women reported their husbands were not supportive. Another study showed that more than 40 percent of the participants identified family members as both the most and least helpful people in their weight-management efforts. Studies suggest that spouses who are taught to provide support for their partner's weight-loss efforts can become effective allies.

If you decide you would like to enlist an individual for support, you have to pick the right person and train that person about how to be supportive. How can you get what you need? As trite as it may sound, you have to communicate. As a case in point, Jordan F. talked about how, when he was on the liquid diet, he had to travel with superiors who were into wining and dining. "I was afraid to go, so I talked with my boss, who talked with his boss. They were very supportive and told me to do whatever I needed to do. There was no ridicule."

What Should You Look For in a Support Person?

- Someone with whom you feel comfortable talking about your weight and problems having to do with your weight.
- Someone who compliments you, for instance, when you do something well or look nice.
- Someone who reassures you when things are not going your way.
- Someone who, in a pinch, would help you — say, with child-care or transportation.
- Someone who is honest with you in a nice way and will give you feedback.
- Someone who is available to you most of the time.
- Someone to whom you can talk even when you are not doing well with weight control.
- Someone who offers good advice and helps you through crises.
- Someone who shares feelings and problems.
- Someone who supports your taking responsibility for your weight problem.

What Don't You Want in a Support Person?

- Someone who hassles you or makes too many demands on you.
- Someone who doesn't understand having a weight problem.
- Someone who offers you food or pushes it on you when it's clear you are watching your weight.
- Someone who says critical things about you and your weight or about overweight people.
- Someone who is jealous of you or competitive with you.
- Someone who is self-righteous and/or who thinks he or she has all the answers.
- Someone who is also struggling with weight and who encourages you to indulge with him or her.
- Someone who offers simplistic advice like, "Just eat less," "Push yourself away from the table" or "Simply cut your portions in half."
- Someone who makes you feel as if you're constantly being watched.

To sum up, if you choose not to go it alone, you have to find the support system that works for you. If, like Paul A., your spouse is not supportive enough, you may want to turn to a group or professional. He told me, "My wife doesn't have a weight problem. After I lost weight, I felt like I needed support, so I became a Weight Watchers leader." Some people combine support systems. At various times, Muriel F. has had all three: professional, group and family. But like Muriel, you may find that what is right for you at one time doesn't suit you at another, so you need to switch support systems. For example, if you lost weight through a group program, the group may suit you just fine for a while. But with time, you may tire of sitting in the same room with the same people, or you may find you don't want to be with folks at earlier stages of weight control. At that point, you could hook up with a professional for "as-needed" support.

Dealing with Nonsupport

The word "sabotage" frequently creeps up among weight-control experts. You have control over sabotage and can often put a stop to it.

A common form of sabotage described by many masters is performed at the hands of the "food pusher," someone who tries to force food upon you. Jim J. says he encounters this all the time. "I might be sipping Perrier at a bar, and someone will say, 'Are you going to be on a diet your whole life?'" Jim may tell him, "I'd rather save my calories for something later." He adds, "You have to speak your mind and be up-front about what you need." Likewise, Muriel F., who has found that she "can't eat just one" of certain foods, deals with food pushers by firmly letting them know, "This is not what I care to do or want to do." (She admits that sometimes she will take the unwanted item "to get the person off my back." But she leaves the food on her plate.)

The importance of these skills is reinforced by preliminary results from a study of 224 women and men who completed the Nutri/System Weight Loss Program. Yale University researchers studied these people to determine what strategies they used to maintain weight 2 years after they finished the program. Individuals who said others tried to interfere with their efforts to keep weight off — for instance, by encouraging them to eat high-calorie foods — were less successful in maintaining their weight losses than were those who reported no interference.

However, another critical determinant of success was the way people handled interference. Researcher Michaela Kiernan, Ph.D., who is now at Stanford University, reported that even in the face of interference, people maintained their weight loss as well as those who had no interference if they took two steps: 1) they refused to give in, and 2) they explicitly said, "No."

Mary S. has learned to be assertive in order to keep off her 71 pounds. She is a school secretary who finds that coworkers often bring "their excess fatty food to work." They tend to place it by the office coffeepot, which is near her desk. "I asked them to move it elsewhere. Once I got a little too excited and told them, 'I'm allergic to fat; I break out!'"

Another form of sabotage can occur within your social circle, particularly if it tends to be food-centered. Note how Muriel F. "stood her ground" in order to get her friends to go to more healthful restaurants. As in her case, you don't have to cut yourself off from your friends: just communicate and make compromises with them.

Certain cultural philosophies about how you should eat or how thin you should be can interfere with your weight-loss efforts. Rosemary O., for instance, is of Lebanese/Italian heritage, cultures that tend to place high value on the connection between food and affection. Not surprisingly, her mother is a "food pusher" and an "exceptionally fine cook and baker." When Rosemary refuses food or leaves something on her plate at the end of a meal, her mother takes it personally. How does Rosemary respond? "I am just very firm. I tell her, 'If you ask me again, I'll just have to keep saying no.'" She adds, "It is still hard for me; it leads to confrontation."

Sometimes sabotage comes from within, from our "shoulds" about food and relationships. Don M. states, "I wanted to be loved, and food equaled love. I couldn't say no when something was given to me."

Jennifer P. sometimes has to deal with her overweight sister who feels it is an affront to a host or hostess not to eat everything offered. "Somehow, to my sister, it's saying 'I'm important and you're not,'" observes Jennifer. If you suspect a loved one is threatened by your weight loss — for example, your husband because you look more attractive at your new weight — talk with him about what he's feeling and offer reassurance.

Whatever the sabotaging situation, psychologist Joyce Nash advises that you give the saboteur a coherent message. In *Now*

That You've Lost It, she warns, "Avoid saying no with your voice, but yes with your eyes." She also suggests making it clear in your tone of voice and body posture that you really mean what you say.

Let the person know you appreciate the offer, but be direct and open, firmly stating what your decision is. In the face of a persistent saboteur, tell him or her to stop asking you, then change the subject.

A Word About Not Going It Alone for Exercise

Support can also be important for making exercise a part of your life. One study showed that the dropout rate from an exercise program was three times higher when spouses were negative or indifferent to the program compared with when spouses were supportive. A number of masters mentioned that they exercise with a spouse, relative or friend. As Mary Ann K. says of her exercise partnership with her husband, "There are days he doesn't want to exercise, but I'm going, so he does, too, and vice versa. We don't want to disappoint each other."

Certainly the popularity of group exercise programs attests to our dependence on others for support and motivation. There is evidence that beginning exercisers tend to prefer working out with others. Some studies suggest that people who exercise in groups are more likely to stick with it. A number of studies indicate that finding friendships within programs motivates people to continue — so if you do join an exercise group, try to stay with it long enough to form some relationships.

Maintaining Your Independence

None of this is to say that if you do choose to go it alone for overall weight control or exercise, you're doomed to remain heavy. In fact, strong independence characterizes many masters. Bear in mind that if you do choose to use a support system, weight control is ultimately up to you and is in your power. Consider Mary Ann K., who has family support, who enjoyed weight-loss classes at a commercial organization and who still goes back if she feels like she's slipping. Ultimately, however, "the support comes from inside myself. I don't look to the outside."

Muriel and Jordan F. seem to have struck a balance between self-reliance and support from others. As Jordan states, "We don't sit and watch each other all day. I know it has to come from me."

Epilogue

It *can* be done. People can — and do — become thin for life. Admittedly, when I began the research for this book, I had doubts. Would I find a significant number of masters at weight control? Would there be similarities in their strategies to keep off weight? After locating hundreds of masters and getting to know them, I am convinced more than ever that despite the "failure talk" about the odds against losing weight and keeping it off, plenty of people manage to do so — many more than we've been led to believe. Since I wrote the first edition of *Thin for Life,* there's far more research evidence supporting my premise.

There are striking common threads in how the masters have found success:

◆ **To lose weight once and for all, the masters accepted that no one could do it for them.** They realized that they must lose weight for themselves — not for their spouses, parents or anyone else. However, although they have assumed ultimate responsibility for their weight, the masters know when to seek support from others — whether from friends, family, groups or professionals.

◆ **The masters give themselves permission to be imperfect.** That is, they accept themselves — bodily flaws and all — many at a higher weight than the so-called "ideal." They allow themselves treat foods that others might view as "forbidden." As part of the process, they talk to themselves positively, pick themselves up when they fall short of their goals and focus on triumphs rather than on shortcomings.

◆ **The masters have changed their attitudes about weight control.** They've stopped viewing the strategies to *lose* weight as separate from those used to *maintain* weight. For example, the vast majority make exercise a way of life but not in a fanatic manner. And most adopt and enjoy new, low-fat eating habits.

◆ **The masters view what they do to control their weight as lifelong change.** They accept that they cannot return to their old ways, but they neither regret their choices nor feel sorry for themselves. They understand that weight maintenance takes effort and determination. Yet the masters make it clear that any hardships associated with maintenance are far less troublesome than the difficulties endured when they were overweight.

◆ **The masters immediately deal with small weight gains before the extra pounds seem insurmountable.** They set upper weight limits that trigger action until they reestablish a comfortable weight.

◆ **The masters stop using food as a shield from problems and learn to handle life's ups and downs more effectively.** They develop confidence in themselves — either before they lose weight or as they are losing — and they extend that confidence to other areas of their lives so they can be proud of more than just being thinner.

◆ **The masters believe in themselves.** Somewhere along the way, they started to have faith in their own ability to conquer their weight problems. They stopped seeing themselves as failures who had repeatedly lost and regained and began to view themselves as people who could take control and be successful.

Using the examples of the masters at weight control, you, too, can start to believe in your own ability to conquer your weight problem, be it large or small. Give yourself time and realize that your new behaviors and attitudes will take practice and continued attention. After all, if you were treated for high blood pressure or diabetes for just three months, would you expect to see beneficial effects three years later? For that to happen, you would have to continue to follow a special diet, take medication and/or exercise in order to stay well. Likewise, with weight control, you must keep taking action if you want to become a master.

Finally, look beyond the weight-loss phase and accept that the real challenge is *maintenance*. If you've made up your mind that you want to make permanent changes in order to lose weight and keep it off, you're off to a great start. Then, if you practice the Keys to Success, you'll come to find, as most masters have, that your old way of life is no longer an option. As they reveal, the payoff is well worth it. Shirley C., who has kept off 26 pounds for 12½ years, exclaims, "No one takes me for 69, and I *feel* 15 years younger." Connye Z., master of a 34-pound loss for 5½ years, says, "I don't feel I'm a better, smarter or more capable person than before. But I feel I look better, and that's important to *me*." Finally, Michael F. sums up his 7 years of living at 160 pounds lighter: "I enjoy my life 100 percent more now."

Who would ever want to go back?

Recipes from the Masters

Some of the following recipes stem from the masters' own "from-scratch" creations; others are the masters' adaptations of high-fat recipes. You'll find most of them simple to make from readily available ingredients. The recipes are clustered into three groups: "Soups, Salads and Accompaniments," "Main Dishes — Light to Hearty" and "Satisfying Sweets."

Each recipe contains nutrition information per serving for calories, fat, cholesterol, sodium, protein and carbohydrate. The recipes were analyzed by nutritionist Mary Jane Laus with the Massachusetts Nutrient Data Bank at the University of Massachusetts, Amherst.

The emphasis in these recipes is on lowering fat and calories, but not on lowering sodium. If you are on a low-sodium or other special diet, you may want to make some additional modifications according to your physician's and/or dietitian's advice. Sodium values of commercial tomato products are particularly high. Homemade versions can be much lower in sodium.

Note that when an ingredient option is listed for a recipe — for instance, "jam or preserves" — the first ingredient was used to calculate nutritional data. Optional ingredients in recipes are not included in the analyses. If a range is given for an ingredient amount, the average was analyzed. Nutritional data for recipes are approximate.

A few words about specific foods:

♦ When eggs are used in a recipe, they are always large.

♦ A number of masters submitted recipes with ground turkey, which can be deceptively high in fat. In recipes calling for it, we purchased skinless turkey breast and had it ground at the supermarket. The taste was much preferred to that of regular ground turkey.

◆ Nonstick cooking spray, such as Pam, is used in many recipes and is not noted in the ingredient lists for recipes.

◆ When reduced-fat cheese is used in a recipe, it should contain no more than 5 grams of fat per ounce. (For the nutritional analyses, reduced-fat cheeses with 5 grams of fat per ounce were used.)

◆ Salad dressing should have no more than 25 calories per tablespoon.

◆ Hamburger for these recipes should be at least 85 percent lean.

Soups, Salads and Accompaniments

Thick and Hearty Bean Soup

Jordan F.

It was love at first taste with this satisfying soup, which makes plenty for leftovers. Says Jordan F., "This freezes well in individual servings. Take a serving of soup, a piece of bread and fruit for an excellent lunch."

1	pound mixture assorted dried beans
1	large carrot, sliced (1 cup)
1	large onion, chopped (about 1 cup)
1	cup sliced celery (about 2 stalks)
1	28-ounce can whole, peeled tomatoes, chopped (save juice)
1	tablespoon minced garlic
4	teaspoons chicken bouillon granules
3	quarts water
½	teaspoon dried basil
½	teaspoon dried oregano
¾	teaspoon ground cumin
1	6-ounce can tomato paste
	Tabasco sauce to taste (optional)

1. Soak beans overnight in enough water to cover and drain. Place in a large soup kettle.

2. Add carrot, onion, celery, tomatoes and their juice, garlic, bouillon granules, water, basil, oregano and cumin. Bring to a boil. Reduce heat and simmer for about 2 hours.

3. Stir in tomato paste and cook for ½ hour longer. Season with Tabasco, if using.

Makes about 14 servings.

PER SERVING: CALORIES: 147; FAT: NEGLIGIBLE; CHOLESTEROL: 0 MG.; SODIUM: 450 MG.; PROTEIN: 9 G.; CARBOHYDRATE: 28 G.

Sweet and Sour Cabbage Soup

Don Mauer

Don says, "When icy Chicago winds are really roaring, this soup can truly warm me up from the inside out." The recipe makes a large quantity and keeps well.

2	quarts fat-free chicken broth
1	pound skinless, boneless turkey breast, cut into ½-inch cubes (about 3 cups)
1½	pounds green cabbage, coarsely chopped (6–7 cups)
2	medium-size ripe tomatoes, peeled and chopped (about 2 cups)
1	medium-size onion, chopped (about ⅔ cup)
1	small green bell pepper, finely diced (about ¾ cup)
1	large stalk celery, strings removed, thinly sliced (about ¾ cup)
1	large carrot, scraped and thinly sliced (about ¾ cup)
⅓	cup tomato paste
1¼	cups catsup
¼	cup light brown sugar
⅓	cup freshly squeezed lemon juice (about 1½ lemons)
1	teaspoon salt
½	teaspoon freshly ground black pepper

1. Place chicken broth in a large soup kettle over medium-high heat. Add cubed turkey and bring to a boil. Lower heat and simmer, skimming from time to time, for about 30 minutes.

2. Add cabbage, tomatoes, onion, green pepper, celery and carrot. Stir in tomato paste, catsup, brown sugar, lemon juice, salt and black pepper. Cover and simmer gently for 1½ hours.

Makes about 14 servings.

PER SERVING: CALORIES: 101; FAT: 1 G.; CHOLESTEROL: 20 MG.; SODIUM: 729 MG.; PROTEIN: 12 G.; CARBOHYDRATE: 11 G.

Summer Garden Gazpacho

Karen S.

A great way to use up your end-of-summer garden overflow. Thick but light-tasting, this soup is great as an appetizer or a meal in itself when served with bread and low-fat cheese.

Hint: It's easiest to chop the first three ingredients in a food processor.

2½	cups diced fresh tomatoes (about 1 pound)
1½	cups finely chopped green bell pepper (1 large)
¾	cup finely chopped onion (1 medium-large)
3	small cloves garlic, minced
2	tablespoons snipped chives
1	teaspoon paprika
1	teaspoon salt
½	teaspoon sugar
	Freshly ground black pepper to taste
2	cups tomato or V-8 juice
1	medium-size cucumber, peeled, cut lengthwise, seeded and shredded with a grater (about 1 cup)
	Juice from ½ fresh lemon (about 2½ tablespoons)
	Tabasco sauce or horseradish to taste (optional)

1. In a large bowl, combine tomatoes, green pepper, onion, garlic, chives, paprika, salt, sugar and black pepper.

2. Stir in remaining ingredients. (If too chunky, process briefly in food processor.) Cover and chill at least 2 hours.

Serves 6 as an appetizer.

PER SERVING: CALORIES: 53; FAT: NEGLIGIBLE; CHOLESTEROL: 0 MG.; SODIUM: 656 MG.; PROTEIN: 12 G.; CARBOHYDRATE: 12 G.

Snow Peas and Carrots

Pat Baird

Turn peas and carrots into a side dish festive enough for a holiday meal. The microwave brings out the natural flavors of the vegetables, so no one will notice that there is less butter than would normally be used. (Adapted from *Quick Harvest: A Vegetarian's Guide to Microwave Cooking* by Pat Baird, Prentice Hall Press, 1991.)

1	medium onion, thinly sliced
4	teaspoons olive oil or butter
2	medium carrots, peeled and cut into 2-×-¼-inch strips
½	pound snow peas, strings removed
3	tablespoons chopped fresh or 2 teaspoons dried dill
	Salt and freshly ground black pepper to taste

1. In a 2-quart microwavable casserole or oval dish, combine onion and oil or butter, stirring well to coat. Microwave on high for 1 minute.

2. Stir in carrots; cover tightly with lid or vented plastic wrap. Microwave on high for 2 minutes.

3. Stir in snow peas and dill. Re-cover and microwave on high for 6 to 8 minutes, or until vegetables are tender-crisp. Let stand, covered, for 3 minutes. Add salt and pepper.

Makes 4 servings.

PER SERVING: CALORIES: 86; FAT: 5 G.; CHOLESTEROL: 0 MG.; SODIUM: 22 MG.; PROTEIN: 2 G.; CARBOHYDRATE: 9 G.

Weequahic Slaw

Karen S.

Pronounced "week-wake," this salad is a nice, light switch from traditional mayonnaise-laden coleslaw. It was inspired by a more oily version served at Karen's childhood country club. It keeps for days in the refrigerator.

1   16-ounce package coleslaw mix (about 7–8 cups shredded cabbage and carrots)
1   small onion, chopped (about ⅓ cup)
1   medium-size green pepper, diced (about 1 cup)
1   medium-size cucumber, peeled and thinly sliced (about 2 heaping cups)

Dressing
3–4   tablespoons apple-cider vinegar
3   tablespoons vegetable oil
1   tablespoon sugar
1   teaspoon salt

1. Mix vegetables in a large bowl.
2. In a small bowl, whisk together the dressing ingredients.
3. Toss dressing and vegetables together. Cover tightly. Refrigerate for at least 1 hour. (The mixture "shrinks" as it sits.)

Serves 6 generously.

PER SERVING: CALORIES: 107; FAT: 7 G.; CHOLESTEROL: 0 MG.; SODIUM: 375 MG.; PROTEIN: 2 G.; CARBOHYDRATE: 11 G.

Sensibly Thin Vegetable Salad

Sam Eukel

For a change of pace, this light, crunchy and attractive salad is a great alternative to a traditional tossed salad. It's also a good company salad because it's made hours in advance. (This recipe is adapted from one in *Sensibly Thin Low-Fat Living and Cooking* by Sam Eukel.)

3	cups broccoli florets (bite-size pieces)
3	cups cauliflower florets
1	cup sliced celery
½	cup pitted black olives (about 18 medium), sliced
1	16-ounce can button mushrooms, drained
1	8-ounce can sliced water chestnuts, drained
¾	cup fat-free Italian salad dressing

1. Combine all ingredients in a large bowl. Stir or cover and gently shake several times to coat vegetables.

2. Chill for at least several hours before serving.

Serves 8.

PER SERVING: CALORIES: 59; FAT: 1 G.; CHOLESTEROL: 0 MG.; SODIUM: 451 MG.; PROTEIN: 3 G.; CARBOHYDRATE: 12 G.

New-Fashioned Creamy-Style Potato Salad

Don Mauer

This is so good it's hard to believe it's no-fat. The red skins add color, and the celery gives it plenty of crunch. It makes a large batch — great picnic fare. This recipe is adapted from one first published in Don's Chicago-area *Daily Herald* column.

3	pounds medium-size red-skinned potatoes
4	stalks celery, diced (about 1¼ cups)
1	medium-size onion, chopped fine (about ⅔ cup)
1½	cups fat-free mayonnaise
1	tablespoon Dijon-style mustard
2	tablespoons chopped fresh parsley
1	teaspoon salt
	Generous grating black pepper
3	hard-cooked egg whites, chopped (optional)

1. Scrub potatoes under cold water. Bring a large pot of water to a boil; cook potatoes in it for 25 minutes. Drain, cool and refrigerate.

2. After potatoes are cold, coarsely chop them with skins still on. Place in a large bowl along with celery and onion.

3. In a small bowl, whisk together mayonnaise, mustard, parsley, salt and pepper.

4. Pour dressing over potato mixture and toss gently to combine. Cover and refrigerate.

Serves 10.

PER SERVING: CALORIES: 126; FAT: 0 G.; CHOLESTEROL: 0 MG.; SODIUM: 535 MG.; PROTEIN: 4 G.; CARBOHYDRATE: 33 G.

Pasta Salad

Kelly S.

This hearty, healthful pasta salad is a breeze to prepare. Make it in a large bowl and cover, and it keeps for days.

> 1   12-ounce package pasta (such as rotini, small or medium shells, spirelli or fusilli), cooked according to package directions and drained
>
> 4   cups frozen-vegetable mixture (such as cauliflower, broccoli and carrots)
>
> 1½   cups drained, canned kidney beans or chickpeas
>
> ¾   cup low-fat or fat-free Italian salad dressing (no more than 16 calories per tablespoon)
>
> 1   tablespoon Dijon-style mustard
>   Generous grating black pepper

1. Combine pasta, vegetable mixture and kidney beans or chickpeas in a large bowl.

2. Mix together salad dressing, mustard and black pepper in a small bowl.

3. Toss dressing with pasta mixture gently to combine. Refrigerate overnight, or until vegetables are thawed. Stir again before serving.

Serves 8.

PER SERVING: CALORIES: 244; FAT: 3 G.; CHOLESTEROL: 1 MG.; SODIUM: 392 MG.; PROTEIN: 9 G.; CARBOHYDRATE: 45 G.

Yellow Squash Custard

Bonnie R.

A tasty and filling rendition of an otherwise plain vegetable, this casserole can be served as a side dish with a light meal or as a main course with a large salad and bread.

7 medium-size or 12 small yellow summer squash (about 1½ pounds), sliced ¼ inch thick
1 medium-size onion, sliced
1 10¾-ounce can reduced-fat, reduced-sodium condensed cream soup (any flavor)
1 egg plus 2 egg whites, beaten
1 cup unseasoned bread crumbs plus 2 tablespoons for topping
¼ pound grated reduced-fat Colby, mild Cheddar or Monterey Jack cheese (about 1 cup), lightly packed

1. Preheat oven to 350 degrees F. Steam squash and onion until very tender, about 20 minutes. Place in a large bowl and mash with a fork or potato masher.

2. With a wire whisk, mix soup and beaten eggs into squash mixture. Add 1 cup bread crumbs and mix well.

3. Coat an 8-×-8-inch baking pan with nonstick cooking spray. Spoon in squash mixture. Bake for 25 minutes. Sprinkle cheese evenly across top, then remaining 2 tablespoons bread crumbs. Bake for another 5 to 10 minutes, or until firm in the middle and piping hot.

Serves 6 as a side dish; 4 as a main course.

PER SIDE-DISH SERVING: CALORIES: 212; FAT: 6 G.; CHOLESTEROL: 50 MG.; SODIUM: 525 MG.; PROTEIN: 12 G.; CARBOHYDRATE: 27 G.

Creamy Leek Dip

Joanna M.

Joanna adapted this from a recipe given to her by a former exercise teacher. Even nondieters enjoy it.

2   cups 1% fat or fat-free small-curd cottage cheese
¼   cup skim milk
1   packet Knorr's leek soup mix
1   cup fresh parsley sprigs

1. In a food processor fitted with the metal blade, combine cottage cheese, skim milk and leek soup mix until smooth.

2. Add parsley and process until it is finely chopped. Place in a medium bowl and refrigerate for at least 2 hours. Serve with raw vegetables.

Makes about 2½ cups or 10 servings.

PER SERVING: CALORIES: 65; FAT: 1 G.; CHOLESTEROL: 3 MG.; SODIUM: 588 MG.; PROTEIN: 7 G.; CARBOHYDRATE: 6 G.

Rosy Red Beet Dip

Pat Baird

This low-calorie and almost fat-free dip has a stunning look that brightens any hors d'oeuvre tray. Use the microwave to cook the beets for about 10 minutes; then serve the dip in the center of steamed vegetables like broccoli, mushrooms and green and yellow squash. (Adapted from *Quick Harvest: A Vegetarian's Guide to Microwave Cooking* by Pat Baird, Prentice Hall Press, 1991.)

4	medium beets, scrubbed, stems and roots trimmed
¾	cup fat-free ricotta cheese
2	tablespoons apple-cider vinegar or rice vinegar
2	tablespoons minced scallions
1	teaspoon Dijon-style mustard
½	teaspoon dried basil
½	teaspoon dried tarragon
	Salt to taste

1. Place beets in a shallow 1-quart microwavable casserole dish. Cover tightly with a lid or vented plastic wrap. Microwave on high for 10 to 12 minutes, or until beets are tender. Let stand, covered, for 3 minutes.

2. Drain and cool beets. Slip off skins under cold running water. Cut beets into 1-inch chunks.

3. In the workbowl of a food processor, process beets and all remaining ingredients except salt until mixture is smooth, stopping occasionally to scrape down the sides of the bowl. Add salt.

Makes about 2 cups or 8 servings.

PER SERVING: CALORIES: 25; FAT: NEGLIGIBLE; CHOLESTEROL: 1 MG.; SODIUM: 30 MG.; PROTEIN: 3 G.; CARBOHYDRATE: 3 G.

Buttermilk Salad Dressing

Don Mauer

Most commercial salad dressings, especially buttermilk-based dressings, are stratospherically high in fat, with as much as 90 percent of their calories from fat. This recipe has practically no calories from fat. The dressing is not only good for green salads but also makes a delicious dip for raw vegetables, baked tortilla chips and nonfat potato chips. You can double it to make enough to last a week or more, since its flavor only improves over time. (Adapted from a recipe in *Lean and Lovin' It* by Don Mauer, Houghton Mifflin Company, 1996.)

1	cup fat-free buttermilk
1	cup fat-free sour cream
¼	cup fat-free mayonnaise
1	tablespoon grated Parmesan cheese
2	small cloves garlic, minced
1	tablespoon minced fresh parsley
1	teaspoon grated onion
½	teaspoon freshly ground white pepper
¼	teaspoon dry mustard
¼	teaspoon salt

1. In a nonaluminum mixing bowl, combine all ingredients. Whisk together until completely combined.

2. Cover and chill.

Makes approximately 1¾ cups.

PER 2-TABLESPOON SERVING: CALORIES: 33; FAT: NEGLIGIBLE; CHOLESTEROL: 1 MG.; SODIUM: 113 MG.; PROTEIN: 2 G.; CARBOHYDRATE: 5 G.

Donny's Zippy Tartar Sauce

Don Mauer

"Regular tartar sauce is dangerous stuff for people like me," says master Don Mauer. "It's virtually all mayonnaise, which means something close to a whopping 99 percent of the calories come from fat. Yikes!" This is a fiery and virtually fat-free version. (Adapted from a recipe in *Lean and Lovin' It! — A Lean Cook's Book* by Don Mauer, published by Don Mauer and Associates, 1993.)

1¾	cups fat-free mayonnaise
2	tablespoons Dijon-style mustard
1	teaspoon Worcestershire sauce
½	teaspoon reduced-sodium soy sauce
¼	cup finely chopped fresh parsley leaves
2	tablespoons chopped fresh dill
2	tablespoons finely chopped dill pickle or dill-pickle relish
1	tablespoon chopped scallion, white part only
1	tablespoon drained capers
½	teaspoon cayenne pepper
½–1	teaspoon Tabasco sauce to taste

1. Place all ingredients in the bowl of a food processor fitted with the plastic blade.

2. Pulse several times, or until mixture is well combined. Place in a bowl or jar, cover and refrigerate for a few hours to allow the flavors to blend.

Makes approximately 2 cups.

PER 2-TABLESPOON SERVING: CALORIES: 21; FAT: 0 G.; CHOLESTEROL: 0 MG.; SODIUM: 269 MG.; PROTEIN: 0 G.; CARBOHYDRATE: 6 G.

Blueberry Yogurt Muffins

Don Mauer

Although low in fat, these muffins literally burst with the fresh flavor of blueberries. If you don't have a nonstick muffin pan, use a standard metal one sprayed with nonstick cooking spray. (Adapted from a recipe in *Lean and Lovin' It* by Don Mauer, Houghton Mifflin Company, 1996.)

2	cups all-purpose flour
1	tablespoon baking powder
½	teaspoon salt
1	cup fresh blueberries, rinsed and picked over, plus 12 whole berries for garnish (frozen may be substituted)
4	egg whites, at room temperature
1½	cups plain fat-free yogurt, at room temperature
½	cup granulated sugar plus 3 teaspoons for sprinkling over tops
1	teaspoon vanilla

1. Preheat oven to 400 degrees F.

2. Sift together flour, baking powder and salt. Add blueberries to sifted dry ingredients. Stir lightly to coat. Set aside.

3. Place egg whites in the bowl of an electric mixer. Beat them at high speed until they hold soft peaks. Add yogurt, ½ cup sugar and vanilla. Mix for 30 to 45 seconds until combined. Add liquid mixture to dry ingredients and fold together just until flour is moistened. Batter should not be smooth. Do not overmix.

4. In a nonstick 12-cup muffin pan, divide batter evenly between the cups. Place 1 blueberry in the center of each muffin. Sprinkle ¼ teaspoon sugar evenly over each muffin. Bake for 20 minutes, or until tops are golden. Remove from the tins immediately and allow to cool.

Makes 12 muffins.

PER MUFFIN: CALORIES: 137; FAT: NEGLIGIBLE; CHOLESTEROL: 0 MG.; SODIUM: 245 MG.; PROTEIN: 5 G.; CARBOHYDRATE: 29 G.

Zucchini Bread

Don Mauer

Don Mauer transformed this zucchini bread from one containing as much fat as he normally allows himself for six days into an almost fat-free version. It also makes a delightful dessert when topped with a scoop of nonfat pineapple sorbet.

3	cups all-purpose flour
2	teaspoons baking soda
1½	teaspoons ground cinnamon
1	teaspoon salt
¾	teaspoon nutmeg, preferably freshly grated
¼	teaspoon baking powder
2	cups granulated sugar
1	cup unsweetened applesauce
1	egg plus 4 egg whites
2	teaspoons vanilla
2	cups shredded zucchini
1	8-ounce can crushed pineapple, well drained
1	cup chopped pitted dates
1	cup Grape-Nuts cereal

1. Preheat oven to 350 degrees F.

2. Sift together twice: flour, baking soda, cinnamon, salt, nutmeg and baking powder. Set aside.

3. In the large bowl of an electric mixer, beat sugar, applesauce, egg, egg whites and vanilla until sugar has dissolved. At low speed, add flour mixture and mix until dry ingredients are just moistened. (Batter will appear lumpy.) By hand, fold in zucchini, pineapple and dates.

4. Lightly spray the bottom and sides of two 9-×-5-inch loaf pans with nonstick cooking spray. Divide batter equally between the loaf pans. Sprinkle Grape-Nuts over the top of batter.

5. Bake 1 hour, or until a toothpick inserted in the center comes out clean. Remove the pans from the oven and set on a cooling rack. Cool 5 minutes, remove from pans and place on rack to cool completely.

Makes 2 loaves or 16 servings.

PER SERVING: CALORIES: 265; FAT: NEGLIGIBLE; CHOLESTEROL: 13 MG.; SODIUM: 367 MG.; PROTEIN: 5 G.; CARBOHYDRATE: 61 G.

Mexican Corn Bread

Bonnie R.

Bonnie's simple adaptations have turned a high-fat recipe into one that's much lower in fat and calories. Serve as a side dish or as a light meal with low-fat sour cream or salsa on the side.

2	cups cornmeal
1½	cups skim milk
4	egg whites
1	15-to-17-ounce can cream-style corn
1	4-ounce can chopped mild green chilies
1	teaspoon baking soda
1	teaspoon salt
¾	pound extra-lean hamburger
1	medium-size onion, chopped (about ⅔ cup)
1½	cups grated reduced-fat Monterey Jack cheese (about 6 ounces)

1. Preheat oven to 350 degrees F. In a large bowl, mix cornmeal, milk, egg whites, corn, chilies, baking soda and salt. Set batter aside.

2. Coat a large nonstick skillet with nonstick cooking spray. Brown hamburger over medium-high heat. Drain, blot with a paper towel and set aside.

3. Coat a 9-×-13-inch baking dish with nonstick cooking spray. Pour half the batter into the dish.

4. Evenly sprinkle onion, cooked hamburger and grated cheese over batter. Pour remaining batter over all and spread to cover filling. Bake for 40 to 50 minutes, or until corn bread is done. (It will be firm to the touch in the center and a toothpick should come out clean.)

Serves 10.

PER SERVING: CALORIES: 261; FAT: 7 G.; CHOLESTEROL: 31 MG.; SODIUM: 740 MG.; PROTEIN: 16 G.; CARBOHYDRATE: 34 G.

Main Dishes — Light to Hearty

Egg and Potato Frittata for One

Jordan F.

This is a tasty, quick one-dish meal. Enjoy it for breakfast, lunch or supper. To further lower cholesterol, replace the whole eggs with a cholesterol-free egg substitute.

1	medium-size potato (about 6 ounces, preferably red or yellow finn variety), partially cooked by boiling or microwaving (it should still be quite firm)
1	medium-size onion, chopped (about ⅔ cup)
¼	cup fat-free chicken broth
2	eggs, beaten
1	tablespoon grated Parmesan cheese
	Salt and freshly ground black pepper to taste

1. Dice the cooked potato, with skin, into ½-inch pieces. Set aside.

2. Coat a large nonstick skillet with nonstick cooking spray. Over medium heat, sauté onion in chicken broth until translucent.

3. Add chopped potato, cover, reduce heat and simmer until pieces are tender.

4. Pour eggs over vegetables and cook like a large pancake.

5. When eggs are firm, slide onto serving plate. Top with cheese and add salt and pepper. (For a kick, Jordan adds a little crushed red pepper.)

Serves 1.

PER SERVING: CALORIES: 338; FAT: 12 G.; CHOLESTEROL: 429 MG.; SODIUM: 705 MG.; PROTEIN: 19 G.; CARBOHYDRATE: 39 G.

Chicken Curried-Rice Salad

Mindy B.

Perfect for lunch or supper, served on a bed of greens. Also delicious as an accompaniment to fresh cut-up fruits.

3	cups cooked white rice (let cool 15–20 minutes)
¾	pound raw chicken breast, cooked, cubed (1½ cups cooked)
⅓	cup currants
1	teaspoon curry powder
½	teaspoon onion powder
¼	teaspoon salt
⅓	cup slivered almonds
½	cup fat-free mayonnaise
½	cup fat-free plain yogurt
1	tablespoon olive oil
1	tablespoon freshly squeezed lime juice

1. Preheat oven to 350 degrees F. In a large bowl, combine rice, chicken, currants, curry, onion powder and salt. Refrigerate for about 30 minutes.

2. Meanwhile, toast almonds in the preheated oven for about 8 minutes, or until lightly browned. Stir into rice mixture. Combine mayonnaise, yogurt, olive oil and lime juice. Gently combine with chilled rice mixture. Refrigerate for several hours or overnight before serving.

Serves 4.

PER SERVING: CALORIES: 403; FAT: 9 G.; CHOLESTEROL: 50 MG.; SODIUM: 437 MG.; PROTEIN: 27 G.; CARBOHYDRATE: 53 G.

Cold Chicken and Pasta Salad

Don Mauer

This foolproof summertime luncheon is delicious served in the hollow of a cantaloupe or on lettuce.

3	cups fat-free chicken broth
3	5-ounce skinless, boneless chicken breasts
5	ounces shell-shaped pasta (2 cups)
1	cup fat-free mayonnaise
½	teaspoon Dijon-style mustard
½	teaspoon celery salt
½	teaspoon freshly ground black pepper
2	ribs celery, cut crosswise into ⅛-inch slices
1	cup baby peas, cooked briefly, drained and cooled
1	cup seedless red grapes, washed, dried and sliced in half

1. In a medium saucepan, bring chicken broth to a simmer and add chicken breasts. Return to a simmer and cook for 20 minutes. Remove breasts, drain and chill. Save broth for another use.

2. Cook pasta according to package directions, drain and rinse under cold water. Set aside.

3. In a medium nonaluminum mixing bowl, whisk together mayonnaise, mustard, celery salt and pepper. Cut chicken breasts into bite-size pieces and add to the mixing bowl, along with pasta, celery, peas and grapes. Toss to combine. Cover and refrigerate.

Makes about 5 to 6 cups; serves 8.

PER SERVING: CALORIES: 185; FAT: 1 G.; CHOLESTEROL: 31 MG.; SODIUM: 461 MG.; PROTEIN: 18 G.; CARBOHYDRATE: 26 G.

Italian-Style Stuffed Zucchini

Carole C.

This makes a super dinner: it tastes as if it were prepared with high-fat Italian sausage. It is pretty enough to serve to company.

2	zucchini (8-to-9-inch)
⅓	cup chopped scallions or shallots
1	clove garlic, minced
2	cups finely chopped fresh mushrooms
½	pound extra-lean ground beef or ground turkey breast
¾	cup 1% fat cottage cheese
1	tablespoon grated Parmesan cheese
1	teaspoon dried basil
½	teaspoon dried oregano
	Generous grating black pepper
⅓	cup grated part-skim mozzarella cheese

1. Preheat broiler. Pierce whole zucchini several times and cook in the microwave, for 4 to 7 minutes on high. Or steam them whole for about 10 minutes on medium-high heat. (Zucchini should still be somewhat firm.) Set aside.

2. Coat a large nonstick skillet with nonstick cooking spray. Over medium-high heat, brown scallions or shallots, garlic, mushrooms and ground beef or turkey.

3. While meat is cooking, make "boats" out of zucchini by cutting them in half and scooping out the soft centers into a small bowl. (Be sure to leave some of the zucchini flesh next to the skin so that they are sturdy enough for stuffing.) Drain and gently squeeze liquid from zucchini insides. Add drained zucchini to meat mixture. Simmer until liquid evaporates.

4. Add cottage cheese, Parmesan, basil, oregano and pepper to meat mixture and stir until cheese is melted.

5. Stuff zucchini boats with meat-cheese mixture. (Use a slotted

spoon so any extra juice drips off.) Evenly distribute mozzarella cheese over tops of boats. Place under broiler until cheese is melted and lightly browned. (You can also bake these for 20 to 25 minutes at 350 degrees F if you want the zucchini softer.)

Serves 4.

PER SERVING: CALORIES: 199; FAT: 9 G.; CHOLESTEROL: 43 MG.; SODIUM: 277 MG.; PROTEIN: 20 G.; CARBOHYDRATE: 11 G.

Note: Zucchini boats can be made ahead and refrigerated. (Reserve mozzarella.) Preheat oven to 350 degrees F. Cover lightly with foil and bake for 30 to 40 minutes, or until centers are piping hot. Remove from oven and preheat broiler. Remove foil. Add mozzarella, return zucchini boats to oven and broil for 5 minutes, or until lightly browned.

Doug's Tuna-Noodle Casserole

Doug S.

A low-fat take-off on what we call in Minnesota "hot dish." A hot dish is basically any casserole, in this case, tuna-noodle.

1 can reduced-sodium, reduced-fat condensed cream of mushroom soup
⅓ cup skim milk
1 cup spiral macaroni (rotini), cooked for the minimum amount of time according to package directions and drained
1 9-ounce package frozen French-cut green beans, cooked according to package directions and drained well (don't overcook)
2 4-ounce cans sliced mushrooms, drained well
1 6-ounce can water-packed white tuna, drained and flaked
1 small onion, finely chopped (about ⅓ cup)
¾ cup crispy chow-mein noodles

1. Preheat oven to 350 degrees F. In a large bowl, whisk together soup and milk.

2. Add all other ingredients, except chow-mein noodles; combine.

3. Coat a small casserole dish with nonstick cooking spray. Bake, covered, for 35 to 40 minutes, or until bubbly. Uncover. If there is excess liquid around edges, carefully drain. Top with chow-mein noodles, and continue baking another 15 minutes.

Serves 4

PER SERVING: CALORIES: 276; FAT: 6 G.; CHOLESTEROL: 22 MG.; SODIUM: 684 MG.; PROTEIN: 19 G.; CARBOHYDRATE: 38 G.

Mindy B.

This filling one-dish meal is a hit with kids and adults alike. If desired, top with salsa and fat-free sour cream or plain yogurt.

½	pound ground turkey breast
1	medium-size onion, chopped (about ⅔ cup)
3	cups salsa or picante sauce
1	16-ounce package flour tortillas
1½	cups 1% fat cottage cheese mixed with 1 egg and 1 egg white
1	16-ounce can pinto beans, drained and rinsed
1	16-ounce can or one 9-to-10-ounce box frozen, thawed corn
1	4-ounce can chopped mild green chilies
1	cup grated reduced-fat Cheddar cheese (about ¼ pound)

1. Preheat oven to 350 degrees F. Spray a large nonstick skillet with nonstick cooking spray. Cook turkey and onion over medium-high heat, mashing with a fork to break up lumps, until turkey is browned. Add salsa or picante sauce and mix. Set aside.

2. Coat a 9-×-13-inch baking dish with nonstick cooking spray. Cover bottom and sides of dish with half the tortillas. (If necessary, cut them to fit and overlap them slightly.)

3. Spread half the turkey mixture over tortillas. Then top with layer of remaining tortillas.

4. Evenly spread cottage cheese–egg mixture over tortillas. Then top with a layer of each of the following: beans, corn and chilies.

5. Top with remaining turkey mixture, distributing it evenly. Sprinkle with grated cheese. Bake 1 hour, or until piping hot in the center. (Lightly cover with foil for first ½ hour, making a tent so it doesn't stick to cheese. Remove foil for second ½ hour.)

Serves 8 generously.

PER SERVING: CALORIES: 429; FAT: 9 G.; CHOLESTEROL: 56 MG.; SODIUM: 1,592 MG.; PROTEIN: 27 G.; CARBOHYDRATE: 63 G.

Mallory's Lean Delight

Don Mauer

This recipe "comes from old family friends who shared the original high-fat version with my family more than 30 years ago." Don's version is filling, yet light on the fat.

1	large onion, chopped (about 1 cup)
1½	pounds ground turkey breast
1	15-to-16-ounce can tomato sauce
20	medium-size pitted black olives, drained and sliced
1	16-ounce can cream-style corn
1	tablespoon chili powder
½	teaspoon salt
1	8-ounce package elbow macaroni, cooked according to package directions and drained
1	cup unseasoned bread crumbs

1. Preheat oven to 350 degrees F. Coat a large nonstick saucepan with nonstick cooking spray. Over medium-high heat, sauté onion for about 2 minutes. Add ground turkey and sauté until no longer pink.

2. Stir in tomato sauce, olives, corn, chili powder and salt. Bring to a simmer and remove from heat.

3. Coat a 9-×-13-inch casserole with nonstick cooking spray. Evenly distribute macaroni across bottom. Top with turkey mixture. Sprinkle bread crumbs over top. Bake for about 45 minutes, or until piping hot.

Makes 8 large servings.

PER SERVING: CALORIES: 333; FAT: 3 G.; CHOLESTEROL: 57 MG.; SODIUM: 862 MG.; PROTEIN: 28 G.; CARBOHYDRATE: 49 G.

Chili-Cheese Casserole

Diane J.

A zesty combination of cheeses, bread, eggs and green chilies. For even more pizzazz, you could top each serving with a dollop of nonfat sour cream and salsa. Serve as a main dish with a shredded carrot salad and a steamed vegetable, such as broccoli.

¼ pound shredded reduced-fat Monterey Jack cheese (about 1 cup, lightly packed)
2 ounces shredded part-skim mozzarella cheese (about ¾ cup)
¼ cup chopped onion
¼ cup canned chopped mild green chilies
6 slices whole-wheat bread
2 tablespoons Dijon-style mustard
3 cups evaporated fat-free milk
4 eggs, lightly beaten
½ teaspoon salt
½ teaspoon freshly ground black pepper

1. Preheat oven to 350 degrees F. In a medium bowl, toss together cheeses, onion and chilies. Set aside.

2. Spread bread with mustard and cut into 1-inch squares. Coat a 1½-quart baking dish with nonstick cooking spray. Cover bottom with half the bread, then half the cheese mixture. Repeat.

3. With a wire whisk, lightly mix milk, eggs, salt and pepper. Pour over cheese and bread. Press bread lightly into liquid to moisten.

4. Put the baking dish into a larger pan and pour 1 inch of hot water into the large pan. Bake 45 to 50 minutes, or until a knife inserted in the center comes out clean.

Serves 6.

PER SERVING: CALORIES: 305; FAT: 10 G.; CHOLESTEROL: 162 MG.; SODIUM: 792 MG.; PROTEIN: 25 G.; CARBOHYDRATE: 30 G.

Vegetable Lasagna

Mindy B.

A meat-free rendition of the traditional version. Serve with Italian bread and a romaine lettuce salad.

1   12-ounce container 1% fat cottage cheese
1   cup part-skim ricotta cheese
1   10-ounce package frozen chopped spinach, cooked according to package directions, drained and squeezed lightly
1   26-ounce jar fat-free spaghetti sauce
8   lasagna noodles, cooked according to package directions and drained
2   cups zucchini (about ½ pound raw), cut in ¼-inch slices, lightly steamed for about 5 minutes and drained
1   16-ounce can Italian green beans, drained, or one 9-to-10-ounce package frozen, cooked and drained
½   pound grated part-skim mozzarella cheese (about 2 cups)

1. Preheat oven to 350 degrees F. In a medium bowl, combine cottage cheese, ricotta and spinach. Set aside.

2. Coat a 9-×-13-inch baking pan with nonstick cooking spray. Spread 1 cup spaghetti sauce on bottom of pan.

3. Top with a layer of 4 cooked noodles, then half the cottage cheese mixture. Spread evenly.

4. Top with a layer of each of the following: all the zucchini, 1 cup spaghetti sauce, all the green beans. Top with 4 more noodles.

5. Spread evenly with remaining cottage-cheese mixture. Top with remaining spaghetti sauce. Bake, lightly covered, for about 30 minutes. Sprinkle with mozzarella cheese and continue baking, uncovered, for another 15 to 20 minutes, or until piping hot in the center.

Serves 8.

PER SERVING: CALORIES: 280; FAT: 8 G.; CHOLESTEROL: 28 MG.; SODIUM: 660 MG.; PROTEIN: 22 G.; CARBOHYDRATE: 31 G.

No-Stir Five-Minute Risotto with Salmon

Pat Baird

Classic risottos normally require about 30 minutes of continual stirring and are often made with lots of oil and cheese. Cooking the rice in a pressure cooker reduces the preparation time to just 5 minutes. This recipe also whittles the oil down to just a table-spoon, yet the results are rich and creamy-tasting. This dish can also be made on the stovetop. (Adapted from *Quick Harvest: A Vegetarian's Guide to Microwave Cooking* by Pat Baird, Prentice Hall Press, 1991.)

Hint: If you're using canned broth — and you can't find a low-sodium one — dilute it with half water so the risotto isn't too salty.

1	tablespoon extra-virgin olive oil
1	cup coarsely chopped onions
1½	cups Arborio or other short-grain rice
3½–4	cups fat-free low-sodium vegetable or chicken broth
¼	cup chopped fresh Italian (flat-leaf) parsley
½	pound salmon fillet, cut in 1-inch pieces
⅓	cup grated Parmesan cheese
	Salt and freshly ground black pepper

Pressure-Cooker Method:

1. In a 6-quart pressure cooker, heat oil over medium heat; stir in onions and cook for 1 minute. Add rice, stirring thoroughly to coat with oil. Stir in 3½ cups broth and parsley.

2. Lock the lid in place and bring to high pressure over high heat. Lower the heat just enough to maintain high pressure; cook 5 minutes longer. Reduce pressure immediately and remove the lid, making sure to tilt the pot away from you to allow excess steam to escape. (The risotto may be quite soupy, but it will continue to absorb liquid. If the risotto is still undercooked and needs more liquid, on the other hand, add a bit more broth.)

3. Over low heat, stir in salmon, cheese, salt and pepper to taste. Cook for 1 minute, until salmon is opaque. Ladle into shallow soup bowls. Sprinkle with more pepper.

Stovetop Method:

In a large heavy skillet, heat oil and stir in onions. Cook for 1 minute. Add rice, stirring thoroughly to coat with oil. Stir in ½ cup of broth, and stir constantly until almost absorbed. Add remaining broth, ½ cup at a time, stirring constantly, until grains are cooked through but not mushy and mixture is soupy. Stir in parsley, salmon and cheese, and salt and pepper to taste and cook 1 minute longer. Serve as directed above.

Serves 4.

PER SERVING: CALORIES: 482; FAT: 12 G.; CHOLESTEROL: 42 MG.; SODIUM: 526 MG.; PROTEIN: 25 G.; CARBOHYDRATE: 64 G.

Tuna and Pasta for Two

Muriel F.

This recipe has a pleasant lemon-garlic taste. Serve with crusty bread and a large spinach salad.

2	teaspoons minced garlic
3	tablespoons fat-free chicken broth
1	14.5-ounce can stewed tomatoes
3	tablespoons freshly squeezed lemon juice
½	teaspoon dried basil
½	teaspoon dried oregano
1	6-ounce can water-packed white tuna, drained and flaked
1	cup elbow macaroni, cooked according to package directions and drained
4	teaspoons grated Parmesan cheese

1. In a large nonstick skillet, over medium-high heat, sauté garlic in chicken broth for a minute or two. (Don't brown.)

2. Add tomatoes, lemon juice, basil and oregano. Bring to a boil, then reduce heat and simmer, uncovered, for about 3 minutes.

3. Stir in tuna. Remove from heat and serve immediately over macaroni. Top with Parmesan cheese.

Serves 2 generously.

PER SERVING: CALORIES: 460; FAT: 5 G.; CHOLESTEROL: 38 MG.; SODIUM: 1,056 MG.; PROTEIN: 35 G.; CARBOHYDRATE: 70 G.

Quick and Spicy Scallops and Peppers

Don Mauer

Not only are scallops sweet and tasty morsels, but they are very low in fat. This is wonderful served over rice. (Adapted from a recipe in *Lean and Lovin' It* by Don Mauer, Houghton Mifflin Company, 1996.)

2	teaspoons extra-virgin olive oil
1	green bell pepper, thinly sliced
1	yellow bell pepper, thinly sliced
1	red bell pepper, thinly sliced
1	jalapeño pepper, seeded and thinly sliced
1	scallion, chopped
2	tablespoons dry white wine
2	tablespoons freshly squeezed lemon juice
2	tablespoons freshly squeezed lime juice
2	teaspoons Tabasco sauce
1	pound bay scallops, cleaned, rinsed and patted dry
1	tablespoon minced fresh basil leaves or 1 teaspoon dried
1	teaspoon salt

1. In a large nonstick skillet, heat olive oil over medium-high heat. Add peppers and scallion and cook, stirring, for 3 minutes.

2. Add wine, lemon juice, lime juice and Tabasco sauce and continue to cook for 1 minute.

3. Add scallops, basil and salt and stir to combine. Cover and cook 3 to 4 minutes over medium heat, or until scallops are cooked through.

Serves 4.

PER SERVING: CALORIES: 159; FAT: 3 G.; CHOLESTEROL: 38 MG.; SODIUM: 720 MG.; PROTEIN: 20 G.; CARBOHYDRATE: 11 G.

Fish with Summer Vegetables

Don Mauer

The best time to prepare this dish is during the summer months when small squash and plum tomatoes are easy to find at your local farmer's market. Serve with steamed baby peas.

3	teaspoons olive oil
2	cups thinly sliced onions
½	teaspoon salt
½	teaspoon freshly ground black pepper
2	pounds firm, white fish fillets (such as red snapper, black bass, halibut or cod), cut into four 8-ounce pieces
1	tablespoon chopped fresh basil (optional)
1	small yellow summer squash (¼ pound), thinly sliced crosswise
1	small zucchini (¼ pound), thinly sliced crosswise
	Juice of 1 lemon
2	ripe plum tomatoes, diced (canned may be substituted)
2	tablespoons chopped shallots

1. Preheat oven to 475 degrees F. Heat 2 teaspoons olive oil over medium heat in a nonstick skillet and add onions. Cook, stirring frequently, for 15 minutes or until lightly browned. Set aside.

2. Spray the bottom and sides of a casserole dish just large enough to hold the 4 pieces of fish with nonstick cooking spray. Sprinkle the bottom with ¼ teaspoon salt and ¼ teaspoon pepper. Place fillets, skin-side down, in the bottom without overlapping them. Distribute basil and cooked onion evenly over fillets.

3. Place squash and zucchini in a medium nonaluminum mixing bowl. Add lemon juice, remaining 1 teaspoon olive oil, and remaining ¼ teaspoon salt and ¼ teaspoon pepper, tossing to combine.

4. Distribute squash mixture evenly over fillets. Pour remaining liquid from the bowl over fillets. Distribute tomatoes and shallots around, not over, fillets. Bake for 15 to 20 minutes, or until fish is just beginning to flake in the center.

5. To serve, slide spatula under each fillet and place on a serving plate; serve tomatoes and shallots on the side.

Serves 4 generously.

PER SERVING: CALORIES: 302; FAT: 7 G.; CHOLESTEROL: 83 MG.; SODIUM: 374 MG.; PROTEIN: 48 G.; CARBOHYDRATE: 11 G.

Summery Swordfish with Vegetables and Cilantro

Jordan F.

A colorful, light way to serve any fish steak — be it swordfish, shark, halibut or fresh tuna. The lime juice and cilantro highlight the taste of the fish and vegetables.

¼   cup fat-free chicken broth
1½ pounds swordfish steak, cut into 1-inch cubes
2   stalks celery, sliced ¼ inch thick on an angle
1   medium-size bell pepper (red, yellow or green), cut in thin strips
1   medium-size tomato, chopped (about 1 heaping cup, drained of excess juice)
2   tablespoons freshly squeezed lime juice
1   teaspoon salt
2   tablespoons dry white wine
2   tablespoons chopped fresh cilantro

1. In a large nonstick skillet, heat chicken broth to a boil over medium-high heat. Add swordfish and sauté for 2 to 3 minutes, turning several times. (Fish will not be done.) With a slotted spoon or spatula, gently remove fish to a plate and set aside.

2. Sauté celery and pepper in remaining broth for about 2 minutes. Drain excess liquid. Add tomato, lime juice and salt. Bring to a boil and cook for another minute or two. Stir in wine.

3. Quickly drain fish of any standing liquid and add fish to vegetable mixture. Cover and cook, stirring once or twice, for another 2 to 3 minutes, or until fish just starts to flake. Remove from the skillet, using a slotted spoon or spatula, topping with some of the juices if desired. Sprinkle with cilantro and serve immediately.

Serves 4.

PER SERVING: CALORIES: 233; FAT: 7 G.; CHOLESTEROL: 66 MG.;
SODIUM: 801 MG.; PROTEIN: 35 G.; CARBOHYDRATE: 5 G.

Pasta-Shrimp Primavera

Gail M.

This dish gets an A+ for color and eye appeal. It is simple to prepare, too.

1   14½-ounce can chunky tomatoes
1   cup fat-free spaghetti sauce
2   cups broccoli florets
2   cups cauliflower florets
2   cups sliced carrots (about 3 large carrots)
1   medium-size red bell pepper, sliced
1   pound medium-size shrimp, shelled, deveined and steamed until done
1   12-ounce package linguine, cooked according to package directions and drained (cover to keep warm)
8   teaspoons grated Parmesan cheese

1. In a medium saucepan, combine tomatoes with spaghetti sauce. Cover and bring to a boil, then reduce heat and simmer.

2. In a large pan, steam broccoli, cauliflower and carrots, covered, for 4 to 5 minutes. Add pepper and steam for another 3 to 4 minutes. (Vegetables should be tender-crisp, not soft.)

3. In a large bowl, combine vegetables, shrimp and linguine. Toss lightly. Divide mixture among four individual serving plates. Ladle on tomato mixture. Sprinkle each serving with 2 teaspoons Parmesan cheese.

Serves 4 generously.

PER SERVING: CALORIES: 538; FAT: 4 G.; CHOLESTEROL: 140 MG.; SODIUM: 903 MG.; PROTEIN: 33 G.; CARBOHYDRATE: 95 G.

Baked Chicken with Orange-Apricot Sauce

Karen S.

Chicken is complemented by an apricot and bread-crumb coating. Serve with brown rice and a marinated green bean salad.

2 whole bone-in chicken breasts (about 2 pounds), split in half and skinned
⅔ cup fat-free Italian salad dressing
1 cup seasoned bread crumbs
½ cup orange juice
¼ cup apricot preserves

1. Marinate chicken in Italian dressing for at least 1 hour, turning occasionally.

2. When chicken is finished marinating, preheat oven to 350 degrees F. One by one, shake excess dressing from each chicken breast and dredge breasts in seasoned bread crumbs.

3. Place chicken on a baking sheet that has been sprayed with nonstick cooking spray. Bake for 40 to 45 minutes.

4. While chicken is cooking, in a blender mix orange juice with apricot preserves until just blended.

5. Remove chicken from oven. Spoon half the orange-juice mixture over chicken. Return chicken to oven and continue baking for 10 minutes. Spoon remaining orange-juice mixture over chicken and bake about 10 minutes more, or until chicken is completely done — when the juices run clear and no pink remains.

Serves 4.

PER SERVING: CALORIES: 338; FAT: 5 G.; CHOLESTEROL: 92 MG.;
SODIUM: 1,021 MG.; PROTEIN: 38 G.; CARBOHYDRATE: 35 G.

Sam's Ham

Sam Eukel

Light, lean ham with fruit and yams makes a colorful, complete meal when served with a salad like Weequahic Slaw (page 314). (This recipe is adapted from one in *Sensibly Thin Low-Fat Living and Cooking* by Sam Eukel.)

1	20-ounce can pineapple rings, in juice
1	15-to-16-ounce can halved pears, in juice
1	15-to-16-ounce can halved peaches, in juice
¼	teaspoon pumpkin-pie spice
¼	cup brown sugar
1	teaspoon dry mustard
2	pounds fully cooked ham, very lean
2	16-to-17-ounce cans unsweetened yams

1. Preheat oven to 350 degrees F. Set aside ½ cup pineapple juice. In a large bowl, combine all fruit, 1½ cups of remaining juice (any type) and pie spice. Set aside.

2. Combine reserved ½ cup pineapple juice, brown sugar and dry mustard. Place ham and yams in a large baking pan that has been coated with nonstick cooking spray. Pour pineapple-juice mixture over hams and yams. Bake, uncovered, for about 50 minutes, or until internal temperature registers 140 degrees F, basting with juice several times while cooking.

3. While ham is cooking, gently stir spiced fruit several times. When ham is done, drain fruit and arrange around ham. Bake 15 minutes longer. Just before serving, "fan" ham by cutting 12 thin slices, but avoid cutting all the way through. Serve with some pan juices.

Serves 6.

PER SERVING: CALORIES: 434; FAT: 8 G.; CHOLESTEROL: 58 MG.; SODIUM: 2,017 MG.; PROTEIN: 32 G.; CARBOHYDRATE: 62 G.

Turkey Meat Loaf

Wendy M.

This hearty meat loaf could easily pass for the hamburger version, were it not for its lighter color. It is great topped with grated horseradish and served with baked potatoes and low-fat coleslaw such as Weequahic Slaw (page 315) or Sensibly Thin Vegetable Salad (page 316).

1½	pounds ground turkey breast
½	cup Italian bread crumbs
½	cup uncooked oatmeal
½	cup catsup
½	cup skim milk
2	tablespoons soy sauce
1	large onion, chopped (about 1 cup)
1	egg
	Generous grating black pepper

1. Preheat oven to 350 degrees F. In a large bowl, thoroughly combine all ingredients.

2. Place mixture in a 9-×-5-inch loaf pan coated with nonstick cooking spray. Bake until internal temperature is at least 160 degrees F, about 1¼ hours. (If you don't have a meat thermometer, toward the end of cooking time, cut a slit in the middle and cook until juices run clear — not pink — and meat has lost its pink or reddish color.)

Serves 8.

PER SERVING: CALORIES: 180; FAT: 2 G.; CHOLESTEROL: 84 MG.; SODIUM: 686 MG.; PROTEIN: 25 G.; CARBOHYDRATE: 16 G.

Donny's Pita Pizza

Don Mauer

Don says that this recipe was born three years ago, while he was in the process of losing weight. As a guest at a small party, he was served wedges of pita smeared with sauce and sprinkled with cheese. The next day, he started experimenting in his kitchen and came up with his own pita pizza. (Adapted from a recipe in *Lean and Lovin' It* by Don Mauer, Houghton Mifflin Company, 1996.)

6	6-to-7-inch pita breads (about 12 ounces)
¾	cup (12 tablespoons) fat-free spaghetti sauce
6–8	fresh mushrooms, cleaned and thinly sliced
3	scallions, trimmed and chopped (including several inches of the green part)
1	medium-size green pepper, seeds and stem removed, chopped coarsely
½	pound Lean-Style Italian Sausage (*recipe follows*), browned in nonstick pan with ½ teaspoon olive oil and crumbled
½	pound part-skim mozzarella cheese, grated (about 2 cups)

1. Preheat oven to 425 degrees F. Place pita breads on baking sheets. Spread 2 tablespoons spaghetti sauce over the surface of each pita, almost to the edge.

2. Divide mushrooms, scallions, pepper and sausage among pitas. Top each with a sprinkling of mozzarella.

3. Bake for 12 to 16 minutes. Remove from oven and cut into fourths. Serve immediately.

Serves 4 as a dinner with a large salad;
serves 10 to 12 as an appetizer.

PER DINNER SERVING: CALORIES: 482; FAT: 14 G.; CHOLESTEROL: 70 MG.; SODIUM: 1,082 MG.; PROTEIN: 36 G.; CARBOHYDRATE: 57 G.

Lean-Style Italian Sausage

Don Mauer

This reduced-fat sausage is very tasty. Don "invented" it to satisfy his past passion for cheese-and-sausage pizza. (Adapted from a recipe in *Lean and Lovin' It* by Don Mauer, Houghton Mifflin Company, 1996.)

2	pounds pork tenderloin, trimmed of all fat
½	medium-size onion, minced
1	medium-size clove garlic, minced
1½	teaspoons salt
1	teaspoon whole fennel seed
1	teaspoon paprika
½	teaspoon freshly ground black pepper
½	small bay leaf, stem removed, crushed
	Pinch dried thyme
¼	cup dry red wine or fat-free chicken stock

Optional for "hot" sausage:
½   teaspoon hot red-pepper flakes

1. Cut pork into 1-inch cubes and feed it through a meat grinder intermittently with onion and garlic. (Pork may also be ground in a food processor by carefully pulsing with the steel blade. Add onion and garlic when meat is almost ground.)

2. Place ground-pork mixture in a large nonaluminum mixing bowl. Add remaining ingredients except wine or chicken stock. Mix well. Add wine or chicken stock. Mix well but do not over-mix or overhandle.

3. Sausage mixture may be divided into 8 equal patties and frozen.

Makes 8 four-to-five-ounce patties.

PER UNCOOKED PATTY: CALORIES: 147; FAT: 4 G.; CHOLESTEROL: 74 MG.; SODIUM: 458 MG.; PROTEIN: 24 G.; CARBOHYDRATE: 1 G.

Dogs in a Blanket

Paul A.

Paul says he adapted this from a low-calorie pancake recipe. He adds, "My family couldn't believe that a low-cal lunch could actually taste like fast food." Serve with mustard and catsup.

4	reduced-fat hot dogs
1	cup plus 2 tablespoons all-purpose flour
1	teaspoon baking powder
½	teaspoon baking soda
1	tablespoon granulated sugar
¼	teaspoon salt
1	cup fat-free plain yogurt
¼	cup water
2	tablespoons plus 2 teaspoons reduced-calorie margarine, melted
2	eggs
1	teaspoon vanilla

1. Preheat oven to 350 degrees F. Boil hot dogs for about 5 minutes or until steaming hot. Set aside. In a large bowl, stir together flour, baking powder, baking soda, sugar and salt. Set aside.

2. In a medium bowl, whisk together yogurt, water, margarine, eggs and vanilla. Whisk this mixture into the dry ingredients just until smooth.

3. Pour half the batter over the bottom of a 1½-quart baking dish or an 8-×-8-inch pan that has been coated with nonstick cooking spray. Evenly distribute batter.

4. Evenly space cooked hot dogs on batter. Cover with remaining batter. Bake for 20 to 25 minutes, or until batter is firm.

Serves 4.

PER SERVING: CALORIES: 297; FAT: 10 G.; CHOLESTEROL: 134 MG.; SODIUM: 1,032 MG.; PROTEIN: 15 G.; CARBOHYDRATE: 35 G.

Satisfying Sweets

Angel Food Berry Trifle

Karen S.

Truly pretty company fare: no one will ever guess how easy it is to prepare. It is refreshing after any meal.

- 1 cup boiling water
- 1 0.6-ounce package sugar-free strawberry-flavored gelatin dessert
- 1 pint low-fat strawberry frozen yogurt (2 cups)
- 1 16-ounce angel food cake, cut into ½-inch slices
- 2 cups sliced strawberries or whole small berries, such as blueberries (or 1 cup each)
- 1 cup "lite" Cool Whip

1. In a medium bowl, add boiling water to gelatin. Stir until dissolved. Add frozen yogurt and stir until melted. Set aside.

2. Layer the following in a glass trifle bowl (or any large bowl): cake, gelatin mixture, berries. Repeat twice, eliminating fruit on the last layer. Chill for at least 3 to 4 hours, or until gelatin mixture is set. Serve each portion with 2 tablespoons Cool Whip.

Serves 8.

PER SERVING: CALORIES: 237; FAT: 2 G.; CHOLESTEROL: 3 MG.; SODIUM: 502 MG.; PROTEIN: 7 G.; CARBOHYDRATE: 48 G.

Diane's Berry-Jam Roll

Diane J.

Simple and elegant, this dessert is easy to make and skimps on fat and calories.

Parchment paper
3 eggs, separated
¼ cup granulated sugar
1 tablespoon cornstarch
1 teaspoon vanilla
½ cup part-skim ricotta cheese
⅓ cup strawberry or raspberry jam or preserves

1. Preheat oven to 375 degrees F. Dampen a 9-×-13-inch cake pan with a little water, then line with parchment paper, making sure the bottom of the pan is covered. Coat paper with nonstick cooking spray. Set aside.

2. In a medium bowl, with an electric mixer, beat egg whites until stiff but not dry. (Peaks should just fold over when beaters are removed.) Set aside.

3. In a large bowl, beat egg yolks until thick and light lemon-colored. Beat in sugar gradually. Continue to beat until thickened. Fold cornstarch and vanilla into egg yolks. (Smooth out any lumps of cornstarch.)

4. Carefully fold egg whites into yolk mixture, then pour batter into prepared pan. Smooth evenly with spatula to edge of pan. Bake for 8 to 10 minutes, or until cake springs back when gently pressed.

5. Turn pan upside down on a towel-covered cooling rack. Cake should come right out, with parchment on top of it. Peel off parchment, then carefully roll cake up in a clean dishtowel. Cool.

6. When cake is cool, unroll and spread lightly with ricotta

cheese, then jam or preserves. Roll cake to enclose filling. Place on plate, seam side down. Refrigerate for 1 to 2 hours, then serve right away.

Serves 4.

PER SERVING: CALORIES: 222; FAT: 6 G.; CHOLESTEROL: 169 MG.; SODIUM: 97 MG.; PROTEIN: 8 G.; CARBOHYDRATE: 34 G.

Peach Cobbler

Sam Eukel

A low-fat but flavorful version of an old favorite. It is especially good topped with a scoop of vanilla ice milk or frozen yogurt. (This recipe was adapted from one in *Sensibly Thin Low-Fat Living and Cooking* by Sam Eukel.)

2	16-ounce cans sliced peaches in juice
¼	cup packed brown sugar
1	tablespoon cornstarch
½	teaspoon ground cinnamon
¼	teaspoon ground nutmeg
1	cup unsifted all-purpose flour
1	tablespoon granulated sugar
2	teaspoons baking powder
¼	teaspoon salt
2	tablespoons margarine
½	cup skim milk

1. Preheat oven to 450 degrees F. Coat an 8-×-8-inch baking dish with nonstick cooking spray. Drain peaches, reserving ¾ cup juice. In a medium saucepan, combine brown sugar, cornstarch, cinnamon and nutmeg. Blend in reserved ¾ cup juice.

2. Bring mixture to a boil over medium-high heat, stirring constantly. Stir in peaches. Pour into the baking dish. Set aside.

3. In medium bowl, combine flour, sugar, baking powder and salt. Cut in margarine until mixture resembles coarse meal. Add milk. Stir to moisten. Drop by tablespoonfuls over fruit mixture. Bake for 15 minutes. Best if served warm.

Serves 6.

PER SERVING: CALORIES: 217; FAT: 4 G.; CHOLESTEROL: 0 MG.; SODIUM: 315 MG.; PROTEIN: 4 G.; CARBOHYDRATE: 43 G.

Apple Charlotte

Diane J.

This dessert is a cross between apple crisp and bread pudding.

3	slices whole-wheat bread
3	teaspoons reduced-fat margarine
3	medium-size apples (about 1⅓ pounds), such as Granny Smith, peeled and very thinly sliced (about 4 cups)
2	tablespoons orange juice concentrate
1	tablespoon plus 1 teaspoon freshly squeezed lemon juice
¼	cup raisins
2	tablespoons light brown sugar
¼	teaspoon ground cinnamon

Topping

½	cup all-purpose flour
¼	cup light brown sugar
½	teaspoon ground cinnamon
3	tablespoons reduced-fat margarine

1. Preheat oven to 425 degrees F. Spread each slice of bread with 1 teaspoon margarine. Cut each slice into ½-inch cubes and set aside.

2. In a medium bowl, combine apple slices with orange juice, lemon juice, raisins, brown sugar and cinnamon. Add bread and toss to combine. Coat a 6-×-10-inch baking dish with nonstick cooking spray and evenly distribute apple-bread mixture in it.

3. *To prepare topping:* combine flour, brown sugar, cinnamon and margarine until crumbly.

4. Crumble topping over surface of apple mixture. Bake 30 to 40 minutes, or until apples are tender.

Serves 6.

PER SERVING: CALORIES: 231; FAT: 7G.; CHOLESTEROL: 0 MG.; SODIUM: 175 MG.; PROTEIN: 3 G.; CARBOHYDRATE: 42 G.

Fat-Free Chocolate Sauce

Diane J.

Diane recommends serving this sauce over fresh fruit, pudding, frozen yogurt, low-fat cheesecake or angel food cake.

¾   cup granulated sugar
¼   cup unsweetened cocoa
1   tablespoon plus 1 teaspoon cornstarch
½   cup evaporated fat-free milk
1   teaspoon vanilla

1. Mix dry ingredients in a small saucepan. Add milk slowly, stirring.

2. Cook over medium heat, stirring constantly until sauce is thickened. Cook for 2 minutes longer, continuing to stir. Remove from heat and add vanilla.

Makes about ¾ cup or 6 servings.

PER SERVING: CALORIES: 131; FAT: NEGLIGIBLE; CHOLESTEROL: 1 MG.; SODIUM: 26 MG.; PROTEIN: 2 G.; CARBOHYDRATE: 31 G.

Black Bottom Cupcakes

Don Mauer

The original version of this recipe contained ⅓ cup vegetable oil, a whole egg, 6 ounces chocolate chips and lots of pecans, according to Don Mauer. "Hating to give up this cupcake confection, I made several changes that retained the moisture and rich flavor but removed almost all the fat." (Adapted from a recipe in *Lean and Lovin' It* by Don Mauer, Houghton Mifflin Company, 1996.)

Chocolate Chip Filling

2	egg whites, at room temperature
8	ounces fat-free cream cheese, at room temperature
⅓	cup granulated sugar
½	teaspoon vanilla
1	ounce mini-morsel semisweet chocolate chips (scant ¼ cup)

Cupcake Batter

1½	cups all-purpose flour
¼	cup unsweetened cocoa
1	teaspoon baking soda
1	teaspoon baking powder
½	teaspoon salt
1	cup granulated sugar
1	cup water
½	cup fat-free plain yogurt
1	teaspoon vanilla
	Foil cupcake cups
2	tablespoons finely chopped pecans

1. Preheat oven to 350 degrees F. *To prepare filling:* in a small bowl, with an electric mixer, beat egg whites until foamy. Blend in cream cheese, sugar and vanilla until smooth. Stir in chocolate chips. Set aside.

2. *To prepare batter:* into a large bowl, sift together flour, cocoa, baking soda, baking powder and salt. Set aside.

3. In another large bowl, with an electric mixer, combine sugar, water, yogurt and vanilla. Mix until smooth, about 1 minute. Add dry ingredients and mix at low speed until barely moistened. Do not overmix.

4. Line cupcake pans with 20 foil cupcake cups. Spray lightly with nonstick cooking spray. Fill each cup about half-full with batter. Top each with 1 tablespoon filling. (Add any leftover filling to less-full cups.) Sprinkle each cupcake with pecans.

5. Bake for 25 to 28 minutes, or until tops spring back when gently pressed. Cool. (Cupcakes will sink a little after cooling.)

Makes 20 cupcakes.

PER CUPCAKE: CALORIES: 117; FAT: 1 G.; CHOLESTEROL: 2 MG.; SODIUM: 230 MG.; PROTEIN: 4 G.; CARBOHYDRATE: 23 G.

Too-Tasty-to-Be-No-Fat Chocolate Cake

Don Mauer

Don recalls, "Once low-fat was a permanent way of life for me, the search for great low- or no-fat chocolate treats began. This recipe is high on my favorites list." (Adapted from a recipe in *Lean and Lovin' It* by Don Mauer, Houghton Mifflin Company, 1996.)

Batter

⅓   cup plus 1 tablespoon unsweetened cocoa plus more for dusting pan
1   cup all-purpose flour
1   teaspoon baking powder
1   teaspoon baking soda
6   egg whites, at room temperature
1⅓   cups firmly packed dark brown sugar
1   cup fat-free plain yogurt
1   teaspoon vanilla

Topping

1   tablespoon unsweetened cocoa
1   tablespoon confectioners' sugar

1. Preheat oven to 350 degrees F. Assemble a 10-inch springform pan. Spray bottom and sides with nonstick cooking spray. Dust pan with cocoa; tap out excess.

2. *To prepare batter:* into a medium bowl, sift together cocoa, flour, baking powder and baking soda. Set aside.

3. In a large bowl, with an electric mixer, beat egg whites, brown sugar, yogurt and vanilla until blended, about 1 to 2 minutes on medium speed. Mix in dry ingredients by hand or on low mixer speed until just moistened. Do not overmix. (This is not a smooth batter.)

4. Pour batter into prepared pan and bake for about 35 min-

utes, or until a toothpick inserted in the center comes out clean. (If the pan is of different size, cooking time may vary.) Cool in the pan on a wire rack for 15 minutes. Then use a knife to loosen sides of cake from the pan. Remove ring and cool completely on a rack. Serve cake on the metal bottom of the pan.

5. *To prepare topping:* in a small bowl, combine cocoa with confectioners' sugar. Place mixture in a small fine sieve and dust top of cake before serving.

Serves 10.

PER SERVING: CALORIES: 188; FAT: NEGLIGIBLE; CHOLESTEROL: 0 MG.; SODIUM: 231 MG.; PROTEIN: 5 G.; CARBOHYDRATE: 43 G.

Bonnie R.

When I first tasted this wonderful-looking coffee cake, I couldn't believe that it had next to no fat in it. It's delicious, either for breakfast or as a dessert.

1   cup unsweetened applesauce
1   cup granulated sugar
1   egg plus 4 egg whites
3   cups all-purpose flour
1   tablespoon baking powder
2   teaspoons baking soda
1   cup fat-free sour cream
1   tablespoon vanilla
1   teaspoon almond extract
1   20-ounce can light pie filling (any flavor)
2   teaspoons ground cinnamon mixed with 2 tablespoons granulated sugar

1. Preheat oven to 350 degrees F. In a large bowl, mix applesauce and sugar with an electric mixer. Beat in egg and egg whites, one at a time.

2. In a separate bowl, sift flour, baking powder and baking soda. Beat these dry ingredients into applesauce mixture, alternating with sour cream. Add vanilla and almond extracts. Mix until combined, but don't overmix.

3. Spray a 12-cup Bundt pan with nonstick cooking spray, then lightly flour. Evenly distribute half the batter in pan.

4. Evenly distribute pie filling over batter. Top with remaining batter and sprinkle with cinnamon-sugar mixture. Bake for 50 to 60 minutes, or until a tester comes out clean. Let cool on a rack for 20 to 25 minutes before inverting and removing from pan. Cool completely on a rack. It keeps best in the refrigerator.

Serves 12.

PER SERVING: CALORIES: 271; FAT: NEGLIGIBLE; CHOLESTEROL: 18 MG.; SODIUM: 392 MG.; PROTEIN: 7 G.; CARBOHYDRATE: 59 G.

Banana Rum Crepes

Diane J.

Bananas Foster in a crepe: a sensational low-fat dessert.

Crepes
1½   cups evaporated fat-free milk
1   cup all-purpose flour
1   egg plus 1 egg white
½   teaspoon finely grated lemon rind
2   tablespoons dark rum

Filling
¼   cup reduced-fat margarine
3   tablespoons light brown sugar
1   teaspoon finely grated lemon rind
½   teaspoon ground cinnamon
5–6   ripe bananas, peeled and sliced
¼   cup dark rum

Topping
¾   cup 1% fat cottage cheese
3   tablespoons light brown sugar
1   teaspoon vanilla
½   teaspoon ground cinnamon
⅛   teaspoon ground nutmeg

1. *To make crepes:* combine all ingredients in a food processor and process until smooth. Let stand 1 hour. Heat a small nonstick pan coated with nonstick cooking spray and measure out enough batter to cover the base of the pan (about ¼ cup). Cook until small bubbles appear and surface is dull, then turn and cook other side for 1 minute. Transfer cooked crepe to a clean dish-towel and cover. Repeat with remaining batter, stacking cooked crepes on top of each other, keeping them covered with a towel.

2. *To make filling:* melt margarine in medium nonstick skillet. Add brown sugar, lemon rind and cinnamon. Stir until bubbling. Add bananas and toss lightly. Carefully averting face, add rum and ignite mixture; shake the pan gently until the flames die down, being careful not to spill mixture. When all flames are extinguished, divide banana mixture evenly among crepes, spooning mixture over one-fourth of crepe. Fold crepe in half over filling and in half again.

3. *To make topping:* combine all ingredients except nutmeg in blender and blend until smooth. Pour into a small serving bowl and dust with nutmeg.

4. Spoon warm or room-temperature topping over crepes.

Makes 12 crepes.

PER CREPE: CALORIES: 180; FAT: 4 G.; CHOLESTEROL: 20 MG.; SODIUM: 146 MG.; PROTEIN: 7 G.; CARBOHYDRATE: 29 G.

Berry-Cheese Torte

Diane J.

A cheesecake-like torte minus much of the fat and calories. Topped with the sweetened berries, each bite melts in your mouth.

1   cup fat-free ricotta cheese
1   8-ounce package Neufchâtel cheese, at room temperature
3   eggs
½   cup plus 3 tablespoons granulated sugar
¼   cup cornstarch
1   teaspoon baking powder
1   teaspoon lemon rind
1   tablespoon freshly squeezed lemon juice
¼   cup jelly, jam or preserves (of a similar flavor to berries)
1½   cups blueberries, raspberries or sliced strawberries

1. Preheat oven to 350 degrees F. In a large bowl, with an electric mixer, cream together ricotta cheese and Neufchâtel. Beat in eggs, then sugar, until mixture is smooth.

2. In a small separate bowl, stir together cornstarch and baking powder. Beat into cheese mixture along with lemon rind and lemon juice.

3. Pour into a 9-to-10-inch springform pan, coated with nonstick cooking spray. Bake about 45 minutes, or until firm in the middle. Let cool for 10 to 15 minutes, loosen and remove sides of pan, then refrigerate torte until chilled.

4. Shortly before serving, place jelly or preserves in a small microwavable bowl and microwave for a short time, until melted, or heat in a small saucepan over low heat. Pour over berries and stir gently. (With blueberries, you may need to add several teaspoons hot water to thin jelly.) When jelly mixture is cool, top each serving of torte with an equal amount of berry mixture.

Serves 8.

PER SERVING: CALORIES: 244; FAT: 9 G.; CHOLESTEROL: 103 MG.; SODIUM: 216 MG.; PROTEIN: 9 G.; CARBOHYDRATE: 33 G.

The Jump-Start Diet

The Jump-Start Diet is one means of getting started on the business of weight loss. It gives you a "jump start" because, in its early stages, it is quite aggressive so you lose some weight quickly and become motivated to proceed. Women may lose as many as 2 to 4 pounds the first week and 1 to 2 pounds a week thereafter; men may lose more. Part of that loss will be water. In addition, your rate of weight loss will be influenced by your age, the amount of exercise you engage in, your metabolic rate and the size of your body frame.

The calorie level for Week 1 is somewhat low. Thus I stress that Week 1 be followed for *no more than 7 days*. Still, provided that the guidelines below are followed, all stages of the Jump-Start Diet are designed to be safe for healthy people. The Jump-Start Diet is recommended for people who, like many of my former patients, do well on a fairly strict diet that initially limits choices and is easy to follow.

In accord with the masters who lost weight *their* way, the Jump-Start Diet soon becomes "customizable," so you can tailor it to meet your own needs and preferences.

If you've had it with diets, the Jump-Start Diet is not for you. This is particularly true if you struggle with a relatively small amount of weight — say, 10 to 20 pounds — or have a history of compulsive dieting or any type of eating disorder. In these cases, it's advisable to try one of the nondieting approaches to weight control, such as the 6-Week Nondieting Weight-Control Plan (page 128). Quite honestly, as a dietitian, I prefer that people lose weight by making an effort to increase exercise and cut back on fat and calorie intake. But many masters did find success with structured low-calorie diets, and you may find the Jump-

Start Diet helpful to get you started. The important point is to realize that, in the long run, you have to come up with your own food plan for maintenance. Chapter 4 offers guidelines for doing so.

Before starting this or any diet, be sure to get your physician's approval. If you currently have any medical problems and/or more than 20 pounds to lose, you should be monitored by your physician while on the diet. (Certain medication needs can change with weight loss.) If you feel weak or experience any physical changes while on the diet, such as constipation or diarrhea, stop the diet and consult your physician. (This diet is not meant for pregnant or breast-feeding women, children or teenagers, or people with serious medical problems such as diabetes.)

Approximate calorie levels for the Jump-Start Diet are as follows:

Week 1: women = 1,000 calories per day
men = 1,400 calories
Do not follow Week 1 for any longer than 7 days.
Week 2: women = 1,100 calories per day
men = 1,550 calories
Week 3: women = 1,200 calories per day
men = 1,600 calories
(women and men add 300 optional calories per week from Special Foods)
Week 4: women = 1,250 calories per day
men = 1,700 calories
(women and men add 500 optional calories per week from Special Foods)

If, at any time, you are uncomfortable or feel deprived with your calorie level, move to the next level of the diet (the level of the following week). It is important that you weigh or measure foods. Be sure to eat all recommended food servings from each food group. Foods may be distributed throughout the day as you please, but it is advised that you divide them among three meals or several meals and several snacks. (See sample meal plans starting on page 379.) *Be sure to increase your foods and calorie levels as recommended each week.* Once you complete Week 4, it would be wise to shift to a plan that focuses less on calorie counting and more on healthful, low-fat eating. Ultimately, most masters found it best to fill up on fruits, vegetables and grains, and cut back on fatty foods and flesh foods like red meat. Men in particular can cut back from 8 to 6 ounces of protein.

The logistics of the diet are quite simple:

◆ On Week 1, your choices are a limited selection of foods from various food groups. (Within any one food group, you can substitute foods in the portion size shown for each other.) Each day, you choose several small servings (6 to 8 ounces total) of protein foods, 4 to 5 servings of vegetables, 2 to 4 servings of complex-carbohydrate foods, 3 to 4 servings of fruit, 2 servings of milk products and up to several "extras," such as reduced-fat margarine or mayonnaise. (The number of servings depends on your gender.) Some serving sizes for fruits and vegetables used in the Jump-Start Diet differ from the "looser" serving sizes in the 6-Week Nondieting Weight-Control Plan. The purpose of the strict portion sizes is to ensure precise weekly caloric levels. For the same reason, a few vegetables appear on the list of complex-carbohydrate foods. Once you finish the Jump-Start Diet, however, you needn't be as rigid with fruit and vegetable serving sizes.

◆ On Week 2, for each day, you add a complex carbohydrate and an "extra," and the selection of foods on these lists expands so you have more options.

◆ On Week 3, for each day, you add an extra complex carbohydrate; the Fruits list choices expand as well, and you get to add 3 weekly "treats" from the Special Foods lists.

◆ On Week 4, for each day, you add yet another complex carbohydrate or an extra fruit, and there are more meat choices. In addition, you can add 5 Special Foods per week.

While you're on the diet . . .

◆ Take a daily multivitamin/mineral supplement.

◆ To meet the recommended calcium intake, you may need to take a supplement containing about 400 milligrams of calcium for ages 19 to 50 and 600 milligrams for ages 51-plus.

◆ Be sure to drink at least 8 cups of water each day.

◆ Make a grocery list of foods you need to have on hand and stock up.

◆ Plan meals at least 1 day in advance.

◆ Read package labels to see if products you choose have the same calorie levels as those on various Jump-Start Diet lists.

(Note that when terms like "reduced-fat," "low-fat" and "reduced-calorie" are used in this diet, they refer to products that are lower in fat and/or calories than their regular counterparts. Use of these terms does not necessarily conform to current U.S. government labeling definitions.)

WEEK 1

Choose foods from Lists 1–8 according to the amounts recommended for women or men. Any combination is acceptable.

List 1: Protein Foods

(average 50 calories per ounce)

Women: 6 ounces per day
Men: 8 ounces per day

1 ounce protein =

1   ounce skinless, boneless chicken or turkey meat (breast or leg)
1   ounce fish or shellfish, any type, fresh or frozen, unbreaded

1   ounce tuna, water-packed
1   ounce lean meat (beef eye of round, top round or tip round/
     pork tenderloin, boneless sirloin chop or boneless loin roast/
     veal chops or roast)
1   ounce low-fat luncheon meat (no more than 50 calories per
     ounce)
1   large egg or 3 egg whites
¼   cup no-cholesterol egg substitute
¼   cup cottage cheese or ricotta cheese (1% or fat-free)
½   cup cooked dry beans (also known as legumes: kidney
     beans, chickpeas, white beans, split or black-eyed peas, len-
     tils or low-fat baked beans*)

Note: All meats, poultry and fish are weighed after cooking and are boneless and trimmed of all visible fat (4 ounces of raw meat will yield about 3 ounces of cooked meat). All foods are cooked without added fat by baking, roasting, steaming, grilling, broiling or pan-broiling in a nonstick pan with nonstick cooking spray.

List 2: Vegetable "A" List

(20 calories or less per serving)

Women: 2 to 3 servings per day
Men: 3 servings per day

1 serving =

1   cup raw or ½ cup cooked shredded cabbage (any type, in-
     cluding Chinese)

---

*Dried beans contain about 80 to 100 calories per ½ cup cooked. But un-like most of the other protein foods, beans contain only a trace of fat, making them an excellent substitute for flesh foods. Most people will find ½ to 1 cup of beans — the protein equivalent of 1 to 2 ounces of meat — extremely filling.

1	cup celery
½	large cucumber
2	cups shredded lettuce (any type, preferably dark green)
1	cup raw or ½ cup cooked, sliced mushrooms
1	green, red or yellow bell pepper
20	radishes
1½	cups raw or ½ cup cooked, chopped spinach
1	cup raw or ½ cup cooked bean sprouts
1	cup raw or ½ cup cooked, sliced zucchini

List 3: Vegetable "B" List

(approximately 25 calories per serving)

Women: 2 servings per day
Men: 2 servings per day
Vegetables may be fresh, frozen or canned (which are higher in sodium). Do not use any added fats or sauces, other than allowed fats. Unless noted otherwise, 1 serving = 1 cup raw or ½ cup cooked of any of the following vegetables:

Artichoke (*½ medium*)	Cauliflower	Tomato juice or
Asparagus	Eggplant	vegetable-juice
Beans (*green, yellow,*	Okra	cocktail (*½ cup*)
Italian)	Onions	Tomato sauce (*⅓ cup*)
Beets	Pea pods	Fat-free spaghetti
Broccoli	Sauerkraut	sauce (*¼ cup*)
Brussels sprouts	Summer squash	Turnips
Carrots	Tomato (*1 large*)	Water chestnuts

List 4: Complex-Carbohydrate Foods

(approximately 80 calories per serving)

Women: 2 servings per day
Men: 4 servings per day

1 serving =

1	slice (1 ounce) regular bread (preferably whole-grain)
2	slices "light" bread (no more than 40 calories per slice)
¾	cup flake-type cereal, preferably high-fiber and not presweetened
1½	cups puffed cereal
½	cup shredded wheat
½	cup cooked cereal (unsweetened)
1	small potato, baked, boiled or mashed
½	cup cooked pasta
2	rice cakes

List 5: Fruits

(approximately 60 calories per serving)

Women: 3 servings per day
Men: 4 servings per day

1 serving =

1	apple, 2 inches across
½	banana (9-inch)
	cantaloupe, one-third of a 5-inch melon or 1 cup cubes
½	medium grapefruit
15	small grapes
1	orange (2½-inch)
1	peach or nectarine (2¾-inch)
½	large or 1 small pear
¾	cup raw pineapple or ⅓ cup canned (in its own juice)
1	cup raw, whole strawberries
½	cup juice: apple, grapefruit, orange or pineapple

List 6: Milk Products

(approximately 100 calories per serving)

Women: 2 servings per day
Men: 2 servings per day

1 serving =

1   cup skim or 1% milk
½   cup evaporated fat-free milk (some people prefer this to skim milk in coffee)
1   cup fat-free plain yogurt or "light" yogurt (about 100 calories per container)
1½–2   ounces reduced-fat cheese (no more than 50 calories per ounce)

List 7: Extras

(approximately 35–45 calories per serving) Since reduced-fat products vary, check labels for equivalent portion sizes.

Women: 1 serving per day
Men: 3 servings per day

1 serving =

1   tablespoon reduced-fat margarine
1   teaspoon regular margarine or mayonnaise
1   tablespoon reduced-fat mayonnaise
4   tablespoons fat-free mayonnaise (free, up to 2 tablespoons)
    35-to-45-calorie portion of reduced-fat liquid salad dressing
4   tablespoons fat-free liquid salad dressing (no more than 10 calories per tablespoon; free, up to 2 tablespoons)
1   teaspoon vegetable or olive oil

List 8: Free Foods

Unlimited amounts allowed. (Check labels to make sure specific items have few or no calories.)

Beverages

>   water
>   sugar-free soft drinks
>   carbonated or sparkling water
>   black coffee or tea
>   sugar-free drink mixes
>   bouillon or broth (preferably reduced-sodium), fat-free

Flavoring agents

>   sugar substitutes (aspartame, saccharin)
>   low-calorie butter-flavoring products
>   lemon or lime juice
>   flavoring extracts (vanilla, almond, etc.)
>   herbs and spices
>   horseradish
>   marinades (not as a sauce — just to marinate protein foods)
>   salsa (up to ⅓ cup)
>   soy or Worcestershire sauce (high in sodium, but there are
>   reduced-sodium soy sauces)
>   mustard
>   vinegar
>   garlic

Miscellaneous

>   nonstick cooking spray
>   sugar-free gelatin dessert (no more than 1 envelope per day)
>   sugar-free gum (up to 5 sticks per day)
>   unsweetened pickles (high in sodium)

WEEK 2

Now, the Jump-Start Diet becomes more customizable, with choices in the Complex-Carbohydrate List and Extras List expanding. Continue to eat recommended servings from all food groups for Week 1, but add 1 additional Complex Carbohydrate per day plus 1 additional Extra per day.

Additional Complex Carbohydrates
You may add the following choices to List 4, page 371.

1 serving =

½   bagel (1 ounce)
½   English muffin
½   hamburger or hot dog roll (or 1 low-calorie roll — no more than 80 calories)
1   small pita bread (1 ounce)
1   slice raisin bread
1   pancake (4-to-5-inch)
1   frozen fat-free waffle
1   6-inch tortilla
3   graham cracker squares
¾   ounce matzoh
5   slices melba toast
24   oyster crackers
¾   ounce pretzels
6   Saltines
2–4   (¾ ounce) reduced-fat whole-wheat crackers
½   cup cooked white or brown rice
½   cup cooked bulgur
½   cup cooked grits
3   tablespoons wheat germ
½   cup corn
1   ear corn (6-inch)

½   cup lima beans

½   cup peas

1   cup winter squash

⅓   cup yam or sweet potato

Additional Extras

You may add the following choices to List 7, page 373.

1 serving =

⅛   medium avocado

10   small or 5 large olives

35–45   calories' worth reduced-fat or fat-free sour cream

35–45   calories' worth cream-cheese product (e.g., Neufchâtel or fat-free cream-cheese product)

2   tablespoons reduced-calorie maple-flavored syrup

1   tablespoon jam, jelly or preserves

2   tablespoons grated Parmesan cheese

WEEK 3

Continue to eat all the foods from Weeks 1 and 2, but add 1 additional Complex Carbohydrate per day.

Additional Fruits

You may add the following choices to List 5, page 372.

1 serving =

½   cup applesauce (no sugar added)

4   apricots

¾   cup blackberries or blueberries

12   large cherries

⅛   medium or 1 cup cubed honeydew melon

1   large kiwi

½   small mango

1   cup papaya

2   plums (each 2-inch)

1   cup raspberries

2   tangerines

1¼   cups watermelon cubes

        dried fruit: 4 apple rings, 7 apricot halves, 2½ medium

        dates, 3 medium prunes, 2 tablespoons raisins

Optional (women and men): You may have 3 Special Foods this week (see below), or you may have an additional 300 calories' worth of foods from any of the Jump-Start food lists.

Special Foods Lists

On Weeks 3 and 4, you may have some Special Foods. The foods on these lists, in the amounts shown, have between 70 and 100 calories each. Check product labels to be certain of 100-calorie (or less) serving sizes. If desired, you may save up your weekly 300- or 500-calorie allotments of Special Foods and spend them in one or two sittings each week.

For Your Sweet Tooth

1   ounce jelly beans

1   ounce marshmallows

1   ounce Good n' Plenty

1   ounce candy corn

1   ounce licorice (any type)

1   ounce gum drops

3   Hershey's Kisses

3   Tootsie Roll Midgies

½   ounce sweet or semisweet chocolate chips

8   animal crackers

1   ounce slice fat-free pound cake

4   ounces reduced-calorie pudding

1   low-calorie popsicle or ice cream sandwich

½   cup frozen fat-free dessert or ice cream

½   cup frozen fat-free yogurt

⅓   cup sherbet

1   Fig Newton
3   ginger snaps
5   vanilla wafers
2   half-ounce chocolate chip cookies

For Your Salty Tooth
10 reduced-fat potato chips
    pretzels (100-calorie portion)
⅓   cup chow-mein noodles
3   cups reduced-fat microwave popcorn
10 Wheat Thins
33 Pepperidge Farm Goldfish
18 regular cheese snack crackers (or a 100-calorie portion of a
    reduced-fat brand)

Alcoholic Beverages
1   light beer
1   shot hard liquor (80-proof)
4   ounces dry white or red wine

Note: Items on Special Foods lists are representative of products available at time of writing. You may substitute 100-calorie portions of similar foods.

WEEK 4

Continue to eat all foods from Weeks 1, 2 and 3, but add 1 additional Complex Carbohydrate OR 1 additional Fruit per day.

Additional Protein Foods
You may add the following choices to List 1, page 369. Follow preparation guidelines from Week 1.

1 ounce protein =

1   ounce sirloin steak
1   ounce flank steak
1   ounce beef tenderloin

1 ounce extra-lean ground beef

1 ounce lean ham

1 ounce Canadian bacon

1 ounce of reduced-fat hot dog (no more than 50 calories per ounce)

2 medium sardines, canned in tomato sauce or mustard

2 tablespoons peanut butter (100 calories per tablespoon — it's wise to limit yourself to no more than 4 tablespoons per week)

Optional (women and men): You may have 5 Special Foods this week, or you may have an additional 500 calories' worth of foods from any of the Jump-Start food lists.

Sample Meal Plans

WEEK 1

(example for 1 day)

Breakfast	Food List
¾ cup bran flakes	1 carbohydrate
1 cup skim milk	1 milk
½ banana, sliced	1 fruit
½ cup orange juice	1 fruit
Men: add 1 slice whole-wheat toast	1 carbohydrate
1 teaspoon margarine	1 extra

Lunch	
Open-faced sandwich:	
1 slice whole-wheat bread	1 carbohydrate
3 ounces smoked turkey breast	3 protein
Dijon-style mustard to taste	free
½ sliced tomato	½ vegetable B
1 yellow or red bell pepper, cut in strips	1 vegetable A
Men: use 2 slices bread	2 carbohydrate

increase turkey to 4 ounces	4 protein
add 2 tablespoons reduced-fat dressing for dipping pepper	1 extra

Snack (anytime)

½ cup plain fat-free yogurt mixed with	½ milk
½ cup strawberries, sliced,	½ fruit
and sugar-free sweetener	free

Supper

Baked cod with cheese and tomatoes:

4 ounces uncooked cod	3 protein (when cooked)
1 ounce reduced-fat grated or sliced cheese	½ milk
½ tomato, sliced	½ vegetable B
2 cups shredded romaine lettuce	1 vegetable A
with 2 tablespoons reduced-fat ranch dressing	1 extra
½ cup steamed spinach with lemon juice and nutmeg	1 vegetable A
½ cup steamed carrots	1 vegetable B
<u>Men:</u> increase cod to 5 ounces (raw)	4 protein (when cooked)

Dessert or Bedtime Snack

<u>Women:</u> 8 grapes	½ fruit
in sugar-free gelatin dessert	free
<u>Men:</u> 23 grapes	1½ fruit
in sugar-free gelatin dessert	free

WEEK 2

(example for 1 day)

Breakfast	Food List
½ English muffin topped with	1 carbohydrate
1 tablespoon strawberry jam	1 extra
1 poached egg	1 protein
½ medium grapefruit	1 fruit
<u>Men:</u> increase English muffin to 1 whole	2 carbohydrate
add 1 teaspoon margarine	1 extra

Lunch

Slim sub:

1 low-calorie hot dog roll	1 carbohydrate
1½ ounces reduced-fat cheese	1 milk
1 ounce low-fat luncheon meat	1 protein
½ sliced tomato	½ vegetable B
lettuce leaves	free
sprinkling of chopped onion	free
dill pickle chips	free

Crunchy salad:

⅓ cup celery, ¼ large cucumber (sliced), ⅓ cup bean sprouts	1 vegetable A
½ cup chickpeas	1 protein
tossed with 2 tablespoons reduced-fat Italian salad dressing	1 extra

<u>Men:</u> use regular hot dog roll	2 carbohydrate
increase lunch meat to 3 ounces	3 protein
add 1 tablespoon reduced-fat mayonnaise to sub	1 extra

Snack (anytime)

Banana shake — whip in blender until smooth:

½ banana	1 fruit
1 cup skim milk	1 milk
sugar-free sweetener to taste	free
½ teaspoon vanilla	free
several ice cubes	

Supper

Steak stir-fry:

4 ounces top round steak, cut in strips	3 protein (when cooked)
and sautéed with 1 crushed garlic clove	free
in 3 tablespoons fat-free beef broth	free

<u>When meat is almost done, add raw vegetables:</u>

1 cup Chinese cabbage	1 vegetable A
1 cup sliced mushrooms	1 vegetable A

1 cup broccoli florets	1 vegetable B
½ cup pea pods	½ vegetable B
Cover and steam until vegetables are tender-crisp — just a few minutes. Sprinkle with soy sauce to taste.	
½ cup cooked white or brown rice	1 carbohydrate

Bedtime snack or dessert

| Women: 1 small pear | 1 fruit |
| Men: 1 large pear | 2 fruit |

WEEK 3

(example for 1 day)

Breakfast	Food List
2 pancakes (4-to-5-inch) with	2 carbohydrate
2 tablespoons reduced-calorie maple syrup	1 extra
⅓ cantaloupe	1 fruit
1 cup skim milk	1 milk
Men: increase maple syrup to 4 tablespoons	2 extra
add ½ cup egg substitute scrambled in nonstick pan	2 protein

Lunch	
Tuna sandwich:	
1 slice oatmeal bread	1 carbohydrate
3 ounces water-packed tuna	3 protein
1 tablespoon reduced-fat mayonnaise	1 extra
chopped celery and onion to taste	free
1 cup mixed raw carrot coins and	1 vegetable B
cauliflower florets	
dipped in Dijon-style mustard	free
1 tangerine	½ fruit
Men: use 2 slices bread	2 carbohydrate
increase mayonnaise to 2 tablespoons	2 extra
have 1 orange instead of tangerine	1 fruit

Snack (anytime)

Crunchy cucumber hors d'oeuvres — serve one on top of the next:

1 ounce reduced-fat Cheddar cheese, sliced thin	½ milk
½ cucumber, sliced	1 vegetable A
10 Wheat Thins	1 special food

Supper

Chicken tortilla:

4 ounces boneless, skinless chicken breast cut in strips, marinated in fat-free Italian salad dressing and sautéed in nonstick skillet with no-stick cooking spray.	3 protein (when cooked)

When chicken is done, add raw vegetables:

1 green bell pepper, cut in strips	1 vegetable A
1 cup sliced onion	1 vegetable B

Cover and steam until vegetables are done to your liking.

Serve open-face on

1 tortilla with	1 carbohydrate
1 ounce shredded reduced-fat Monterey Jack cheese	½ milk
salsa to taste	free
1½ cups spinach salad with	1 vegetable A
2 tablespoons fat-free French dressing	free
Men: increase tortillas to 2	2 carbohydrate

Bedtime Snack or Dessert

Women: 18 bing cherries	1½ fruit
Men: 24 bing cherries	2 fruit

WEEK 4

(example for 1 day)

Breakfast	Food List
1 cup cooked oatmeal made with	2 carbohydrate
½ cup skim milk and	½ milk
1 tablespoon raisins	½ fruit
⅛ honeydew melon	1 fruit
Men: increase raisins to 2 tablespoons	1 fruit

Lunch

2-ounce reduced-fat hot dog	2 protein
1 low-calorie hot dog roll <u>with</u>	1 carbohydrate
mustard	free
½ cup low-fat baked beans	1 protein
<u>(no more than 1 gram of fat per ½ cup)</u>	
1 cup raw, shredded cabbage <u>mixed with</u>	1 vegetable A
2 tablespoons reduced-fat ranch dressing	1 extra
1 cup skim milk	1 milk

Snack (anytime)

Fruit kebabs — alternate on toothpicks:	
1 ounce reduced-fat Cheddar cheese, in small cubes	½ milk
8 grapes	½ fruit
1 nectarine, cubed	1 fruit
<u>Men:</u> increase grapes to 15	1 fruit

Supper

4 ounces raw flank steak, marinated in teriyaki sauce, grilled or broiled, sliced thin	3 protein (when cooked)
Ratatouille:	
<u>Cut all vegetables in ½-inch-thick slices and marinate in</u> <u>fat-free Italian salad dressing.</u>	
1 cup zucchini	1 vegetable A
3 slices eggplant	½ vegetable B
1 large tomato	1 vegetable B
½ large onion	½ vegetable B
Broil or grill, then serve layered.	
Pesto pasta:	
1 cup cooked pasta spirals	2 carbohydrate
seasoned with basil and crushed garlic or garlic powder	free
2 cups shredded Bibb or leaf lettuce with	1 vegetable A
2 tablespoons reduced-fat blue-cheese dressing	1 extra
<u>Men:</u> increase flank steak to 6 ounces	5 protein
increase pasta to 1½ cups <u>and add</u>	3 carbohydrate

1 teaspoon olive oil	1 extra
add 5 large olives to salad	1 extra

Bedtime snack or dessert

8 animal crackers	1 special food
½ cup vanilla fat-free ice cream	1 special food

Internet Resources for Slimming Down and Healthful Eating

When the masters lost their weight many years ago, today's plethora of Internet resources for weight management was not around. Now, the Internet combines dissemination of written information about weight with the opportunity for interaction through e-mail, bulletin boards and chat rooms. A growing number of Web sites provide personalized advice and counseling as well.

There's not much research on Internet weight-loss programs, but a study published in a 2001 issue of the *Journal of the American Medical Association* found that dieters who received a behavior-modification program by e-mail along with weekly advice and feedback from doctoral-level behavioral therapists lost 3 times as much weight in 6 months as those who just had access to information about diet and exercise on the Internet — 9 pounds compared to 3 pounds. The authors of this Brown University study concluded, "Thus, the Internet and e-mail appear to be viable methods for delivery of structured behavioral weight loss programs." The study also suggests that a structured program with continued contact and individualized feedback may work better than just giving people access to information online.

The problem is, not everything on the Internet is reliable. So how do you tease out the good from the not-so-good? For starters, find out who runs the site and what their credentials are. Is the site reviewed by health professionals such as experts in the field, medical centers or nationally respected organizations? If personalized diets or exercise plans are offered, do the prescribers have appropriate credentials — for instance, are diets formulated by registered dietitians? Are exercise plans devised by exercise physiologists? Can you ask questions of a professional? Are chat sessions monitored by experts in the field? What's the privacy policy? Also, beware that chat sessions with lay members of an online community may not offer legitimate advice. Finally, take into consideration the site's sources of funding and — for sites at which you pay for services — read the terms of the contract carefully before committing. (You can also apply the guidelines set out in Chapter 3, "Finding the Right Match" and "Is It Legit?")

Following is a sampling of Web sites with useful information.

Note: This list of Web sites is by no means exhaustive — there are many other good sites on the Net. I cannot vouch for the validity of information on Web sites mentioned in Thin for Life *or on other Web sites to which they are linked. Because Web sites commonly go out of business, merge with other sites or move without leaving a forwarding address, some of the Web addresses in this book may no longer be accessible — or the content of sites may have changed. The content herein reflects information gathered in mid-2002.*

http://www.navigator.tufts.edu The Tufts University Nutrition Navigator helps you sort through the large volume of nutrition information on the Internet to find accurate, useful nutrition information. Web sites are reviewed by Tufts nutritionists, who apply rating and evaluation criteria developed by a prestigious panel of experts. Site reviews are updated every three months. At this writing, they rate the following six weight-related Web sites as "better than most" and describe them as follows:

http://www.fitday.com "Takes the food and exercise diary to a new level . . . This site is perfect for those who like to track progress visually or analytically . . . The activity list is one of the most specific we've seen."

http://www.thedietchannel.com "Think of this as a 'Yellow Pages' of online nutrition information." It provides hundreds of links that have been chosen with good judgment as credible sources of information.

http://www.shapeup.org This is the "Shape Up America!" Web site, created by former U.S. Surgeon General Dr. C. Everett Koop to combat obesity in the United States. "This is the place to find unbiased information about weight loss that's based on sound science." (Registration and a fee are required to access most of the interactive resources, but there's some free information as well.)

http://www.weight.com Run by a medical doctor with many years of experience treating obesity, this site has lots of background information about obesity and eating disorders. The Tufts review indicates that the site's bias is toward very-low-calorie diets (with behavior modification). The review adds, "Visitors can find plenty of good answers to weight loss and obesity questions here."

http://www.niddk.nih.gov/health/nutrit/win.htm This is the Web site of the Weight-control Information Network, or WIN, which offers thorough and clearly written articles along with resources on various aspects of weight management. "Because this information comes from the National Institutes of Health, it can be considered authoritative coverage of weight issues."

http://www.nutrio.com Positioning itself as an online "weight-loss community," this Web site "has an impressive crew of health experts" who offer advice and interactive tools for weight management. For a fee, personalized meal plans, recipes and a suggested exercise routine are available. Nutrio.com also has a section for children.

http://www.cyberdiet.com This site comes recommended by any number of nutrition experts. Cofounded by a registered dietitian, the site says of itself, "Unlike many other diet sites on the web, Cyberdiet offers its visitors the unique benefits of real live, accredited dietitians, offering sound nutritional advice." It allows users to customize their own weight-loss program and provides meal plans in different calorie ranges, as well as shopping lists, recipes and live chat rooms that give visitors the opportunity to mingle and support each other. Cyberdiet also offers exercise plans with tracking tools and an activity calculator. This site charges a fee.

http://www.healthyeating.net One of the masters recommended this Web site, which describes itself as "an award-winning site with one of the largest collections of nutrition/fitness links." Indeed, this Web site has a myriad of links to a myriad of resources on such subjects as listings of books by registered dietitians, fitness and food experts, healthy eating checklists, BMI and other weight calculators, fat intake calculators and fitness readiness quizzes.

http://www.dietitian.com This highly acclaimed, award-winning "Ask the Dietitian" Web site is a question-and-answer forum of nutrition advice that contains more than 90 different topics, including weight-related subjects. The site's Healthy Body Calculator will determine a healthy body-weight range, BMI and personalized information for calories, fat grams, vitamins and minerals.

http://www.foodfit.com Founded by a former top U.S. government nutrition official, this site offers personalized e-mail newsletters, menu planners, weight calculators, calorie burner calculators, a food and exercise diary and customizable recipes.

http://www.nutricise.com This registered-dietitian-run site offers a compendium of free and fee-based services. (Its free services even include a "healthy restaurant locator.") For a fee, the Nutricise Weight Loss Program combines nutrition, exercise, behavior modification and motivational techniques with personalized one-on-one coaching by a registered dietitian via e-mail. Counselors provide *live* counseling — clients do not receive automated responses.

http://www.ediets.com This subscription-based online diet, fitness and counseling network has an impressive-looking staff of experts. For a monthly fee, this site creates custom diet plans based upon individual members' personal goals, food preferences and lifestyles. In addition, eDiets.com publishes biweekly diet and fitness e-mail newsletters. The site states, "Each eDiets.com member enjoys the convenience and privacy of 24/7 access to their personalized online eDiets.com program that includes customized weekly menus, recipes and grocery shopping lists, interactive tools, online meetings, support boards, chats, fitness tips, professional advice and more through their desktop computers."

http://www.wfubmc.edu/nutrition/in.html From Wake Forest University Baptist Medical Center, this Web site, titled "Count Your Calories Because Calories Count," features a number of interactive assessments, such as a "Fit or Not Quiz" and a "Calorie Calculator," which allows you to track calories and other nutrients in your meals.

http://www.caloriecontrol.org From the Calorie Control Council, a nonprofit association representing the low-calorie and reduced-fat food and beverage industry, this Web site offers useful weight-loss information and aids, including exercise and calorie calculators, recipes and a weekly news-update section that features current news stories related to weight control.

Here are some additional Web sites worth checking out:

http://www.judyfields.com — a Web site of one of the "masters" who's a registered dietitian.

http://www.nat.uiuc.edu/mynat — an online no-cost nutrition analysis program launched by a university professor. Features an energy calculator.

http://www.dietwatch.com — this fee-based Web site provides users with meal plans, shopping lists, fitness workouts, weekly progress reports, chat meetings, support groups and more.

http://miavita.com — a fee-based Web site that provides customized diet and wellness services plus recipes and interactive tools to track progress.

The *Tufts University Health & Nutrition Letter* (March 2001) listed the following Web sites as helpful sources for healthful recipes:

http://www.intelihealth.com (under "Healthy Lifestyle," click on "Weight Management" — then go to "Healthful Recipes" under "InteliTools")

http://www.cookinglight.com (*Cooking Light* magazine's Web site)

http://www.deliciousdecisions.org (from the American Heart Association)

http://www.nhlbi.nih.gov (Web site of the National Heart, Lung, and Blood Institute — click on "Health Information, then on "Heart and Vascular Diseases," then on "Stay Young at Heart Recipes")

http://www.allrecipes.com (has a section for diabetes)

http://www.mealsforyou.com

Resources Recommended
by the Masters

For this new edition of *Thin for Life,* I went back to the masters for a list of resources that they've found to be helpful. The following list of recommendations includes everything from general inspirational books to cookbooks to nutrient counters to magazines. (Some of these books may be available in other editions. If any of these resources has gone out of print, you may be able to find it at a public library or through an Internet bookseller.)

Inclusion in this list does not necessarily indicate an endorsement. Readers need to assess whether resources suit their circumstances.

Books

Books About Weight Loss

Gentle Eating/Permanent Weight Loss Through Gradual Life Changes by Stephen Arterburn, Mary Ehemann and Vivian Lamphear. 1994. Nashville, TN: Thomas Nelson.

The Solution: 6 Winning Ways to Permanent Weight Loss by Laurel Mellin. 1998. New York: Regan Books.

Ultimate Fit or Fat: Get in Shape and Stay in Shape with America's Best-Loved and Most Effective Fitness Teacher by Covert Bailey. 1999. Boston: Houghton Mifflin.

Write Yourself Thin!: Writercises to Release the Thin Person Within by Toni Lynn Allawatt. 1991. Minneapolis: CompCare Publishers.

The Zen of Eating: Ancient Answers to Modern Weight Problems by Ronna Kabatznick. 1998. New York: Berkley Pub. Group.

Motivational Books

The Body Image Workbook: An 8-Step Program for Learning to Like Your Looks by Thomas F. Cash. 1997. Oakland, CA: New Harbinger.

Breaking Free from Compulsive Eating by Geneen Roth. 1993. New York: Plume.

Clear Your Clutter with Feng Shui by Karen Kingston. 1999. New York: Broadway Books.

Dr. Wayne Dyer's 10 Secrets for Success and Inner Peace by Wayne W. Dyer. 2001. Carlsbad, CA: Hay House.

Feeding The Hungry Heart: The Experience of Compulsive Eating by Geneen Roth. 2002, 1993, 1982. New York: Plume.

The Feeling Good Handbook by David D. Burns. 1999. New York: Plume.

Intuitive Eating: A Recovery Book for the Chronic Dieter: Redis-cover the Pleasures of Eating and Rebuild Your Body Image by Evelyn Tribole. 1996. New York: St. Martin's Paperbacks.

It's Not About the Bike: My Journey Back to Life by Lance Arm-strong. 2001. New York: Berkley Books.

Making Peace with Food: Freeing Yourself from the Diet/Weight Obsession by Susan Kano. 1989. New York: Perennial Library.

Moving Away from Diets by Karin Kratina. 1996. Lake Dallas, Texas: Helm Seminars & Publishing (http://www.helmnutrition. com).

Self Matters: Creating Your Life from the Inside Out. Phillip C. McGraw. 2001. New York: Simon & Schuster Source.

Stand Up for Your Life: Develop the Courage, Confidence, and Character to Fulfill Your Greatest Potential by Cheryl Richard-son. 2002. New York: Free Press.

Take Time for Your Life: A Personal Coach's Seven-Step Program for Creating the Life You Want by Cheryl Richardson. 1999. New York: Broadway Books.

The Tao of Eating: Feeding Your Soul Through Everyday Experi-ences with Food by Linda R. Harper. 1998. Philadelphia: Innisfree Press.

What Are You Hungry For?: Women, Food, and Spirituality by Lynn Ginsburg. 2002. New York: St. Martin's Press.

What's Your Sabotage: The Last Word in Overcoming Self-Sabotage by Alyce Cornyn-Selby. Portland, OR: Beynch Press, 1999.

You Can't Afford the Luxury of a Negative Thought by Peter McWilliams. 1995. Los Angeles: Prelude Press.

Books About Food, Cooking and Healthy Eating

Bowes & Church's Food Values of Portions Commonly Used by Anna de Planter Bowes. 1998. Philadelphia: Lippincott.

The Complete Book of Food Counts by Corinne T. Netzer. 2000. New York: Dell.

Eat, Drink, and Be Healthy: The Harvard Medical School Guide to Healthy Eating by Walter C. Willett. 2001. New York: Simon & Schuster Source.

Fabulous Fat-Free Cooking: More Than 225 Dishes — All Delicious, All Nutritious, All with Less Than 1 Gram of Fat! by Lynn Fischer. 1997. Emmaus, PA: Rodale Press.

Fat-Free Holiday Recipes by Sandra L. Woodruff. 1995. Garden City Park, NY: Avery Publishing Group.

500 Fat-Free Recipes: A Complete Guide to Reducing the Fat in Your Diet: 500 Recipes from Soup to Dessert Containing One Gram of Fat or Less by Sarah Schlesinger. 1994. New York: Villard.

A Guy's Guide to Great Eating by Don Mauer. 1999. Boston: Houghton Mifflin Company.

Lean and Lovin' It by Don Mauer. 1996. Boston: Houghton Mifflin Company.

Lickety-Split Meals: For Health Conscious People on the Go! by Zonya Foco. 1998. Walled Lake, MI: ZHI Publishing.

Low Fat, Low Calorie, Low Cholesterol Light Cooking. 1994. Lincolnwood, IL: Publications International.

Mediterranean Light: Delicious Recipes from the World's Healthiest Cuisine by Martha Rose Shulman. 2000. New York: William Morrow & Company.

Moosewood Restaurant Low-Fat Favorites: Flavorful Recipes for Healthful Meals. 1996. New York: C. Potter.

A Potful of Recipes by JoAnna M. Lund. 2001. New York: Berkley Publishing Group.

The Quick and Easy Fat Gram & Calorie Counter by Lynn Sonberg 1992. New York: Avon Books.

Saved by Soup: More Than 100 Delicious Low-Fat Soup Recipes to Eat and Enjoy Every Day by Judith Barrett. 1999. New York: William Morrow & Company.

Stealth Health: How to Sneak Nutrition Painlessly into Your Diet. 1998. New York: Penguin Books.

Weight Watchers New Complete Cookbook by Nancy Gagliardi. 1999. New York: Macmillan.

The Whole Soy Cookbook: 175 Delicious, Nutritious, Easy-To-Prepare Recipes Featuring Tofu, Tempeh, and Various Forms of Nature's Healthiest Bean by Patricia Greenberg. 1998. New York: Three Rivers Press.

Compact Disc

A Meditation to Help You with Weight Loss by Belleruth Naparstek. 1997. NY: Time Warner AudioBooks.

Magazines

Cooking Light. Customer Service, PO Box 62376, Tampa, FL 33662-3768. Telephone: 1-800-336-0125. Web site (recommended by the masters): cookinglight.com.

EatingWell. 823A Ferry Rd, Charlotte, VT 05445. Telephone: 1-800-337-0402. Web site: eatingwell.com.

Prevention. Customer Service, PO Box 7319, Red Oak, IA 51591-0319. Telephone: 1-800-813-8070. Web site: prevention.com/magazine.

Vegetarian Journal. The Vegetarian Resource Group, PO Box 1463, Baltimore, MD 21203. Telephone: 410-366-8343. Web site: vrg.org/journal.

Selected References

Anderson, J. W., Konz, E. C., Frederich, R. C., & Wood, C. L. (2001). Long-term weight-loss maintenance: A meta-analysis of US studies. *American Journal of Clinical Nutrition, 74,* 579–584.

Astrup, A. (1999). Dietary approaches to reducing body weight. *Baillière's Clinical Endocrinology and Metabolism,* 13(1), 109–119.

Astrup, A., Gøtzsche, P. C., van de Werken, K., Ranneries, C., Toubro, S., Raben, A., & Buemann, B. (1999). Meta-analysis of resting metabolic rate in formerly obese subjects. *American Journal of Clinical Nutrition, 69,* 1117–1122.

Beliard, D., Kirschenbaum, D. S., & Fitzgibbon, M. L. (1992). Evaluation of an intensive weight control program using *a priori* criteria to determine outcome. *International Journal of Obesity, 16,* 505–517.

Bray, G. A., York, B., & DeLany, J. (1992). A survey of the opinions of obesity experts on the causes and treatment of obesity. *American Journal of Clinical Nutrition, 55,* 151S–154S.

Brownell, K. D. (2000). *The LEARN program for weight management — 2000.* Dallas: Brownell & Hager Publishing Company.

Brownell, K. D., & Jeffery, R. W. (1987). Improving long-term weight loss: Pushing the limits of treatment. *Behavior Therapy, 18,* 353–374.

Brownell, K. D., Marlatt, G. A., Lichtenstein, E., & Wilson, G. T. (1986). Understanding and preventing relapse. *American Psychologist,* 41(7), 765–782.

Brownell, K. D., & Rodin, J. (1990). *The weight maintenance survival guide.* Dallas: Brownell & Hager Publishing Company.

Brownell, K. D., & Wadden, T. A. (1992). Etiology and treatment of obesity: Understanding a serious, prevalent, and refractory disorder. *Journal of Consulting and Clinical Psychology,* 60(4), 505–517.

Colvin, R. H., & Olson, S. C. (1983). A descriptive analysis of men and women who have lost significant weight and are highly successful at maintaining the loss. *Addictive Behaviors, 8*, 287–295.

Colvin, R. H., & Olson, S. C. (1984). Winners revisited: An 18-month follow-up of our successful weight losers. *Addictive Behaviors, 9*, 305–306.

Colvin, R. H., & Olson, S. C. (1989). *Keeping it off.* Arkansas City, KS: Gilliland.

Cooper, Z., & Fairburn, C. G. (2001). A new cognitive behavioural approach to the treatment of obesity. *Behaviour Research and Therapy, 39*, 499–511.

Cornyn-Selby, A. P. (1989). *Alyce's fat chance.* Portland, OR: Beynch Press Publishing Co.

Ferguson, K. J., Brink, P. J., Wood, M., & Koop, P. M. (1992). Characteristics of successful dieters as measured by guided interview responses and restraint scale scores. *Journal of the American Dietetic Association, 92*(9), 1119–1121.

Foreyt, J. P., & Goodrick, G. K. (1992). *Living without dieting.* Houston: Harrison Publishing.

Foster, G. D. (1990). Causes of obesity: Genetics. *The Weight Control Digest, 1*(1), 11–12.

Foster, G. D. (1991). Causes of obesity: Resting metabolic rate. *The Weight Control Digest, 1*(3), 42–44.

Foster, G. D., Wadden, T. A., Phelan, S., Sarwer, D. B., & Sanderson, R. S. (2001). Obese patients' perceptions of treatment outcomes and the factors that influence them. *Archives of Internal Medicine, 161*, 2133–2139.

Foster, G. D., Wyatt, H. R., Hill, J. O., McGuckin, B. G., Brill, C., Mohammed, B. S., Edman, J., & Klein, S. (2001). Evaluation of the Atkins diet: A randomized controlled trial. *Obesity Research, 9*(3), 85S.

Ganley, R. M. (1989). Emotion and eating in obesity: A review of the literature. *International Journal of Eating Disorders, 8*(3), 343–361.

Gavin, J. (1992). *The exercise habit.* Champaign, IL: Leisure Press.

Grilo, C. M., & Brownell, K. D. (1993). Relapse: Why, how, and what to do about it. *The Weight Control Digest, 3*(1), 217, 220–224.

Grilo, C. M., Shiffman, S., & Wing, R. R. (1989). Relapse crises and coping among dieters. *Journal of Consulting and Clinical Psychology, 57*(4), 488–495.

Hebl, M. R., & Xu, J. (2001). Weighing the care: Physicians' reactions to the size of a patient. *International Journal of Obesity, 25,* 1246–1252.

Heppner, P. P. (1983). Strategies for facilitating client's personal problem solving. In P. A. Keller & L. G. Ritt (Eds.), *Innovations in clinical practice: A source book. Volume 2* (pp. 73–85). Sarasota, Florida: Professional Resource Exchange, Inc.

Home exercise equipment. (1992, December). *University of California at Berkeley Wellness Letter,* pp. 4–5.

Jeffery, R. W., Bjornson-Benson, W. M., Rosenthal, B. S., Lindquist, R. A., Kurth, C. L., & Johnson, S. L. (1984). Correlates of weight loss and its maintenance over two years of follow-up among middle-aged men. *Preventive Medicine, 13,* 155–168.

Jeffery, R. W., Mayer, R. R., & Wing, R. R. (1998). Are smaller weight losses or more achievable weight loss goals better in the long term for obese patients? *Journal of Consulting and Clinical Psychology, 66*(4), 641–645.

Kayman, S., Bruvold, W., & Stern, J. S. (1990). Maintenance and relapse after weight loss in women: Behavioral aspects. *The American Journal of Clinical Nutrition, 52,* 800–807.

Kennedy, E. T., Bowman, S. A., Spence, J. T., Freedman, M., & King, J. (2001). Popular diets: Correlation to health, nutrition, and obesity. *Journal of the American Dietetic Association, 101*(4), 411–420.

Kirschenbaum, D. S., Fitzgibbon, M. L., Martino, S., Conviser, J. H., Rosendahl, E. H., & Laatsch, L. (1992). Stages of change in successful weight control: A clinically derived model. *Behavior Therapy, 23,* 623–635.

Klem, M. L., Wing, R. R., Lang, W., McGuire, M. T., & Hill, J. O. (2000). Does weight loss maintenance become easier over time? *Obesity Research, 8*(6), 438–444.

Klem, M. L., Wing, R. R., McGuire, M. T., Seagle, H. M., & Hill, J. O. (1997). A descriptive study of individuals successful at long-term maintenance of substantial weight loss. *American Journal of Clinical Nutrition, 66,* 239–246.

Klem, M. L., Wing, R. R., McGuire, M. T., Seagle, H. M., & Hill,

J. O. (1998). Psychological symptoms in individuals successful at long-term maintenance of weight loss. *Health Psychology*, 17(4), 336–345.

Losing weight: What works. What doesn't. (1993, June). *Consumer Reports*, pp. 347–359.

Ludwig, D. S. (2002). The glycemic index. *Journal of the American Medical Association*, 287(18), 2414–2423.

Mahoney, M. J., & Mahoney, K. (1976). *Permanent weight control: A total solution to the dieter's dilemma*. New York: W. W. Norton & Company.

McGuire, M. T., Wing, R. R., & Hill, J. O. (1999). The prevalence of weight loss maintenance among American adults. *International Journal of Obesity*, 23, 1314–1319.

McGuire, M. T., Wing, R. R., Klem, M. L., Lang, W., & Hill, J. O. (1999). What predicts weight regain in a group of successful weight losers? *Journal of Consulting and Clinical Psychology*, 67(2), 177–185.

Nash, J. D. (1992). *Now that you've lost it*. Palo Alto: Bull Publishing Co.

National Institutes of Health (1998). *Clinical guidelines on the identification, evaluation, and treatment of overweight and obesity in adults: The evidence report*. U.S. Department of Health and Human Services.

National Task Force on the Prevention and Treatment of Obesity (2000). Dieting and the development of eating disorders in overweight and obese adults. *Archives of Internal Medicine*, 160, 2581–2589.

"No sweat" guide to designing a fitness plan. (1992, April). *Tufts University Health & Nutrition Letter*, pp. 3–6.

North American Association for the Study of Obesity (2001). Popular diets: A scientific review. *Obesity Research*, 9 (Supplement 1).

Peele, S., & Brodsky, A. (1991). *The truth about addiction and recovery*. New York: Simon & Schuster.

Perri, M. G., Sears, S. F., & Clark, J. E. (1993). Strategies for improving the maintenance of weight loss: Toward a continuous care model of obesity management. *Diabetes Care*, 16(1), 200–209.

Polivy, J., & Herman, C. P. (1983). *Breaking the diet habit*. New York: Basic Books, Inc.

Rand, C. S. W., & Macgregor, A. M. C. (1991). Successful weight loss following obesity surgery and the perceived liability of morbid obesity. *International Journal of Obesity,* 15, 577–579.

Ravussin, E., Lillioja, S., Knowler, W. C., Christin, L., Freymond, D., Abbott, W. G. H., Boyce, V., Howard, B. V., & Bogardus, C. (1988). Reduced rate of energy expenditure as a risk factor for body-weight gain. *The New England Journal of Medicine,* 318(8), 467–472.

Ross, S. T. (1985). *The process of personal change: A case study of adults who have maintained weight loss.* Unpublished doctoral dissertation, Northern Illinois University.

Schachter, S. (1982). Recidivism and self-cure of smoking and obesity. *American Psychologist,* 37(4), 436–444.

Schoenborn, C. A., and Barnes, P. M. (2002). Leisure-time physical activity among adults: United States, 1997–98. *Advance Data from Vital and Health Statistics,* Number 325.

Should you be choosing foods by their glycemic index? (2000, November). *Tufts University Health & Nutrition Letter,* pp. 4–5.

Tate, D. F., Wing, R. R., & Winett, R. A. (2001). Using Internet technology to deliver a behavioral weight loss program. *Journal of the American Medical Association,* 285 (9), 1172–1177.

The truth about dieting (2002, June). *Consumer Reports,* pp. 27–31.

U.S. Department of Health and Human Services (2001). The Surgeon General's call to action to prevent and decrease overweight and obesity. Rockville, MD: U.S. Department of Health and Human Services, Public Health Service, Office of the Surgeon General.

Wadden, T. A., & Stunkard, A. J. (1988). Three year follow-up of the treatment of obesity by very-low-calorie diet, behavior therapy, and their combination. *Journal of Consulting and Clinical Psychology,* 56, 925–928.

Wadden, T. A., & Stunkard, A. J., Eds. (2002). *Handbook of Obesity Treatment.* New York: The Guilford Press.

Weight-control Information Network publications niddk.nih.gov/health/nutrit/pubs:
Binge Eating Disorders (2001)
Gastrointestinal Surgery for Severe Obesity (2001)
Prescription Medications for the Treatment of Obesity (2001)

Wesley, S. M. (1992). *Overcoming an addiction*. El Sobrante, CA.

Willis, J. D., & Campbell, L. F. (1992). *Exercise psychology*. Champaign, Illinois: Human Kinetics Publishers.

Wing, R. R. (1992). Weight cycling in humans: A review of the literature. *Annals of Behavioral Medicine*, 14(2), 113–119.

Wolfe, B. L., & Marlatt, G. A. (1992). Reframing relapse: From endpoint to turning point. *The Weight Control Digest*, 2(5), 185, 188–193.

Wyatt, H. R., Grunwald, G. K., Mosca, C. L., Klem, M. L., Wing, R. R., & Hill, J. O. (2002). Long-term weight loss and breakfast in subjects in the National Weight Control Registry. *Obesity Research*, 10(2), 78–82.

Yanovski, J. A., Yanovski, S. Z., Sovik, K. N., Nguyen, T. T., O'Neil, P. M., & Sebring, N. G. (2000). A prospective study of holiday weight gain. *The New England Journal of Medicine*, 342(12), 861–867.

Zelasko, C. J. (1995). Exercise for weight loss: What are the facts? *Journal of the American Dietetic Association*, 95(12), 1414–1417.

Index

Recipe Index

ALSO AVAILABLE

THIN FOR LIFE DAYBOOK
A Journal of Personal Progress

The best-selling inspirational journal that has helped thousands make healthful changes in their lifestyle, one week at a time

ISBN 0-618-34424-1 $16.00 PA

"It's a perfect tool for people who want to take positive steps, not just to lose weight but to incorporate better eating and exercise patterns into their lives." — *USA Today*

EATING THIN FOR LIFE
Food Secrets and Recipes from People Who Have Lost Weight and Kept It Off

122 favorite low-fat recipes   **ISBN 1-576-30062-5 $14.00 PA**

"Both a low-fat cookbook and a trove of weight-control secrets."
— *Seattle Times*

OTHER TITLES BY ANNE M. FLETCHER

SOBER FOR GOOD
New Solutions for Drinking Problems — Advice from Those Who Have Succeeded   **ISBN 0-618-21907-2 $14.00 PA**

SOBER FOR GOOD
(audiocassette)   **ISBN 0-618-23303-2 $29.00**

 Available from Houghton Mifflin